Gastrointestinal emergencies

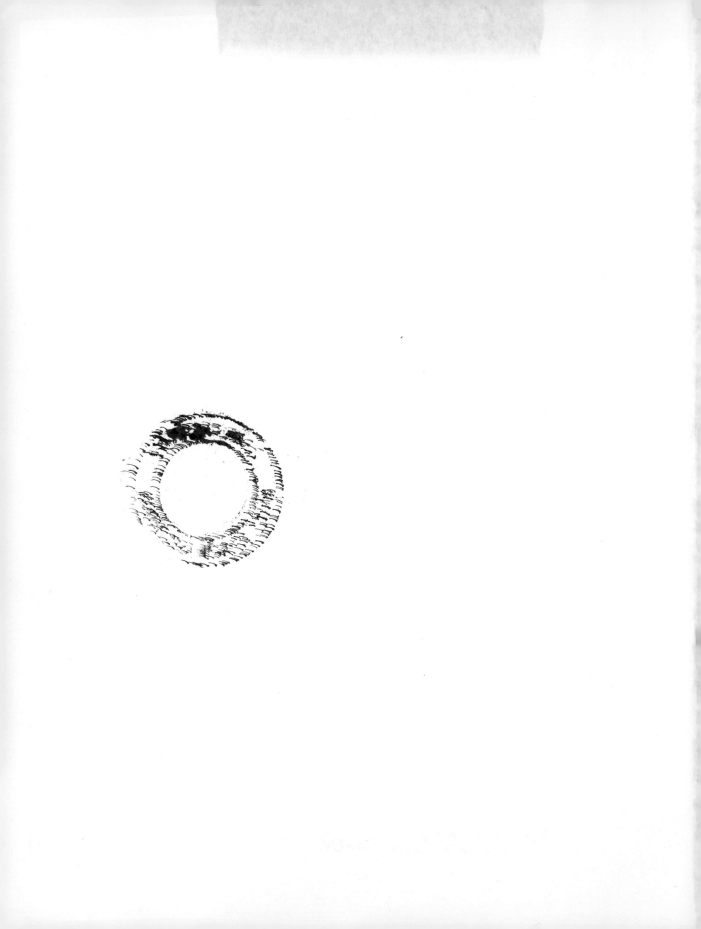

Gastrointestinal emergencies

EDITED BY

Tony C. K. Tham

Consultant Gastroenterologist,
Ulster Hospital,
Dundonald, Belfast,
Northern Ireland, UK

John S. A. Collins

Associate Postgraduate Dean,
Northern Ireland Medical and Dental Training Agency
Formerly Consultant Gastroenterologist,
Royal Victoria Hospital,
Belfast, Northern Ireland, UK

Roy Soetikno

Chief, GI Section,
Veterans Affairs Palo Alto Health Care System,
Palo Alto;
Associate Professor,
Stanford University,
Stanford, CA, USA

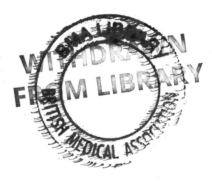
THIRD EDITION

WILEY Blackwell

This edition first published 2016 © 2016 by John Wiley & Sons, Ltd
Second edition published 2009
First edition published 2000
© 2000, 2009 by Blackwell Publishing Ltd

Registered Office
John Wiley & Sons, Ltd, The Atrium, Southern Gate, Chichester, West Sussex, PO19 8SQ, UK

Editorial Offices
9600 Garsington Road, Oxford, OX4 2DQ, UK
The Atrium, Southern Gate, Chichester, West Sussex, PO19 8SQ, UK
111 River Street, Hoboken, NJ 07030-5774, USA

For details of our global editorial offices, for customer services and for information about how
to apply for permission to reuse the copyright material in this book please see our website at
www.wiley.com/wiley-blackwell.

Library of Congress Cataloging-in-Publication Data

Gastrointestinal emergencies (Tham)
   Gastrointestinal emergencies / edited by Tony C.K. Tham, John S.A. Collins, Roy Soetikno. – Third edition.
      p. ; cm.
   Includes bibliographical references and index.
   ISBN 978-1-118-63842-2 (pbk.)
I. Tham, Tony C. K., editor.   II. Collins, John S. A., editor.   III. Soetikno, Roy, editor.   IV. Title.
[DNLM: 1. Gastrointestinal Diseases–therapy.   2. Emergency Treatment.   3. Endoscopy, Gastrointestinal.
WI 140]
   RC801
   616.3'3–dc23

                                        2015024791

A catalogue record for this book is available from the British Library.

Wiley also publishes its books in a variety of electronic formats. Some content that appears in print may
not be available in electronic books.

Cover image: © Paul Bradbury/GettyImages

Set in 8.5/12pt Meridien by SPi Global, Pondicherry, India
Printed and bound in Malaysia by Vivar Printing Sdn Bhd

1   2016

Contents

Notes on contributors

Seiichiro Abe
National Cancer Center Hospital, Tokyo, Japan

Aijaz Ahmed MD
Division of Gastroenterology and Hepatology, Stanford
University School of Medicine, Stanford, CA, USA

Patrick B. Allen MB, FRCP, BSc
Consultant Gastroenterologist, Ulster Hospital, Belfast,
Northern Ireland, UK

Constantinos P. Anastassiades MBBS (Lond), FACP
Consultant, Division of Gastroenterology & Hepatology,
Khoo Teck Puat Hospital, Singapore
Adj. Assistant Professor of Medicine, Case Western Reserve
University School of Medicine, Cleveland, OH, USA

Stephen Attwood MCh, FRCS, FRCSI
Consultant Upper GI and Laparoscopic Surgeon, Honorary
Professor, Durham University, Durham, UK

Andrés Cárdenas MD, MMSc, PhD, AGAF
Faculty Member/Senior Specialist, GI Unit, Institute of
Digestive Diseases, Hospital Clinic, IDIBAPS, University
of Barcelona, Barcelona, Spain

David L. Carr-Locke MB, Bchir, FRCP, FASGE
Chief, Division of Digestive Diseases, Associate Chair of
Medicine, Mount Sinai Beth Israel Medical Center,
New York, USA
Professor, Icahn School of Medicine, New York, USA

W. Johnny Cash MD, FRCP
Consultant Hepatologist, Royal Victoria Hospital, Belfast,
Northern Ireland, UK

John S. A. Collins MD
Associate Postgraduate Dean, Northern Ireland Medical and
Dental Training Agency
Formerly Consultant Gastroenterologist, Royal Victoria
Hospital, Belfast, Northern Ireland, UK

Wallace Dinsmore MD, FRCP, FRCPI, FRCPEd
Professor of Medicine, Department of GU Medicine, Royal
Victoria Hospital, Belfast, UK

Shai Friedland MD
Assistant Professor, Stanford University School of Medicine
and VA Palo Alto, Stanford, CA, USA

Subrata Ghosh MD, FRCP, FRCPE, FRCPC, FCAHS
Professor of Medicine, Microbiology & Immunology,
University of Calgary, Alberta, Canada

Pere Ginès MD, PhD
Chief of Hepatology, Liver Unit, Institute of Digestive Diseases
Hospital Clinic, IDIBAPS, Professor of Medicine, University
of Barcelona, Spain

Isabel Graupera
Institut de Malalties Digestives i Metabolisme, Hospital Clinic,
IDIBAPS, University of Barcelona, Barcelona, Spain

Philip S. J. Hall MRCP, MB, BCh
Specialty registrar in Gastroenterology, Gastroenterology
training program, Altnagelvin Hospital, Londonderry,
Northern Ireland, UK

Paul Kevin Hamilton BSc (Hons), MD, FRCPE
Specialty Registrar, Department of Clinical Biochemistry;
Formerly Consultant Physician and Clinical Pharmacologist;
Belfast Health and Social Care Trust, Belfast, Northern
Ireland, UK

Brian J. Hogan
Specialty Registrar, Sheila Sherlock Liver Centre, Royal
Free London NHS Foundation Trust, Royal Free Hospital,
London, UK

Marietta Iacucci MD, PhD
Clinical Associate Professor of Medicine Division of
Gastroenterology, University of Calgary, Alberta, Canada

Tonya Kaltenbach MD, MS
Veterans Affairs Palo Alto Health Care System, Clinical
Assistant Professor of Medicine (Affiliated), Stanford
University, Palo Alto, CA, USA

Joseph K. N. Kim
Icahn School of Medicine, New York, USA

Jennifer M. Kolb MD
Icahn School of Medicine at Mount Sinai, Internal Medicine,
New York, NY, USA

Bee Chan Lee MB, MRCP
Consultant Gastroenterologist, Warwick Hospital,
Warwicks, England, UK

David R. Lichtenstein MD
Director of Endsocopy & Associate Professor of Medicine,
Boston Medical Center, Boston University School of Medicine,
Boston, MA, USA

Ian McAllister MD
Consultant Surgeon, Ulster Hospital, Dundonald, Belfast,
Northern Ireland, UK

Daniel F. McAuley
Professor and Consultant in Intensive Care Medicine, Royal
Victoria Hospital and Queen's University of Belfast, Belfast,
Northern Ireland, UK

Kevin McCallion
Consultant Surgeon, Ulster Hospital, Dundonald, Belfast,
Northern Ireland, UK

Emma McCarty
Consultant in Genitourinary Medicine, Royal Victoria Hospital,
Belfast, Northern Ireland, UK

James J. McNamee FCARCSI, FRCA, FCICM, FFICM
Consultant in Intensive Care Medicine, Royal Victoria
Hospital, Belfast, Northern Ireland, UK

Graham Morrison MB, MRCP
Consultant Gastroenterologist, Altnagelvin Hospital,
Londonderry, Northern Ireland, UK

Ichiro Oda MD
National Cancer Center Hospital, Tokyo, Japan

Khalid Osman FRCS
North Tyneside General Hospital, Tyne & Wear, UK

Kelvin Palmer FRCP(Edin)
Formerly Consultant Gastroenterologist, Western General
Hospital, Edinburgh, UK

Ioannis S. Papanikolaou
Department of Internal Medicine and Research Unit, "Attikon"
University General Hospital, University of Athens, Greece

David W.M. Patch MBBS, FRCP
Consultant Hepatologist, Department of Hepatology, Royal
Free Hospital, London, UK

Ryan B. Perumpail MD
Stanford Hospital and Clinics, Stanford, CA, USA

Aarti K. Rao MD
Resident Physician, Department of Internal Medicine, Stanford
University; Department of Gastroenterology, Veterans Affairs
Palo Alto Health Care System, CA, USA

Michele B. Ryan
Brigham and Women's Hospital, Harvard Medical School,
Boston, MA, USA

Andres Sanchez-Yague MD, PhD
Chief, Gastroenterology Unit, Vithas Xanit International
Hospital, Benalmadena, Spain
Consultant, Gastroenterology Unit, Hospital Costa del Sol,
Marbella, Spain

Allison R. Schulman
Brigham and Women's Hospital, Harvard Medical School,
Boston, MA, USA

Reza Shaker MD, FACP
Professor and Chief, Division of Gastroenterology and
Hepatology; Director, Digestive Disease Center, Medical
College of Wisconsin, Milwaukee, WI, USA

Peter D. Siersema MD, PhD
Professor of Gastroenterology and Chief, Department of
Gastroenterology and Hepatology, University Medical Center,
Utrecht, The Netherlands

Maria Cecilia M. Sison-Oh
Medical Center Manila, Manila, Philippines

Roy Soetikno MD, MS (Health Service Research)
Chief, GI Section, Veterans Affairs Palo Alto Health Care System,
Palo Alto
Associate Professor, Stanford University, Stanford, CA, USA

Daniel J. Stein MD
Assistant Professor of Medicine, Division of Gastroenterology and
Hepatology, Medical College of Wisconsin, Milwaukee, WI, USA

Matthias Steverlynck
Centre Hospitalier de Mouscron, Belgium

Haruhisa Suzuki
National Cancer Center Hospital, Tokyo, Japan

Tony C. K. Tham MD, FRCP, FRCPI
Consultant Gastroenterologist, Dundonald, Ulster Hospital,
Belfast, Northern Ireland, UK

Christopher C. Thompson
Brigham and Women's Hospital, Harvard Medical School,
Boston, MA, USA

Philip Toner MRCP
Specialty Registrar, Department of General Medicine, Belfast
Health and Social Care Trust, Belfast City Hospital, Belfast, UK

George Triadafilopoulos MD, DSc
Clinical Professor of Medicine, Division of Gastroenterology
and Hepatology, Stanford University School of Medicine,
Stanford, CA, USA

Jo Vandervoort MD
Department of Gastroenterology, Onze-Lieve-Vrouw
Ziekenhuis, Aalst, Belgium

Barbara Willandt
KU Leuven, Netherlands

Richard C. K. Wong BSc, MBBS(Lond), FASGE, FACG,
AGAF, FACP
Professor of Medicine, Case Western Reserve University School
of Medicine, Cleveland, OH, USA
Medical Director, DHI Endoscopy Unit, University Hospitals
Case Medical Center, Cleveland, OH, USA

Robert J. Wong MD, MS
Stanford University School of Medicine, Stanford, CA, USA

SECTION 1
Approach to specific presentations

CHAPTER 1
Approach to dysphagia

John S. A. Collins

Northern Ireland Medical and Dental Training Agency, Royal Victoria Hospital, Belfast, UK

Definitions

Dysphagia refers to a subjective sensation of the obstruction of swallowed solids or liquids from mouth to stomach. Patients most frequently complain that food "sticks" in the retrosternal area or simply will "not go down." Patients may complain of a feeling of choking and chest discomfort. In some cases food material is rapidly regurgitated to relieve symptoms.

Dysphagia can be divided into two types:
- *oropharyngeal dysphagia,* where there is an inability to *initiate* the swallowing process and may involve disorders of striated muscle. There may be a sensation of solids or liquids left in the pharynx.
- *esophageal dysphagia,* which involves disorders of the smooth muscle of the esophagus and results in symptoms within seconds of the initiation of swallowing.

Odynophagia is the sensation of pain on swallowing which is usually felt in the chest or throat. *Globus* is the sensation of a lump, fullness or tightness in the throat.

Differential diagnosis

The causes of the above types of dysphagia are shown in Tables 1.1 and 1.2.

History and examination

Acute dysphagia is a relatively uncommon, but dramatic, presenting symptom and constitutes a gastrointestinal emergency. The patient will complain of difficulty initiating swallowing or state that food is readily swallowed but results in the rapid onset of chest discomfort or pain, which is only relieved by passage or regurgitation of the swallowed food bolus. The latter sensation can result after swallowing a mouthful of liquid. In the acute case it is important to ask the patient about the presence of other neurological symptoms.

If oropharyngeal dysphagia is suspected, the following points are important:
- The patient may complain of nasal regurgitation of liquid, coughing or choking during swallowing or a change in voice character which may indicate nasal speech due to palatal weakness.
- Patients may describe repeated attempts at the initiation of swallowing.
- Symptoms are noticed within a second of swallowing.
- Patients with cerebrovascular disease may give a history of symptoms of transient ischemic attacks (TIA) – these would include visual disturbance, dysphasia, or transient facial or limb weakness.
- There may be progressive muscular weakness and dysphagia is only part of the symptom complex, in contrast to esophageal dysphagia where swallowing disorder is the most prominent symptom.
- Patients should have a careful neurological examination and evaluation of the pharynx and larynx including direct laryngoscopy.
- In cases of esophageal dysphagia, the following points are important:
- Is the sensation of dysphagia worse with liquids or solids? If a progressive obstructive lesion is the cause of symptoms, the patient will notice difficulty

Gastrointestinal Emergencies, Third Edition. Edited by Tony C. K. Tham, John S. A. Collins, and Roy Soetikno.
© 2016 John Wiley & Sons, Ltd. Published 2016 by John Wiley & Sons, Ltd.

Table 1.1 Etiology of oropharyngeal dysphagia.

Neurological disorders
Cerebrovascular disease
Amyotrophic lateral sclerosis
Parkinson's disease
Multiple sclerosis
Bulbar poliomyelitis
Wilson's disease
Cranial nerve injury
Brainstem tumors

Striated muscle disorders
Polymyositis
Dermatomyositis
Muscular dystrophies
Myasthenia gravis

Structural lesions
Inflammatory – pharyngitis, tonsillar abscess
Head and neck tumors
Congenital webs
Plummer–Vinson syndrome
Cervical osteophytes

Surgical procedures to the oropharynx
Pharyngeal pouch (Zenker diverticulum)
Cricopharyngeal bar

Metabolic disorders
Hypothyroidism
Hyperthyroidism
Steroid myopathy

Table 1.2 Etiology of esophageal dyphagia.

Neuromuscular/dysmotility disorders
Achalasia
CRST syndrome
Diffuse esophageal spasm
Nutcracker esophagus
Hypertensive lower esophageal shincter
Nonspecific esophageal dysmotility
Chaga disease
Mixed connective tissue disease

Mechanical strictures – intrinsic
Peptic related to GERD
Carcinoma
Esophageal webs
Esophageal diverticula
Lower esophageal ring (Schatzki)
Benign tumors
Foreign bodies
Acute esophageal mucosal infections
Pemphigus/pemphigoid
Crohn's disease

Mechanical lesions – extrinsic
Bronchial carcinoma
Mediastinal nodes
Vascular compression
Mediastinal tumors
Cervical osteoarthritis/spondylosis

swallowing solids initially and liquids later. Difficulty with both solids and liquids suggests dysmotility.
- Is the dysphagia intermittent or progressive? Intermittent dysphagia may indicate a motility disorder such as diffuse esophageal spasm whereas a progressive course is more characteristic of an esophageal tumor.
- How long have symptoms been present? A long history usually greater than 12 months suggests a benign cause, whereas a short history less than 4 weeks suggests a malignant etiology.
- Has the patient a history of heartburn suggesting gastroesophageal reflux disease (GERD)? While a history of heartburn does not rule out gastroesophageal cancer as a cause of dysphagia, a long history in the presence of slow onset, non-progressive symptoms may point to a benign peptic stricture as the cause.

A diagnostic algorithm for the symptomatic assessment of the patient with dysphagia is shown in Fig. 1.1.

The etiology of esophageal dysphagia is summarized in Table 1.2.

While acute dysphagia may be painful, especially in relation to foreign body or food bolus impaction above an existing stricture, a history of odynophagia usually suggests an inflammatory condition or disruption of the esophageal mucosa leading to the irritation of pain receptors. The causes of odynophagia are:
- *Candida*
- herpes simplex
- cytomegalovirus
- pill-induced ulceration
- reflux disease/stricture
- radiation esophagitis
- caustic injury
- motility disorders stimulated by swallowing
- cancer
- graft-versus-host disease
- foreign body.

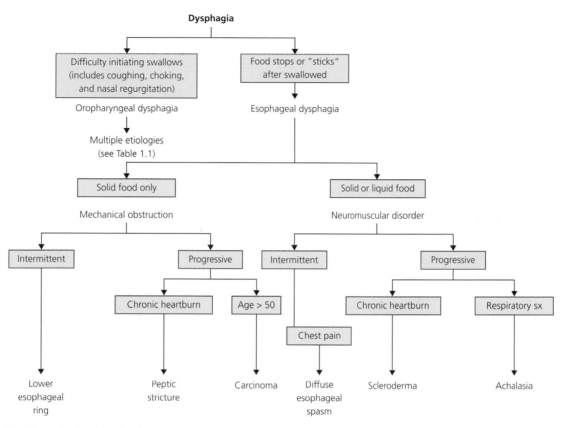

Fig. 1.1 Diagnostic algorithm for the symptomatic assessment of the patient with dysphagia. Source: Yamada 1995. Reproduced with permission of Wiley.

Clinical signs in patients who present with dysphagia are uncommon. On examination, the following signs should be noted:
• loss of weight
• signs of anemia
• cervical lymphadenopathy
• hoarseness
• concomitant neurological especially bulbar signs
• respiratory signs if history of cough/choking
• hepatomegaly
• oral ulcers or signs of *Candida*
• goiter.

Investigation

Dysphagia is considered to be an "alarm symptom" and should be investigated as a matter of urgency in all cases. Upper gastrointestinal endoscopy is a safe investigation in experienced hands provided the intubation is carried out under direct visualization of the oropharynx and upper esophageal sphincter. The endoscopist should be alert to the possibility of a high obstruction and the likelihood of retained food debris or saliva if dysphagia has been present for some time. If there is a history of choking, the patient should have a liquid-only diet for 24 hours followed by a 12-hour fast prior to the procedure. In some cases, the careful passage of a naso-esophageal tube to aspirate retained luminal contents may be necessary. At endoscopy, obstructing lesions can be biopsied and peptic strictures can be dilated with a balloon or bougie.

The presence of a dilated food and saliva-filled esophagus in the absence of a stricture raises the possibility of achalasia.

Barium studies are not a prerequisite for endoscopy but should be considered complementary in dysphagia. Barium swallow may give additional information in the following situations:
• in cases of suspected oropharyngeal dysphagia, especially if videofluoroscopy is employed;

• where a high esophageal obstruction is suspected prior to endoscopy;
• where a motility disorder is suspected as a method to assess lower esophageal relaxation.

In some cases, a barium swallow may be a useful investigation in certain circumstances:

• Where there is suspected proximal obstruction, e.g. laryngeal cancer, Zenker's diverticulum;
• Following a negative endoscopy or obstructive symptoms as lower esophageal rings may be more easily detected at fluoroscopy.

Esophageal manometry is indicated if both endoscopy and barium studies are inconclusive in the presence of persistent symptoms. Manometry requires intubation of the esophagus with a multilumen recording catheter attached to a polygraph. Pressure changes are recorded during water bolus swallows along the esophageal body and at the upper and lower esophageal sphincters.

Management of dysphagia

The management of dysphagia depends on the underlying cause. In a patient presenting with total dysphagia who is unable to swallow even small amounts of liquid or saliva, urgent treatment is indicated (Fig. 1.2).

The management of oropharyngeal dysphagia can be treated by control of the underlying neurological

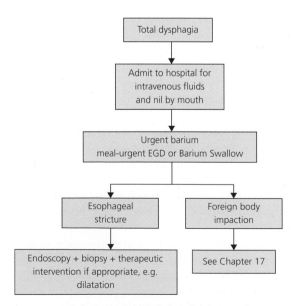

Fig. 1.2 Approach to management of total dysphagia.

or metabolic disorder. Dietary modification under the supervision of a speech and language therapist may maintain oral swallowing and avoid gastrostomy tube placement in patients with stroke and pseudobulbar or bulbar palsy. Gastrostomy tube placement may be the only management option in patients with inoperable mouth or throat tumors, or in cases where recurrent pulmonary aspiration is life threatening.

Peptic stricture

When the endoscopic appearances are characteristic of a benign peptic stricture, dilatation can usually be carried out at the time of the procedure using either wire-guided bougies or a balloon. If the stricture is complex, very tight or associated with esophageal scarring, it may be safer to carry out wire-guided dilatation using graded bougies. The majority of patients will gain symptomatic relief and the risk of complications is low (see Chapter 21, Esophageal Perforation).

It is essential that all patients are treated with an adequate dose of a proton pump inhibitor to prevent recurrence. Repeat dilatations are necessary in some cases and repeat inspection and biopsy is advised if there is any concern about mucosal dysplasia or malignancy.

Esophageal carcinoma

Suspected carcinoma, which is detected at endoscopy, requires biopsy confirmation and subsequent staging so that a management plan can be formulated. The most accurate modality for staging is endoscopic ultrasound which can assess depth of local invasion and regional lymph node status. Chest and abdominal computerized tomography (CT) is a less accurate technique but CT/positron emission tomography (PET) scanning enhances staging accuracy, especially in adenocarcinomas.

Surgery offers the only chance of cure but only 30% of tumors are resectable and 5-year survival is 10% in European studies. Contraindications to surgery include invasion of vascular structures, metastatic disease and patients with comorbidity and high operative risk.

Palliative management will be indicated in 70% of patients following staging. Esophageal dilatation, followed by the endoscopic placement of a metal stent, gives adequate swallowing relief in the majority of cases. In situations where there is complete obstruction of the esophageal lumen by tumor, endoscopic laser therapy can provide adequate palliation of dysphagia. The prognosis is poor with a mean survival of 10 months after diagnosis with a 5-year survival of 5%. Where surgical resection is completed after staging and selection, 5-year survival can be up to 25%.

Radiation injury

Following radiotherapy to the thorax or head and neck, some patients develop esophagitis, which may progress to stricturing and fibrosis. The diagnosis is confirmed by endoscopy and biopsy. Treatment consists of balloon or bougie dilatation and may have to be repeated in severe cases.

Esophageal webs and rings

Both of these esophageal lesions can result in dysphagia or lead to food bolus impaction. Webs are typically composed of thin mucosal tissue covered with squamous epithelium. They tend to occur proximally in the upper cervical esophagus and may be missed or ruptured at endoscopy, which is both diagnostic and therapeutic in these cases. They have been associated with chronic iron deficiency anemia. Rings are mucosal circular structures associated with dysmotility and seen at the esophagogastric junction. A Schatzki ring is a solitary thin rim of mucosa usually seen in the distended lower oesophagus. They are usually treated by dilatation and may be recurrent.

Food bolus Impaction

See Chapter 20, Foreign Body Impaction in the Esophagus.

Eosinophilic esophagitis

This is an increasingly recognized cause of dysphagia and is diagnosed by characteristic endoscopic appearances and the finding of a dense eosinophilic infiltrate in esophageal mucosal biopsies (>15 per high power field). Dilatation is rarely required and the condition responds to low-dose swallowed topical steroids, administered by a metered inhaler.

Further reading

American Gastroenterology Association medical position statement on management of oropharyngeal dysphagia. *Gastroenterology* 1999; **116**:452.

Castell DO. Approach to the patient with dysphagia. In *Textbook of Gastroenterology*, Yamada T, Alpers DH, Owyang C, Powell DW, Silverstein FE (eds). Lippincott, Philadelphia, 1995.

Falk GW, Richter JE. Approach to the patient with acute dysphagia, odynophagia, and non-cardiac chest pain. In *Gastrointestinal Emergencies 2nd edition*, Taylor MB (ed.). Williams & Wilkins, Baltimore, 1997:65–84.

Kahrilas PJ, Smout AJ. Esophageal disorders. *Am. J. Gastroenterol.* 2010;**105**:747.

Prasad GA, Talley NJ, Romero Y, et al. Prevalence and predictive factors of eosinophilic esophagitis in patients presenting with dysphagia: a prospective study. *Am. J. Gastroenterol.* 2007; **102**:2627.

Yamada T, Alpers DH, Owyang C, Powell DW, Silverstein FE (eds). *Textbook of Gastroenterology*. Lippincott, Philadelphia, 1995.

CHAPTER 2

Approach to vomiting

Bee Chan Lee[1] and John S. A. Collins[2]

[1] Warwick Hospital, Warwick, UK

[2] Northern Ireland Medical and Dental Training Agency, Royal Victoria Hospital, Belfast, UK

Definition

Acute nausea with or without vomiting is a common symptom. Nausea is described as an unpleasant sensation of imminent vomiting. Vomiting is defined as the forceful expulsion of gastric contents through the mouth and it should be differentiated from retching and regurgitation. Retching is the term that describes the labored, rhythmic respiratory activity and abdominal muscular contractions, which usually precede vomiting. Regurgitation is the effortless propulsion of gastric contents into the mouth without abdominal diaphragmatic muscular contractions.

The act of vomiting is initiated by the vomiting center in the medulla or the chemoreceptor trigger zone (CTZ) in the floor of the fourth ventricle, via a combination of motor and autonomic responses. Vomiting starts with salivation and then reverse peristalsis in the small intestines and a relaxed pyloric sphincter. Subsequent glottis closure (to prevent aspiration), abdominal and gastric muscular contractions and relaxation of the lower esophageal sphincter result in the final act of vomiting.

Etiology

The causes of acute nausea and vomiting are extensive and are summarized in Table 2.1.

- **Visceral (gut and peritoneum)** – visceral pain from a variety of intra-abdominal causes is often associated with an acute abdomen, including sepsis and mechanical obstruction. Gastric outlet obstruction leads to prolonged vomiting of the projectile nature.
- **CNS causes** – these include head injuries, intracranial infections/inflammation and raised intracranial pressure. Stimulation or disorders of the vestibular system such as motion sickness should not be overlooked.
- **Drugs** – nausea and vomiting are common side effects of chemotherapeutic agents, antibiotics, analgesics, and narcotics but the list of other offending drugs is endless. It is also important to enquire about recreational druguse, of which the commonest is alcohol abuse. Acetaminophen/paracetamol and salicylate toxicity also result in nausea or vomiting, and this needs to be excluded.
- **Infections** – food poisoning (bacterial and viral) is the commonest. Others include epidemic viral infections, e.g. Norwalk agent and non-gastrointestinal infections such as otitis media and urinary tract infection.
- **Endocrine and metabolic** – commoner ones are hypercalcemia and uremia; less common cause includes acute intermittent porphyria.
- **Miscellaneous** – pregnancy (hyperemesis gravidarum), postoperation, cardiac causes (myocardial infarction, and congestive cardiac failure), psychogenic vomiting, and cyclical vomiting syndrome.
- **Functional nausea and vomiting.** This is a diagnosis of exclusion in some patients who present with chronic or episodic symptoms in the absence of a positive physical cause and despite full investigation.

Gastrointestinal Emergencies, Third Edition. Edited by Tony C. K. Tham, John S. A. Collins, and Roy Soetikno.
© 2016 John Wiley & Sons, Ltd. Published 2016 by John Wiley & Sons, Ltd.

Table 2.1 Causes of acute vomiting.

Visceral stimuli	Peritonitis
	Small bowel obstruction
	Pseudo-obstruction
	Acute pancreatitis
	Acute cholecystitis
	Acute appendicitis
	Gastric outlet obstruction
	Mesenteric ischemia
CNS	Vestibular disorders
	CNS tumors
	Meningitis
	Cerebral abscess
	Subarachnoid hemorrhage
	Head injury
	Migraine
	Reye's syndrome
Drugs	Chemotherapeutic agents
	Antibiotics/antivirals
	Narcotics
	Analgesics
	Digoxin
Infections	Sporadic viral infections
	Gastroenteritis (bacterial/viral)
	Hepatitis viruses
	Non-gastrointestinal infections
Endocrine/metabolic	Diabetic ketoacidosis
	Adrenal insufficiency
	Hypercalcemia
	Uremia
	Acute intermittent porphyria
Miscellaneous	Psychogenic
Ethanol abuse	Radiotherapy
	Pregnancy
	Carcinomatosis
	Postoperation
	Cyclical (functional) vomiting

History

A detailed history is crucial in elucidating the cause of vomiting. The above causes should be considered. Constitutional symptoms of fever, myalgia, headache, or possible infectious contacts in the family, school, workplace, or institutions should alert the clinicians to an infectious etiology. Foreign travel and ingestion of inadequately cooked meat raise the suspicion of gastroenteritis. In these situations, a stool sample may reveal Norwalk agent, *Salmonella*, *Campylobacter*, *Staphylococcus aureus*, or *Bacillus cereus*.

Any associated abdominal pain with guarding points to an acute abdomen. Bilious vomiting suggests a proximal intestinal obstruction, while feculent vomiting is due to a more distal obstruction. Gastric outlet obstruction usually leads to postprandial projectile vomiting. When vomiting is associated with jaundice, anorexia and nausea, a hepatic etiology should be considered.

If there are no obvious symptoms of infection or acute abdomen, pregnancy should be excluded in female patients who are in their reproductive years. A thorough drug history, including over-the-counter medication and herbal remedies, may reveal the cause. Patients should also be asked about recent relevant CNS symptoms of vertigo, headache, blurred vision, or head injury. If no organic causes are obvious, then consider psychogenic or functional vomiting.

Examination

- Signs of dehydration – dry tongue, decreased skin turgor, postural hypotension.
- Smell of alcohol or ketones on the breath.
- Abdominal examination for signs of peritonism, gastric stasis, or acute intestinal obstruction. A succussion "splash" is suggestive of gastric outlet obstruction.
- CNS signs of meningism, nystagmus or papilledema.
  Other important clinical features to look out for include:
- Signs of uremia – sallow appearance, pericardial rub.
- Signs of hypoadrenalism – pigmentation, postural hypotension.
- Characteristic skin blisters of acute intermittent porphyria.

Investigations

In all cases, basic laboratory tests such as full blood count, urea, electrolytes, and inflammatory markers are essential. A pregnancy test should be performed in any female of reproductive age, preferably before any radiographic studies are performed. Subsequent investigations will be directed towards the suspected cause elicited from the history.

If infection is suspected:
- Liver function tests.
- Viral hepatitis serology.

- Stool culture.
- Urinalysis and urine culture (particularly in elderly patients).

  If a visceral cause is suspected:
- Serum pancreatic enzymes (amylase and lipase) – if acute epigastric tenderness suggests acute pancreatitis.
- Plain abdominal radiographs (erect and supine) – in the presence of peritonism, they may show an ileus, small bowel obstruction or free gas due to perforation.
- Abdominal ultrasound – may show gallstones and a thickened gallbladder wall if biliary signs are present.
- Upper endoscopy or barium meal – to confirm gastric outlet obstruction, preferably *after* the residual gastric contents have been emptied using a nasogastric tube.

  If a central nervous system cause is suspected:
- Computerized tomography or magnetic resonance imaging of brain;
- Lumbar puncture – should be avoided until the presence of raised intracranial pressure has definitely been excluded.
- Vestibular testing.

  Other tests to consider are synacthen test and urinary porphyrins.

Management of acute nausea and vomiting

A three-step approach is advocated:
1 Correction of any complications of vomiting such as dehydration and acid/electrolyte abnormalities.
2 Targeted therapy of identified cause of vomiting.
3 Symptomatic treatment if necessary.

Fluid replacement

If the patient is dehydrated and cannot tolerate oral fluids, intravenous fluid replacement using normal saline should be started. Potassium supplements may be required in patients with gastric outlet obstruction or if the vomiting has been associated with prolonged diarrhea. Management of diabetic ketoacidosis should be tailored according to local hospital guidelines.

Antiemetic drugs

These agents are useful in the acute phase in the majority of cases of acute vomiting where the underlying etiology is not clear but urgent symptomatic relief is necessary. In some cases, more than one agent may be

Table 2.2 Classes of antiemetic drug.

Antimuscarinic	Scopalamine (hyoscine)
Antihistamine	Cyclizine
	Promethazine
	Meclozine
	Cinnarazine
Antidopaminergic	Prochlorperazine
	Domperidone
	Metoclopramide
Antiserotoninergic	Ondansetron
	Granisetron
	Tropisetron

Table 2.3 Clinical uses of different antiemetics.

Antimuscarinic	Motion sickness
Antihistamine	Motion sickness, vestibular causes
Antidopaminergic	
Extensive indications including gastroenteritis, postoperative, chemo/radiotherapy-induced vomiting, medication	
Antiserotoninergic	As above indications

required. The main types of antiemetic drugs are summarized in Table 2.2 and their clinical uses in Table 2.3.
- **Prochlorperazine (Stemetil®):** Particularly effective in vestibular vomiting. Its main side effects are extrapyramidal symptoms. It must be cautiously used in patients with Parkinson disease, narrow angle glaucoma and a history of phenothiazine sensitivity.

  Oral prochlorperazine – 20 mg initially followed by 10 mg after 2 hours. For prevention, give 5–10 mg 2–3 times daily.

  Sublingual (Buccastem®) – a 3 mg tablet can be placed high up between the upper lip and gums and left to dissolve. Recommended dosage is 1–2 tablets twice daily.

  Suppository – a 25 mg suppository can be placed rectally stat, followed by oral dose after 6 hours if necessary.

  Injection – give 12.5 mg stat by deep intramuscular injection, followed by oral dose after 6 hours if necessary.
- **Cyclizine (Valoid®):** This is a histamine H1 receptor antagonist and is effective in patients where there is a contraindication to the above. It can cause drowsiness and should be used with caution in the elderly. For

severe vomiting or in patients who cannot tolerate oral medication, give 50 mg stat either by intramuscular or intravenous injection and this can be repeated 8-hourly. For less severe vomiting, oral dose 50 mg 8-hourly can be given.

- **Domperidone (Motilium®) and metoclopramide (Maxolon®):** These drugs are dopamine receptor antagonists and also function as prokinetic agents. Domperidone has not been approved for use in the USA. Metoclopramide is contraindicated in gastrointestinal obstruction and perforation. Domperidone can be given orally (10–20 mg) or rectally (30–60 mg) every 4–8 hours. Alternatively, give metoclopramide 10 mg, either oral or injections (intramuscular/intravenous) every 8 hours.
- **Ondansetron (Zofran®):** If all above fail, this serotonin 5-HT3 receptor antagonist can be given as a 4 mg dose either by intramuscular or intravascular injection. It can also be given as 16 mg suppositories. If vomiting is controlled after the initial dose, the oral form can be given up to a daily maximum dose of 32 mg in the 4 or 8 mg tablet form. 5-HT3 receptor antagonists are regarded as first line antiemetics for chemotherapy-induced vomiting and they are generally well tolerated.

- **Erythromycin:** This antibiotic can enhance gastric emptying but may not improve nausea. It has been used as a prokinetic agent in cases of gastroparesis, but there is not a clear evidence base for prolonged benefit.
- **Antidepressants:** These drugs have been used in cases of functional nausea and vomiting where conventional antiemetics have been unsuccessful. They should be used in conjunction with psychological supportive therapy. There are few data or strong evidence base from trial to support their efficacy.

Further reading

American Gastroenterology Association medical position statement: nausea and vomiting. Gastroenterology 2001; 120:261.

Tack J, Talley NJ, Camilleri M, et al. Functional gastrointestinal disorders. In Rome III, The Functional Gastrointestinal Disorders, 3rd ed, Drossman DA, et al (eds), Degnon Associates, McLean, VA, 2006.

Flake ZA, Scalley RD, Bailey AG. Practical selection of antiemetics. Am. Fam. Physician 2004;69:1169.

Management of specific causes of acute vomiting is described in detail in relevant chapters in this book.

CHAPTER 3

Approach to upper gastrointestinal bleeding

Patrick B. Allen and Tony C. K. Tham

Ulster Hospital, Dundonald, Belfast, UK

Introduction

Upper gastrointestinal bleeding (UGIB) is a common presentation to emergency departments and associated with higher mortality with in-patients who experience UGIB. It commonly present with hematemesis (vomiting of blood) and/or melena (passage of black and tarry stools). The initial management of patients with UGIB involves an initial assessment, resuscitation if required, and then endoscopy to achieve hemostasis. A small number of patients may be discharged from the emergency department (ED) if they are deemed "low-risk" and an urgent endoscopy can be subsequently arranged; however, this practice varies throughout countries and institutions.

At endoscopy the major aim is to stratify the patients into low, medium, and high risk, depending on their initial findings and to perform therapeutic intervention if required to stop the bleeding and reduce the risk of recurrent bleeding post-endoscopy (rebleeding).

This chapter will summarize the approach and up-to-date management in patients with UGIB. (See also Chapter 22 on Acute Upper Non-variceal Gastrointestinal Hemorrhage and Chapter 25 on Variceal Hemorrhage.)

History

The symptoms and signs of patients presenting with upper gastrointestinal bleeding may include:
- dyspepsia
- epigastric pain
- heartburn
- weakness
- syncope
- hematemesis (e.g. coffee-ground vomitus, bright red vomitus, etc.)
- melena (black stools)
- hematochezia (bright red rectal bleeding)
- weight loss
- dysphagia.

Hematemesis suggests bleeding proximal to the ligament of Treitz. The character of vomitus can assist with the severity of bleeding – frank blood suggests active and more severe bleeding, whereas dark and coffee-ground vomitus suggests less active bleeding. The majority of patients with melena can have bleeding from the upper gastrointestinal tract; however, a small proportion may have bleeding from the small bowel or proximal right colon.

Causes of upper gastrointestinal bleeding

The causes of UGIB are summarized in Table 3.1 [1].

Past medical history

It is necessary to document the recent use of antiplatelet therapies and non-steroidal anti-inflammatory drugs (NSAIDs). Warfarin/low-molecular-weight heparins, and patients receiving newer anticoagulants such as

Gastrointestinal Emergencies, Third Edition. Edited by Tony C. K. Tham, John S. A. Collins, and Roy Soetikno.
© 2016 John Wiley & Sons, Ltd. Published 2016 by John Wiley & Sons, Ltd.

Table 3.1 Causes of upper gastrointestinal bleeding.

Source of bleeding	Frequency (%)
Peptic ulcer	35–62%
Gastroesophageal varices	4–31%
Mallory–Weiss tear	4–13%
Gastroduodenal erosions	3–11%
Erosive esophagitis	2–8%
Malignancy	1–4%
Unidentified source	7–25%

Source: Laine 2001 (1). Reproduced with permission of McGraw-Hill Education.

Dabigatrin (Pradaxa®) and Rivaroxaban (Xarelto®), should be documented.

As peptic ulcers can recur, it is important to elicit a past medical history of peptic ulcer disease. A history of chronic alcohol abuse or likelihood of chronic viral hepatitis (B or C) increases the likelihood of variceal hemorrhage or portal gastropathy.

Examination and assessment

The initial evaluation of a patient with UGIB includes: a full history, physical examination, laboratory tests, and in some centers, nasogastric tube insertion (to estimate the volume and activity of the blood loss).

The benefit of a full initial evaluation is to assess the quantity of the bleed, the severity of the bleed, possible causes of the bleed, and any associated conditions that may be associated with a higher mortality (e.g. chronic liver disease).

In a recent meta-analysis on the indicators for UGIB, the specific indicators include: melena (likelihood ratio LR 5.1–5,9), melena identified on per-rectal exam (LR 25), blood or coffee ground-like vomitus detected during nasogastric lavage (LR 9.6), and a ratio of blood urea nitrogen to serum creatinine greater than 30 (LR 7.5) [2].

Specific factors associated with "severe bleeding" included red blood detected during nasogastric lavage (LR 3.1), tachycardia (LR 4.9), and or hemoglobin less than 8 g/dL (LR 4.5–6.2).

The majority of patients with melena can have bleeding from the upper gastrointestinal tract; however, a small proportion may have bleeding from the small bowel or proximal colon.

Table 3.2 Glasgow-Blatchford Score for upper gastrointestinal bleeding.

Admission risk marker	Score component value
Blood urea	
≥6.5 <8.0	2
≥8.0 <10.0	3
≥10.0 <25.0	4
≥25	6
Hemoglobin (g/L) for men	
12.0 <13.0	1
≥10.0 <12.0	3
<10.0	6
Hemoglobin for women	
≥10.0 <12.0	1
<10.0	6
Systolic blood pressure (mmHg)	
100–109	1
90–99	2
<90	3
Other markers	
Pulse ≥100 (per min)	1
Presentation with melena	1
Presentation with syncope	2
Hepatic disease	2
Cardiac failure	2

Scores of 6 or greater were associated with a greater than 50% risk of requiring an intervention (3,4).
Source: Blatchford 2013 (3) and Rockall 1996 (4). Reproduced with permission of Elsevier and the BMJ.

Initial assessment: risk stratification

See Chapter 22, Acute Upper Non-variceal Hemorrhage, for more details.

An urgent assessment of patients who present with UGIB should allow triage into low, medium-, and high-risk, and patients can be stratified according to risk with various risk calculators. The widely used calculators are the *Glasgow Blatchford Score (GBS)* (Table 3.2) and the *Rockall Score* (pre- and postendoscopy) (Table 3.3), and the *AIMS-65* scoring systems (Table 3.4) (3,4).

The Blatchford Score includes biochemical markers of blood loss and renal failure including: urea and hemoglobin level, whereas the Rockall Score includes age parameters, and also the postendoscopy diagnosis to ascertain the risk of rebleeding and mortality. The AIMS-65 scoring system includes albumin, INR, Glasgow Coma Scale, blood pressure, and age.

Table 3.3 Rockall Score for upper gastrointestinal bleeding.

Variable	Score 0	Score 1	Score 2	Score 3
Age	<60	60–79	>80	
Shock	No shock	Pulse > 100 BP > 100 systolic	Systolic < 100	
Co-morbidity	Nil		CCF, IHD, major morbidity	Renal failure, liver failure, metastatic cancer
Diagnosis	Mallory–Weiss tear	All other diagnoses	GI malignancy	
Evidence of bleeding	None		Blood, adherent clot, spurting vessel	

Source: Rockall 1996 (4). Reproduced with permission of Elsevier and the BMJ.

Table 3.4 Components of the pre-endoscopy AIMS 65 Score.

Albumin less than 30 g/L
INR greater than 1.5
Altered mental status (Glasgow Coma Scale score less than 14)
Systolic blood pressure of 90 mmHg or less
Age older than 65 years
Mortality associated with the number of risk factors in the AIMS 65 Score
- No risk factors 0.3%
- One risk factor 1%
- Two risk factors 3%
- Three risk factors 9%
- Four risk factors 15%
- Five risk factors 25%

Source: Saltzman 2011 (21). Reproduction with permission from Elsevier.

Can "low-risk' patients be discharged from the ED for early outpatient endoscopy?

A small proportion of patients with low GBS may be treated as outpatients with an early endoscopy [5]. In this study the GBS was better in predicting patients' need for hospital-based intervention, 30-day mortality and identifying low-risk patients than the Rockall Score, the Baylor Bleeding score, and the Cedars-Sinai Medical Center predictive index. An age-extended GBS (EGBS) identified a significantly higher proportion of low-risk patients than the GBS ($p = 0.006$); however, this requires further external validation. None of the scoring systems accurately predicted which patients would have rebleeding or mortality at 30 days.

This study is promising, but requires further validation and better scoring systems are required, which can accurately predict rebleeding and medium-term mortality, before they can be reliably utilized.

Medium- to high-risk patients with UGIB

All patients with hemodynamic instability (shock, orthostatic hypotension) or active bleeding should be admitted to a high dependency/intensive care unit for resuscitation and close observation. The majority of patients can be admitted to a gastrointestinal ward that is familiar with managing patients before and after endoscopic therapy.

AIMS 65 is a newly developed and validated score (Table 3.4), and in one US study appeared to be superior to GBS in predicting specifically inpatient mortality from UGIB; however, the GBS was superior for predicting the requirement for blood transfusion. Both risk scores were similar when predicting the composite clinical endpoint of: inpatient mortality, rebleeding, and need for endoscopic, radiological, or surgical intervention, blood transfusion, intensive care admission, rebleeding, length of stay, and timing of endoscopy [6]. The AIMS 65 score requires further validation in different countries, and racial mixes before it can be widely adopted.

Management of UGIB

Resuscitation

The initial resuscitation of patients should include administration of intravenous fluids, supplementary oxygen, and correction of any underlying coagulopathy. Routine blood transfusion in patients with UGIB is controversial, and a Cochrane Review meta-analysis suggested that red blood cell transfusion in patients with

UGIB may be associated with higher mortality and rebleeding rate. This meta-analysis was limited by the small studies included in the analysis and the large quantity of missing data. In addition, the most important confounder was the possibility that patients who presented with more severe bleeding received more rapid and aggressive transfusions [7]. In the recently published UK National Institute for Health and Care Excellence (NICE) guidance, there is agreement with blood transfusion in massive bleeding with blood, platelets, and clotting factors, if certain criteria are met. The guidance advised that platelet transfusions are not to be offered in patients who are "not actively bleeding and are hemodynamically stable," but only offered to patients "actively bleeding with a platelet count less than 50×10^9/L."

It was recommended that fresh frozen plasma should be offered to patients with either a fibrinogen level less than 1 g/L or a prothrombin time (international normalized ratio [INR]) or activated partial thromboplastin time greater than 1.5 times the upper limit of normal range. Those taking warfarin with therapeutic INRs and who are actively bleeding should be offered prothrombin complex concentrate [8].

Patients who receive early intensive resuscitation are more quickly stabilized hemodynamically and the hematocrit corrected quicker, resulting in a lower incidence of myocardial infarction and reduction in mortality.

The approach to a hemodynamically unstable patient begins initially with assessing the airway, breathing, and circulation (ABCs). Some patients who present with severe blood loss and hypovolemic shock can present with mental status changes; in these circumstances the patients are at increased risk for aspiration. This is a potentially preventable complication and one that if present may increase morbidity and mortality in these patients. This situation should be recognized early and patients electively intubated in a controlled setting using cricoid pressure.

When the airway has been secured it is important to obtain intravenous access. It is adequate to obtain bilateral 16-gauge upper extremity intravenous lines for volume resuscitative measures. An estimated guideline for fluid replacement to correct the hypovolemia is the *3-for-1 rule*. This rule aims to replace each milliliter of blood loss with 3 mL of crystalloid (or colloid) fluid. This regime is commonly the initial fluid replacement until cross-matched or type-specific blood becomes available.

Patients with comorbidities (e.g. cardiovascular diseases) may require pulmonary artery catheter insertion to evaluate cardiac performance profiles and resuscitation adequacy in the early stages.

Are there risks with "over-transfusing" patients with UGIB?

It is important to avoid over-transfusing patients with variceal and non-variceal bleeding as it may be associated with worse outcomes. A recent randomized trial included 921 patients with UGIB were assigned to either a "restrictive transfusion strategy" (transfusion to only when the Hb fell to <7 g/dL) or a "liberal transfusion strategy" (transfusion when the Hb fell to less than 9 g/dL) [9]. Patients in the restrictive transfusion group were more likely than those in the liberal group to avoid transfusion (51% vs. 14%, respectively) and received fewer units of blood (mean 1.5 vs. 3.8 units). Mortality was lower in the restrictive group (5% vs. 9%, adjusted hazard ratio 0.55). Patients in the restrictive group were also less likely to have further bleeding or complications. Among patients with cirrhosis, the risk of death and further bleeding were lower with the restrictive group for patients with Childs "A or B" cirrhosis, but were similar for patients with Childs "C" cirrhosis. All patients in this study underwent emergency endoscopy (mean within 5 hours) and endoscopic therapy was given to those with active bleeding, a non-bleeding visible vessel, an adherent clot, or bleeding esophageal varices. This prompt endoscopy cannot be replicated in all units, and therefore the restrictive strategy may not be better for these patients who do not have an early endoscopy within 5 hours of presentation to the ED.

A recent large retrospective study, which included 1677 patients with non–variceal UGIB, reported that if patients received a blood transfusion within 24 hours, this was associated with an increased risk of bleeding after adjusting for factors such as hemodynamic instability, endoscopic therapy, high risk stigmata, or recurrent hemorrhage, initial Hb value and the presence of blood on rectal examination or in the nasogastric tube aspirate (OR 1.8) [10].

How to manage anti-coagulated patients with UGIB?

Endoscopy also appears to be safe in patients with UGIB who are moderately anti-coagulated [11] and therefore our approach is to reverse the INR to less than 3 before endoscopy, whilst continuing the reversal during endoscopy. This level of moderate anticoagulation should not delay the endoscopy.

How to manage patients with UGIB on aspirin or clopidrogel

Patients presenting with acute upper gastrointestinal bleeding whilst taking aspirin or clopidogrel present a clinical dilemma (see also Chapter 22, Acute Upper Non-variceal Hemorrhage). Stopping these drugs may reduce the risk of continuing bleeding but risks vascular events that can prove fatal. Both aspirin and clopidogrel bind irreversibly to platelet receptors, thereby impairing platelet function for 7–10 days. The rationale for discontinuing their use following the onset of bleeding is therefore ill founded, and for patients in whom there is a good indication for their use, it is wise to continue aspirin and clopidogrel despite upper gastrointestinal hemorrhage.

What is the role of proton pump inhibitors?

The use of proton pump inhibitors (PPI) before endoscopy in suspected non-variceal hemorrhage is controversial. The recently published NICE guidelines suggest that PPI should not be offered before endoscopy in patients with non-variceal bleeding [8]. However, in practice it is difficult to predict that patients do not have variceal bleeding, although with a reliable history and examination this accuracy may be improved.

One of the largest studies to evaluate the role of pre-endoscopy proton pump inhibitor therapy randomized 638 patients with UGIB to omeprazole or placebo before endoscopy. Patients randomized to omeprazole had significantly shorter lengths of stay, fewer actively bleeding ulcers (6% vs. 15%) and more ulcers with a clean base. There was no significant difference in the proportion needing surgery or with recurrent bleeding [12]. A Cochrane analysis of six randomized trials of pre-endoscopic PPI therapy found no significant difference between PPI groups and controls in mortality (OR1.12), rebleeding (OR 0.81), or surgery (OR 0.96). However, pre-endoscopic use of PPIs significantly reduced the number of patients with high risk stigmata (OR 0.67) and the need for endoscopic therapy (OR 0.68) compared with patients who received placebo or a histamine-2 receptor antagonist [13]. The 2010 international consensus guidelines on UGIB recommends the use of intravenous PPIs in all patient with high-risk lesions post-endoscopic therapy [14]. High-dose oral PPIs may be used in patients who do not have active bleeding or high risk stigmata for recurrent bleeding and therefore have a low risk for rebleeding.

The optimal prescribing of PPI therapy with dosing, route of administration, and the decision to prescribe prior to endoscopy remains controversial, and practice varies widely between units and countries.

Endoscopy for UGIB
Timing of endoscopy

It is recommended that all hospitals provide adequate resources for an endoscopy service that can provide interventional endoscopy within 24 hours after patient admission. In addition in high risk patients who present with unstable haemodynamic parameters and who present with UGIB, an urgent endoscopy should be performed when the patient has been resuscitated [8]. The benefit for early endoscopy (defined as endoscopy within 24 hours) was reported by a large retrospective study from the USA using a database of hospital inpatient admission (Nationwide Inpatient Sample) [15]. The study included 35 747 adults with acute variceal bleeding and 435 765 adults with non-variceal UGIB. Among patients with variceal hemorrhage, inpatient mortality was 8% for those who underwent upper endoscopy within one day of admission and was 15% who those who did not (OR 1.18). For patients with non-variceal bleeding the corresponding mortality rates were 3 and 7%, respectively (OR 1.32). Another study included 8222 patients with UGIB. In this study, patients who died had a significantly longer waiting time to endoscopy than those who survived (1.65 versus 0.95 days OR 1.10) [16].

Endoscopy for variceal and non-variceal UGIB will be discussed in Chapters 25 and 22, respectively.

What do in cases of rebleeding

In patients with rebleeding a second-look endoscopy is reasonable and has fewer complications than proceeding straight to surgery. However, if hemostasis is not achievable then these patients should be considered for interventional radiology, and if not available then emergency surgery. However, interventional radiology is not as widely available as emergency surgery and this should be delivered where local facilities and expertise exist; this approach was supported in the recently published NICE guidance [8]. Reduceed for surgery, and had fewer complications without an increase in mortality [17][18].

Variceal hemorrhage
Prophylactic antibiotics
Multiple trials have demonstrated the effectiveness of prophylactic antibiotics in cirrhotic patients hospitalized for bleeding and suggest an overall decrease in the risk of infectious complications and mortality. Both the AASLD American Association for Study of Liver Diseases (AASLD) and NICE guidance have recommended antibiotic prophylaxis in any patient with liver cirrhosis and UGIB [8].

Intravenous vasopressin and its analogs
Intravenous vasopressin constricts mesenteric arterioles and decreases portal venous inflow, thereby reducing portal pressures. Terlipressin is a synthetic analogue of vasopressin (not available in the USA) and is widely used in many countries. A meta-analysis of patients prescribed terlipressin for variceal UGIB reported a significant reduction in all-cause mortality with terlipressin compared with placebo (RR 0.66) [19]. Terlipressin is usually administered at a dose of 2 mg every 4 hours and then reduced to 1 mg every 4 hours when haemostasis has been achieved, and the usual treatment period is over 72 hours.

Somatostatin inhibits the release of vasodilator hormones such as glucagon which results in decreased portal inflow and octeotride is a long acting analogue of somatostatin. Octeotride is usually administered as a 50 µg bolus followed by a continuous infusion of 50 µg per hour and is continued for 3–5 days. Somatostatin is more effective for controlling bleeding than placebo or vasopressin and has fewer side effects than vasopressin. Octeotride's effects are less well studied but remains the first line in the many centres in the USA for variceal haemorrhage.

Post-endoscopy management
Patients who have had UGIB in the presence of *Helicobacter pylori* should receive eradication therapy. A large systematic review demonstrated the benefit of *H. pylori* eradication on the rate of rebleeding was greater than antisecretory therapy [20].

If patients receive concomitant antiplatelet medications or NSAIDs the risks and need for therapy should be discussed with the patients and/or cardiologists (in the case of anti-platelets therapies if coronary stents are *in situ*). For patients with UGIB who require a NSAID, a PPI with a cyclo-oxygenase-2 inhibitor is preferred to reduce subsequent rebleeding. Patients with UGIB who require secondary cardiovascular prophylaxis should start receiving acetylsalicylic acid (ASA/aspirin) again as soon as cardiovascular risks outweigh gastrointestinal risks (usually within 7 days); ASA plus PPI therapy is preferred over clopidogrel alone to reduce rebleeding [14].

Summary

UGIB is a common presentation to EDs and in patients who are admitted to hospital. Patients who present to the ED with UGIB should be risk assessed with the GBS at presentation and the Rockall score after endoscopy.

In the initial resuscitation of patients it is important to avoid "over-transfusing" patients with blood products. Patient should receive endoscopy after resuscitation if severe acute upper gastrointestinal bleeding has occurred, and lower-risk patients should receive endoscopy within 24 hours after presentation. When required, therapeutic endoscopy for non-variceal UGIB a combination of techniques (clipping and/or thermocoagulation) is preferable to mono-therapy to achieve hemostasis.

Patients with suspected or confirmed variceal bleeding should receive antibiotics at presentation and those with high-risk/rebleeding after an episode of variceal bleeding should be considered for transjugular intrahepatic portosystemic shunt (TIPSS). After endoscopy in patients who have cardiovascular risk factors, aspirin and PPI therapy should be commenced when the risk of cardiovascular events are greater than the risk of rebleeding. If patients have had recent coronary intervention then discussion with cardiologists is advised and these patients may have a high risk of cardiovascular morbidity and mortality if the antiplatelet therapy is stopped abruptly.

References

1. Laine L. Gastrointestinal bleeding, in Braunwalde E, Fauci A, Kasser D, eds. Harrison's Principles of Internal Medicine 15th edn. McGraw-Hill, New York, p. 252; 2001.
2. Srygley FD, Gerardo CJ, Tran T, Fisher DA. Does this patient have a severe upper gastrointestinal bleed? *JAMA* 2012;**307**(10):1072–9.

3. Blatchford O, Murray WR, Blatchford M. A risk score to predict need for treatment for upper-gastrointestinal haemorrhage. *Lancet.* 2000;**356**(9238):1318–21.

4. Rockall TA, Logan RF, Devlin HB, Northfield TC. Risk assessment after acute upper gastrointestinal haemorrhage. *Gut.* 1996;**38**(3):316–21.

5. Laursen SB, Hansen JM, Schaffalitzky de Muckadell OB. The Glasgow Blatchford score is the most accurate assessment of patients with upper gastrointestinal hemorrhage. *Clin. Gastroenterol. Hepatol.* 2012;**10**(10):1130–1135.e1.

6. Hyett BH, Abougergi MS, Charpentier JP, et al. The AIMS65 score compared with the Glasgow-Blatchford score in predicting outcomes in upper GI bleeding. *Gastrointest. Endosc.* 2013;**77**(4):551–7.

7. Jairath V, Hearnshaw S, Brunskill SJ, et al. Red cell transfusion for the management of upper gastrointestinal haemorrhage. Cochrane Database Syst. Rev. 2010;(9):CD006613.

8. NICE Guidelines Acute upper gastrointestinal Bleeding: management. [Online] Available from http://www.nice.org.uk/nicemedia/live/13762/59549/59549.pdf (accessed 22 June 2015).

9. Villanueva C, Colomo A, Bosch A, et al. Transfusion strategies for acute upper gastrointestinal bleeding. *N. Engl. J. Med.* 2013;**368**(1):11–21.

10. Restellini S, Kherad O, Jairath V, Martel M, Barkun AN. Red blood cell transfusion is associated with increased rebleeding in patients with nonvariceal upper gastrointestinal bleeding. *Aliment. Pharmacol. Ther.* 2013;**37**(3):316–22.

11. Wolf AT, Wasan SK, Saltzman JR. Impact of anticoagulation on rebleeding following endoscopic therapy for nonvariceal upper gastrointestinal hemorrhage. *Am. J. Gastroenterol.* 2007;**102**(2):290–6.

12. Lau JY, Leung WK, Wu JCY, et al. Omeprazole before endoscopy in patients with gastrointestinal bleeding. *N. Engl. J. Med.* 2007;**356**(16):1631–40.

13. Sreedharan A, Martin J, Leontiadis GI, et al. Proton pump inhibitor treatment initiated prior to endoscopic diagnosis in upper gastrointestinal bleeding. Cochrane Database Syst. Rev. 2010;(7):CD005415.

14. Barkun AN, Bardou M, Kuipers EJ, et al. International consensus recommendations on the management of patients with nonvariceal upper gastrointestinal bleeding. *Ann. Intern. Med.* 2010;**152**(2):101–13.

15. Wysocki JD, Srivastav S, Winstead NS. A nationwide analysis of risk factors for mortality and time to endoscopy in upper gastrointestinal haemorrhage. *Aliment. Pharmacol. Ther.* 2012;**36**(1):30–6.

16. Tsoi KKF, Chiu PWY, Chan FKL, Ching JYL, Lau JYW, Sung JJY. The risk of peptic ulcer bleeding mortality in relation to hospital admission on holidays: a cohort study on 8222 cases of peptic ulcer bleeding. *Am. J. Gastroenterol.* 2012;**107**(3):405–10.

17. Aad G, Abbott B, Abdallah J, et al. Search for pair production of a heavy up-type quark decaying to a W boson and a b quark in the lepton + jets channel with the ATLAS detector. *Phys. Rev. Lett.* 2012;**108**(26):261802.

18. Wong TCL, Wong K-T, Chiu PWY, et al. A comparison of angiographic embolization with surgery after failed endoscopic hemostasis to bleeding peptic ulcers. *Gastrointest. Endosc.* 2011;**73**(5):900–8.

19. Ioannou G, Doust J, Rockey DC. Terlipressin for acute esophageal variceal hemorrhage. Cochrane Database Syst. Rev. 2003;(1):CD002147.

20. Gisbert JP, Khorrami S, Carballo F, Calvet X, Gené E, Dominguez-Muñoz JE. *H. pylori* eradication therapy vs. antisecretory non-eradication therapy (with or without long-term maintenance antisecretory therapy) for the prevention of recurrent bleeding from peptic ulcer. Cochrane Database Syst. Rev. 2004;(2):CD004062.

21. Saltzman JR, Tabak YP, Hyett BH, Sun X, Travis AC, Johannes RS. A simple risk score accurately predicts in-hospital mortality, length of stay, and cost in acute upper GI bleeding. *Gastrointest. Endosc.* 2011;**74**(6):1215–24.

CHAPTER 4

Approach to acute abdominal pain

Tony C. K. Tham

Ulster Hospital, Dundonald, Belfast, UK

Introduction

The term "acute abdomen" describes a syndrome of sudden abdominal pain with accompanying symptoms and signs that focus attention on the abdominal region. The causes of an acute abdomen can be abdominal (Table 4.1) or extra-abdominal (Table 4.2). In the majority of cases in adults, the diagnosis of acute abdominal pain can be established on clinical grounds without resort to extensive investigation.

The following pathophysiological mechanisms can cause acute abdominal pain (Table 4.3): peritoneal, obstructive, hemorrhage, and non-specific.

Peritoneal

This symptom complex is a consequence of an inflamed intra-abdominal viscus. The inflamed viscus causes irritation of the visceral peritoneum, initially causing vague central abdominal pain, which may be difficult for the patient to localize. Continued inflammation or localized perforation leads to involvement of the parietal peritoneum. Pain becomes localized and is then associated with tenderness, guarding, and rebound tenderness on local palpation. Spread of infection generally throughout the abdominal cavity leads to generalized abdominal wall rigidity, often associated with a rigid or board-like abdomen. Generalized systemic signs of sepsis are apparent at this stage with pyrexia, tachycardia, and pallor.

Obstructive

In this situation, a hollow viscus has a lumenal blockage which interferes with its normal motility pattern and its ability to deal with lumenal contents or secretions. This often results in severe crampy pain, as in cases of biliary colic where the cystic duct is obstructed by a gallstone or renal colic due to an obstructing ureteric calculus. When the bowel itself is obstructed the result is the classical clinical triad of:

- abdominal colic
- vomiting (due to failure of transit)
- increasing constipation.

Intestinal obstruction, if left untreated, will lead to perforation with signs of an acute abdomen. In the early stages of acute obstruction, bowel sounds are often high pitched or "tinkling" in character, but the sounds disappear when prolonged obstruction leads to perforation and peritonitis.

Hemorrhagic

Although this is not the commonest cause of acute abdominal pain, it must be considered because of its serious and often rapid progression. It is due to bleeding into the peritoneal cavity or retroperitoneum either due to a leaking major vessel (e.g. aortic aneurysm) or a ruptured organ (e.g. spleen or ectopic tubal pregnancy). Onset of the pain may be insidious and poorly localized at first. Soiling of the peritoneum with blood may simulate peritonitis. The bowel sounds may diminish and

Gastrointestinal Emergencies, Third Edition. Edited by Tony C. K. Tham, John S. A. Collins, and Roy Soetikno.
© 2016 John Wiley & Sons, Ltd. Published 2016 by John Wiley & Sons, Ltd.

Table 4.1 Abdominal causes of acute abdomen.

Gastrointestinal	Appendicitis
	Perforated peptic ulcer
	Intestinal obstruction
	Intestinal perforation
	Intestinal ischemia
	Colonic diverticulitis
	Meckel diverticulitis
	Inflammatory bowel disease
Pancreatic, biliary,	Acute pancreatitis
hepatic, splenic	Acute cholecystitis
	Hepatic abscess
	Ruptured or hemorrhagic
	hepatic tumor
	Acute hepatitis
	Acute cholangitis
	Splenic rupture
Urological	Ureteral stone
	Pyelonephritis
Retroperitoneal	Aortic aneurysm
	Retroperitoneal hemorrhage
Gynecological	Ruptured ovarian cyst
	Ovarian torsion
	Ectopic pregnancy
	Acute salpingitis
	Pyosalpinx
	Endometritis
	Uterine rupture
Abdominal wall	Rectus muscle hematoma

Source: Mulholland and Sweeney 2003 [1]. Reproduced with permission from Wiley.

Table 4.2 Extra-abdominal causes of acute abdomen.

Thoracic	Myocardial infarction
	Acute pericarditis
	Lower lobe pneumonia
	Pneumothorax
	Pulmonary infarction
Hematological	Sickle cell crisis
	Acute leukemia
Neurological	Herpes zoster
	Tabes dorsalis
	Nerve root compression
Metabolic	Diabetic ketoacidosis
	Addisonian crisis
	Acute porphyria
	Hyperlipoproteinemia
Drug related	Lead toxicity
	Narcotic withdrawal

Source: Mulholland and Sweeney 2003 [1]. Reproduced with permission from Wiley.

Table 4.3 Causes of abdominal pain based on pathophysiological mechanisms.

Infective/inflammatory	Acute cholecystitis
	Acute pancreatitis
	Acute appendicitis
	Pelvic inflammatory disease
Hemorrhagic	Ruptured aneurysm
	Ruptured ectopic pregnancy
	Mesenteric thrombosis
	Ruptured spleen
Obstructive	Intestinal obstruction
	Biliary obstruction
	Renal colic
Miscellaneous	Referred from chest, spine
	Diabetes
	Porphyria
	Psychogenic

ileus may be present. The patient's circulatory system will show signs of shock and the abdomen will distend as bleeding progresses.

Non-specific acute abdominal pain

This presentation is common and may present with colicky abdominal pain, or even progressive generalized pain. Pain may result from:
- parietal pleura in pneumonia
- subphrenic sepsis
- myocardial ischemia
- diabetic ketoacidosis
- hypercalcemia
- porphyria
- psychogenic factors.

In this scenario, the abdomen is usually generally tender with guarding. Bowel sounds are preserved and there may be no signs of systemic sepsis or bleeding.

History

A careful history can often lead to an accurate diagnosis of abdominal pain. Several important features need to be determined. A comparison of the symptoms of common causes of acute abdominal pain is shown in Table 4.4.

Site
A diagnosis based on site alone is difficult because of the phenomenon of referred pain. However, such an approach is commonly used with most clinicians dividing the abdomen into quadrants (Table 4.5).

Table 4.4 Comparison of symptoms of common causes of acute abdominal pain.

Condition	Onset	Location	Character	Descriptor	Radiation	Intensity
Appendicitis	Gradual	Periumbilical early; RIF late	Diffuse early, localized late	Ache	RIF	11
Cholecystitis	Rapid	RUQ	Localized	Constricting	Scapula	11
Pancreatitis	Rapid	Epigastric, back	Localized	Boring	Midback	11 to 111
Diverticulitis	Gradual	LIF	Localized	Ache	None	1 to 11
Perforated peptic ulcer	Sudden	Epigastric	Localized early, diffuse late	Burning	None	111
Small bowel obstruction	Gradual	Periumbilical	Diffuse	Crampy	None	11
Mesenteric ischemia/infarct	Sudden	Periumbilical	Diffuse	Agonizing	None	111
Ruptured abdominal aortic aneurysm	Sudden	Abdominal, back, flank	Diffuse	Tearing	Back, flank	111
Gastroenteritis	Gradual	Periumbilical	Diffuse	Spasmodic	None	1 to 11
Pelvic inflammatory disease	Gradual	Either LIF, pelvic	Localized	Ache	Upper thigh	11
Ruptured ectopic pregnancy	Sudden	Either LIF, pelvic	Localized	Light headed	None	11

RIF, right iliac fossa; RUQ, right upper quadrant; LIF, left iliac fossa; 1, mild; 11, moderate; 111, severe.
Source: Glasgow and Mulvihill 2003 [2]. Reproduced with permission from Elsevier.

Temporal characteristics

Immediate pain is suggestive of an acute obstruction of a hollow viscus (e.g. bile duct obstruction by a stone), perforation or acute ischemia. The more common situation is a relatively gradual onset of pain, which may take hours or days. This is typical of inflammatory conditions such as appendicitis, diverticulitis, pancreatitis, and cholecystitis. Abrupt spontaneous cessation of pain suggests the relief of an obstructed organ (e.g. passage of a stone). Intermittent, or waxing and waning, pain is typical of colic, which is usually intestinal in origin. Biliary pain actually shows less variability than is commonly thought. Some other causes of intermittent abdominal pain with periodicity (i.e. long duration of pain-free intervals), are shown in Table 4.6.

Character and intensity of pain

Rating the severity or describing the nature of the pain seldom helps in distinguishing the cause of the pain. The pain of colic refers to a characteristic wave-like build-up in intensity, culminating in severe pain often associated with other symptoms such as sweating, nausea and dizziness. Colicky abdominal pain is due to obstructive causes as described above. Causes of colicky abdominal pain are listed in Table 4.3 (obstructive causes).

Relieving and aggravating factors

The pain of duodenal ulcer tends to improve with food or antacids. The pain of gastric ulcer may be worsened by food. Relief after vomiting suggests a pyloric or proximal small bowel lesion. In contrast, recurrent and progressive vomiting usually results from mechanical intestinal obstruction. Colonic pain may be relieved by a bowel movement. Retroperitoneal processes (e.g. pancreatitis), tend to be relieved by maneuvers that increase the volume of this space such as sitting up and bending forward. Obstructive pain tends to induce restlessness. Peritoneal pain is aggravated by motion, coughing, or straining.

Associated symptoms

Anorexia accompanies almost all acute abdominal processes but is not specific to any pathological process. Anorexia is found less frequently with urological or gynecological causes. Abdominal distension usually signifies accumulation of swallowed gas in the bowel as a result of mechanical obstruction or ileus. Constipation

Table 4.5 Localization of common causes of acute abdominal pain.

Right upper quadrant	Acute cholecystitis
	Biliary colic
	Acute hepatic inflammation or distention
Left upper quadrant	Splenic infarct
	Splenic flexure ischemia
Right lower quadrant	Appendicitis
	Infective terminal ileitis
	Crohn's disease
	Tubo-ovarian disorders
	Ectopic pregnancy
	Ruptured ovarian cyst
	Salpingitis
	Renal disorders
	Right ureteric calculus
	Pyelonephritis
	Pyogenic sacroileitis
Left lower quadrant	Acute diverticulitis
	Infectious or inflammatory colitis
	Pyogenic sacroileitis
	Tubo-ovarian disorders
Central abdominal pain	Gastroenteritis
	Peptic ulcer disease
	Small intestinal colic
	Acute pancreatitis
Diffuse abdominal pain	Acute infectious peritonitis
	Appendicitis
	Diverticulitis
	Inflammatory bowel disease and toxic megacolon
	Perforated ulcer
	Spontaneous bacterial peritonitis in cirrhosis
	Ischemic bowel
	Acute non infectious peritonitis
	Familial Mediteranean fever
	Hemorrhagic pancreatitis
	Postoperative pain
	Perforated ulcer

Source: Pasricha 2003 [3]. Reproduced with permission from Wiley.

Table 4.6 Causes of intermittent abdominal pain with periodicity.

Physical or obstructive	Cholelithiasis
	Ampullary stenosis
	Intermittent intestinal obstruction, e.g.:
	– intussusception
	– internal hernia
	– abdominal wall hernia
Metabolic or genetic	Acute intermittent porphyria
	Familial Mediterranean fever
Neurological	Abdominal epilepsy
	Abdominal migraine
	Diabetic and other forms of radiculopathy
	Nerve entrapment syndromes
Miscellaneous	Irritable bowel syndrome
	Endometriosis
	Heavy metal poisoning
	Mesenteric ischemia
	Acute recurrent pancreatitis

Source: Pasricha 2003 [3]. Reproduced with permission from Wiley.

of inflammatory bowel disease, mesenteric ischemia, or mesenteric venous thrombosis.

Other aspects of history

Recent symptoms of dyspepsia, jaundice, amenorrhea, dysuria, or renal colic can suggest a possible etiology. A past history of peptic ulcer, gallstones, abdominal trauma, or peripheral vascular disease can also suggest a possible etiology. A history of peripheral vascular disease could suggest an aortic aneurysm or mesenteric ischemia. Recent non-steroidal anti-inflammatory drug (NSAID) or aspirin use could suggest an ulcer. Other aspects of the history such as presence of diabetes, alcohol, or drug abuse may be relevant in determining the cause.

Examination

Inspection

A patient with serious intraperitoneal disease usually has an anxious, pale face, sweating, dilated pupils, and shallow breathing. The patient should be assessed for pyrexia, signs of shock, fetor, and ketones on the breath. With peritonitis, the patient tends to lie immobile. Knees may be flexed. Inhaling or coughing aggravates the pain. With colic, the patient may appear

may be a sign of previous health habits, a disease process such as obstruction or the development of a complication such as perforation. Obstipation refers to the cessation of intestinal movements or flatus coinciding with the development of acute abdominal pain. Obstipation is associated with mechanical obstruction or ileus. Watery diarrhea suggests acute gastroenteritis. Bloody diarrhea may be associated with exacerbation restless with frequent changes in posture to relieve discomfort. The location of all surgical scars, masses, external hernias and stomas should be determined. Bruising in the flanks will indicate possible acute pancreatitis (Grey Turner's sign). This is due to exudation of fluid stained by pancreatic necrosis into the subcutaneous tissue. Similar discoloration in the periumbilical area is known as the Cullen sign. A distended abdomen should suggest ascites or intestinal obstruction.

Palpation

Light and deep palpation of the abdomen will indicate areas of local tenderness, rebound, or guarding or whether generalized tenderness is present. Point tenderness, caused by the movement of parietal peritoneum against the inflamed surface of a diseased viscus, gives good evidence of a localized inflammatory process. The Carnett test may help to determine whether chronic abdominal pain arises from the abdominal wall or has an intra-abdominal origin. If a tender spot is identified, the patient is asked to raise his or her head, thus tensing the abdominal muscles. If there is greater tenderness on repeat palpation, the Carnett test is positive and suggests a cause in the abdominal wall. The Murphy sign may indicate the presence of an acute cholecystitis. The right upper quadrant is palpated and, during the palpation, the patient is asked to take a deep breath. If the patient complains of increased pain during this maneuver due to the movement of the gallbladder towards the peritoneum, this sign is positive suggesting the presence of an inflamed gallbladder. If a mass is palpable, this could be due to a neoplasm or hernia. A palpable tender mass in the right iliac fossa could also be due to Crohn's disease or an appendix abscess. A pulsatile abdominal mass usually indicates the presence of an abdominal aortic aneurysm.

Auscultation

Bowel sounds will be high pitched in impending obstruction, absent in ileus or the presence of peritonitis. Bowel sounds are considered absent if no tones are heard over a 2-minute period.

A *digital rectal examination* should be performed. If an inflamed appendix lies deep within the pelvis, point tenderness may be elicited by palpation through the right rectal wall.

A *pelvic examination* should be performed if a gynaecological cause is suspected.

Investigation

Investigations should reflect the clinical suspicion raised during the history and clinical examination. They must be tailored to answer specific questions arising from the differential diagnosis.

- **Full blood picture and differential white cell count:** Hemoglobin will be reduced in the presence of acute intra-abdominal bleeding. White cell count will rise in the presence of sepsis with a neutrophilia in cases of bacterial infection
- **Serum amylase** will be elevated in acute pancreatitis (usually three or four times greater than normal), perforated peptic ulcer and in some cases of ruptured abdominal aortic aneurysm, small bowel obstruction and ischemia and ectopic pregnancy.
- **Serum lipase** has a superior sensitivity and specificity for acute pancreatitis and where available is preferable to serum amylase for the diagnosis of acute pancreatitis.
- **Urea, electrolytes and blood glucose:** Sodium will be low in cases of pain associated with prolonged vomiting and decreased fluid intake.
- **Liver function tests:** Should be performed in patients with upper abdominal pain.
- **Urine pregnancy testing:** Should be performed in women of reproductive age with lower abdominal pain.
- **Other blood tests:** These are obtained on the basis of clinical history, e.g. prothrombin time in those with suspected liver disease, blood cultures if pyrexia is present.
- **Plain abdominal radiography (erect and supine)** will demonstrate bowel fluid levels in cases of obstruction, free intra-abdominal gas. It is important to determine if a patient has complete or partial small bowel obstruction. Complete obstruction is characterized by dilated loops of small intestine with air-fluid levels and no gas within the colon. Those with partial obstruction usually show clear evidence of gas in the colon in addition to dilated loops of small intestine. Only 10% of abdominal radiographs reveal diagnostic findings but the examination is readily available, inexpensive, and should be obtained in most circumstances.

- **Chest radiography** may demonstrate a basal pneumonia or a pleural effusion or pneumoperitoneum (air under the diaphragm).
- **Ultrasound of abdomen** if ruptured aortic aneurysm, ectopic pregnancy or acute pancreatitis are suspected. Ultrasound is the preferred initial test for acute cholecystitis. It can detect gallstones with 95% sensitivity and also provides information regarding other abdominal organs, e.g. ectopic pregnancy, ovarian cyst. A positive sonographic Murphy sign in the presence of gallstones predicts acute cholecystitis in 90% of cases.
- **Computerized tomography (CT) abdomen and pelvis:** CT of the abdomen and pelvis provides information about the presence of pneumoperitoneum, abnormal bowel gas patterns and calcifications. CT can also detect inflammatory lesions, e.g. appendicitis, diverticulitis, pancreatitis and abscess. CT can detect neoplastic lesions (e.g. obstructing colon cancer, pancreatic tumors, and trauma such as spleen, liver, and kidney injury). CT also provides information about vascular lesions, e.g. portal vein thrombosis, pyelophlebitis, aneurysms, and intra-abdominal or retroperitoneal hemorrhage. CT is rapidly displacing traditional contrast radiography in the evaluation of small bowel obstruction. CT is useful when diverticular complications are suspected as it can confirm diverticulitis (sensitivity 65%) and also perforation, abscess or fistula (sensitivity 90–100%).
- **Endoscopy:** Endoscopy can be useful in evaluation of the stomach, duodenum and colon for ulceration, neoplasia, and inflammation.
- **Diagnostic laparoscopy:** This is a safe and accurate tool that can be used to rule out acute intra-abdominal disease thus avoiding the need for a laparotomy. This technique is appealing in critically ill patients, in whom the morbidity and mortality associated with a nontherapeutic laparotomy can be substantial. In some cases, definitive therapy can also be undertaken using minimally invasive techniques. Also, if conversion to a laparotomy is required, the information obtained from the laparoscopy allows the surgeon to appropriately place and minimize the size of a laparotomy incision.
- **Laparotomy:** This is reserved for patients with intra-abdominal catastrophe whose diagnosis is obvious from the clinical history and examination, e.g. ruptured aortic aneurysm or patients in extremis, in whom delay in therapy would be life-threatening. The placement of the incision is influenced strongly by the presumed pathological process and by the certainty of diagnosis. In many instances, the precise diagnosis is not known at the time of laparotomy and a vertical midline incision may be performed.

Management

- If the patient is shocked, he or she will need the following:
  - vigorous fluid resuscitation, initially via a peripheral intravenous line with colloid 500 mL over 15–30 minutes and then guided by measurement of the central venous pressure;
  - monitoring of urine output with a urinary catheter;
  - antibiotic therapy directed against gram negative and anaerobic bacteria. Regimens can Include cefotaxime 1 g 8-hourly intravenously or Tazocin (piperacillin/tazobactam) 4.5 g 8 hourly plus gentamicin 80 mg 8-hourly intravenously (reduce dose in renal impairment) plus metronidazole 500 mg 8-hourly intravenously;
  - an urgent surgical consult.
- Give oxygen if the patient has severe pain, is breathless, or if oxygen saturation by pulse oximetry is less than 90%.
- Relieve severe pain with diamorphine or pethidine.
- Further management will be determined by clinical assessment and the results of the investigations. The treatment of specific causes of acute abdominal pain are dealt with in the specific sections relating to intra-abdominal emergencies.

References

1. Mulholland MW, Sweeney JF. Approach to the patient with acute abdomen. In Textbook of Gastroenterology, 4th edition, Yamada T (ed.). Lippincott Williams & Wilkins, Philadelphia, 2003: 813–28.
2. Glasgow RE, Mulvihill SJ. Abdominal pain, including the acute abdomen. In Sleisenger & Fordtran's Gastrointestinal and Liver Disease, 7th edition, Feldman M, Friedman LS, Sleisenger MH (eds). Saunders, Philadelphia, 2003: 71–83.
3. Pasricha PJ. Approach to the patient with abdominal pain. In Textbook of Gastroenterology, 4th edition, Yamada T (ed.). Lippincott Williams & Wilkins, Philadelphia, 2003: 781–801.

CHAPTER 5

Approach to jaundice

Tony C. K. Tham

Ulster Hospital, Dundonald, Belfast, UK

Definition

Jaundice is the abnormal accumulation of bilirubin in body tissues which occurs when the serum bilirubin level exceeds 50 μmol/L (3 mg/dL). Excess bilirubin causes a yellow tinting to the skin, sclera, and mucous membranes. A basic knowledge of bilirubin metabolism is necessary to understand the investigations of jaundice (Fig. 5.1). *Bile acids* or *bile salts* are soluble, amphipathic end products of cholesterol metabolism formed in the pericentral hepatocytes and account for approximately 85% of the constituents of bile. *Cholestasis* is characterized by the constellation of physiological, morphological, and clinical manifestations that result from the impairment of the bile excretory system in the liver and biliary tree. Reduced bile flow results in the accumulation of conjugated bilirubin, bile salts, and cholesterol in the blood. *Obstructive jaundice* usually applies to extrahepatic causes. About 20% of patients with features of cholestasis have hepatocellular disease.

Differential diagnosis

Conditions that cause jaundice can be classified under the broad categories of: [1] isolated disorder of bilirubin metabolism (*prehepatic jaundice*), [2] liver disease (*hepatic jaundice*), and [3] obstruction of the bile ducts (*obstructive/cholestatic jaundice*) (see Table 5.1). A mixed pattern of conjugated and unconjugated bilirubin is usually present. Normally about 95% of bilirubin is conjugated unless there is an enzyme deficiency or transport defect (prehepatic jaundice).

History and examination

When first evaluating a patient with jaundice, a quick assessment of the emergency of the situation must be made. Fever, leukocytosis, and hypotension point to ascending cholangitis, which requires immediate therapy. Asterixis, confusion, or decreased level of consciousness may indicate severe hepatocellular dysfunction or fulminant hepatic failure and requires immediate therapy. After immediate life-threatening causes of jaundice have been excluded, a systematic approach to the patient helps to make the diagnosis. An algorithm for assessing the patient with jaundice is shown in Fig. 5.2 [1]. The history and examination provide important clues regarding the cause of the jaundice (see Table 5.2).

History

A simplified aide memoire for specific questions to ascertain the cause of jaundice is as follows:

A **A**lcohol – ask about alcohol use, present and past.
B **B**lood transfusion – ask about previous transfusions of blood, plasma factors, or tattoos.

Gastrointestinal Emergencies, Third Edition. Edited by Tony C. K. Tham, John S. A. Collins, and Roy Soetikno.

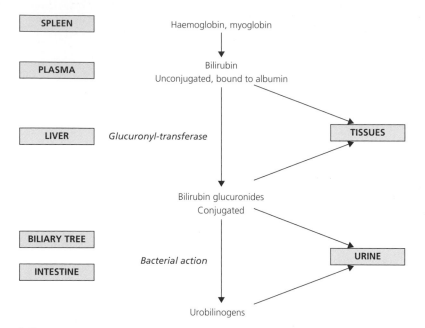

Fig. 5.1 Bilirubin metabolism.

C **C**ontact with jaundice.

D **D**rugs – ask about prescribed, over-the-counter, or alternative medicines such as homeopathic treatment. Hepatotoxicity can be divided into those that occur in most patients given a sufficiently high dose of the drug (dose-related) and idiosyncratic (dose-independent) reactions. Dose-related hepatotoxicity can be due to paracetamol/acetaminophen (0.10 g/24 h, but as little as 6 g/24 h in those with alcoholic liver disease), anabolic steroids, halothane, methotrexate (fibrosis is unusual if total dose is <2 g). Drugs that can cause dose-independent hepatotoxicity are listed in Table 5.3. The diagnosis is suspected if jaundice occurs within 3 months of starting any new drug. Occasionally, liver damage can present 1 year or more after starting the drug (minocycline, methotrexate, methyldopa).

E **E**nvironment – ask about animal contact, e.g. rats; industrial exposure.

F **F**oreign travel – hepatitis-endemic areas, malaria. **F**amily history – e.g. hemochromatosis.

G **G**allstones – ask about right upper quadrant abdominal pain.

H **H**epatitis – ask about intravenous drug abuse and sexual relations.

Ask about associated symptoms. The time sequence of symptoms may be helpful in distinguishing hepatitis from cholestatic causes. Dark urine, pale stools and pruritus indicates cholestasis. Anorexia, nausea, distaste for cigarettes may indicate hepatitis. Weight loss may indicate malignancy or chronic pancreatitis. Pyrexia and rigors suggest cholangitis or abscess.

Examination

Look for signs suggesting acute or chronic liver disease or cholestasis/obstruction (Table 5.2). Physical signs in *chronic liver disease* include [2]:

- leukonychia/telangiectasia
- loss of muscle bulk
- spider nevi
- splenomegaly
- ascites
- peripheral edema
- loss of axillary/pubic hair
- testicular atrophy
- Dupuytren contracture
- small or large liver.

Physical signs in cholestatic/obstructive jaundice include [2]:

- pale stools
- dark urine
- scratch marks (excoriation)
- polished nails (itching)
- xanthelasma (eyelids)

Table 5.1 Differential diagnosis of jaundice*.

Prehepatic jaundice: isolated disorders of bilirubin metabolism
Unconjugated hyperbilirubinemia
1. Increased bilirubin production, e.g. *hemolysis, ineffective erythropoiesis*, blood transfusion, resorption of hematomas
2. Decreased hepatocellular uptake, e.g. rifampicin
3. Decrease conjugation, e.g. *Gilbert syndrome*, Crigler–Najjar syndrome, physiologic jaundice of the newborn
Conjugated or mixed hyperbilirubinemia
1. Dubin–Johnson syndrome
2. Rotor syndrome

Hepatic jaundice: liver disease
Acute or chronic hepatocellular dysfunction
1. Acute or subacute
   - *Viral hepatitis*
   - Toxins (*alcohol*, amanita)
   - Drugs (*paracetamol/acetominophen*, isoniazid, methyldopa)
   - Ischemia (hypotension, vascular occlusion)
   - Metabolic disorders (Wilson disease, Reye syndrome)
   - Pregnancy related (acute fatty liver of pregnancy, pre-eclampsia)
2. Chronic
   - *Viral hepatitis*
   - Toxins (*ethanol*, vinyl chloride, vitamin A)
   - *Autoimmune hepatitis*
   - Metabolic (*hemachromatosis*, Wilson disease, α_1-antitrypsin deficiency)

Obstructive/cholestatic jaundice: obstruction of the bile ducts
Extrahepatic
1. *Choledocholithiasis*
2. Diseases of the bile ducts
   - Neoplasms (*cholangiocarcinoma*)
   - Inflammation/infection (primary sclerosing cholangitis, AIDS cholangiopathy, hepatic arterial chemotherapy, post-surgical strictures)
3. Extrinsic compression of the biliary tree
   - Neoplasms (*pancreatic carcinoma*, metastatic lymphadenopathy, hepatoma)
   - Chronic pancreatitis
   - Vascular enlargement (aneurysm, portal cavernoma)
Intrahepatic: hepatic disorders with prominent cholestasis
1. Diffuse infiltrative disorders
   - Granulomatous diseases (mycobacterial infections, *sarcoidosis, lymphoma*, drug toxicity, Wegener granulomatosis)
   - Amyloidosis
   - Malignancy
2. Inflammation of intrahepatic bile ductules and/or portal tracts
   - *Primary biliary cirrhosis*
   - Graft-versus-host disease
   - Drug toxicity (*chlorpromazine, erythromycin*)
3. Miscellaneous
   - Benign recurrent intrahepatic cholestasis
   - Drug toxicity
   - Estrogens, anabolic steroids
   - Total parenteral nutrition
   - Bacterial infections
   - Uncommon manifestations of viral or alcoholic hepatitis
   - Intrahepatic cholestasis of pregnancy
   - Postoperative cholestasis

* Common disorders are in *italics*
AIDS, acquired immune deficiency syndrome.

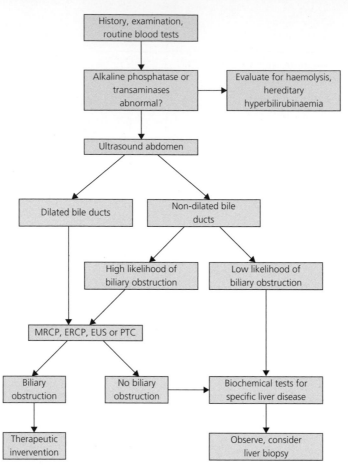

Fig. 5.2 Diagnostic algorithm for assessment of the patient with jaundice. ERCP endoscopic retrograde cholangiopancreatography, EUS endoscopic ultrasound, MRCP magnetic resonance cholangiopancreatography, PTC percutaneous transhepatic cholangiogram. Source: Lidofsky 1998.

Table 5.2 Differentiating obstructive jaundice from hepatic jaundice.

Suggests obstructive jaundice	Suggests hepatic jaundice
History	
Abdominal pain	Anorexia, malaise, myalgias, viral-type illness
Fever, rigors	Known infectious exposure
Prior biliary surgery	Receipt of blood products, use of intravenous drugs
Older age	Exposure to known hepatotoxin
Dark urine and pale stools	Family history of jaundice
Physical examination	
High fever	Ascites
Abdominal tenderness	Stigmata of liver disease (e.g. gynecomastia, spider nevi, Kayser–Fleischer rings)
Palpable abdominal mass	
Abdominal scar	Asterixis, encephalopathy
Urinalysis – large amount of bilirubin with little or no urobilinogen	Urinalysis – mixture of bilirubin and urobilinogen
Laboratory tests	
Predominant elevation of serum bilirubin and alkaline phosphatase	Predominant elevation of serum transaminases
Prothrombin time that is normal or normalizes with vitamin K administration	Prothrombin time that does not correct with vitamin K administration
Elevated serum amylase	Blood tests indicative of specific liver disease, e.g. autoantibodies, positive viral serology

Source: Lidofsky and Scharschmidt 1998 [1].

- xanthomas (rarely palmar creases, tendons)
- hepatomegaly (alcohol, malignancy)
- palpable gallbladder (especially malignancy) – Courvoisier's sign states that if the gallbladder is palpable in the right upper quadrant, then jaundice is unlikely to be due to stones. By implication, it is more likely to be due to malignancy. However, one in four patients has obstruction due to bile duct stones.

Look for other signs:

- Previous biliary surgery may indicate possible obstructive jaundice.

Table 5.3 Drugs that can cause dose-independent hepatotoxicity.

Liver lesion	Common culprits
Hepatitis	Isoniazid
	Sodium valproate
	Rifampicin
	NSAIDs
	Azathioprine
Cholestasis	Co-amoxiclav
	Chlorpromazine
	Prochlorperazine
	Fusidic acid
	Glibenclamide
Chronic hepatitis	Methyldopa
	Nitrofurantoin
	Dantrolene
Alcoholic hepatitis-like	Verapamil
Granulomas	Hydralazine
	Allopurinol
	Phenylbutazone

Source: Travis et al. 2005 [2]. Reproduced with permission from Wiley. NSAID, non-steroidal anti-inflammatory drug.

- Fever – suspect cholangitis although hepatitis and acute cholecystitis may cause a low-grade fever.
- Personality change or confusion may indicate encephalopathy.
- Constructional apraxia may indicate encephalopathy.
- Asterixis – flapping tremor of outstretched hands, with fingers splayed.
- Dilated abdominal veins are rare – flow radiating away from the umbilicus ("caput medusa") indicates portal hypertension. Flow towards the head only indicates inferior vena cava obstruction.
- Arterial bruit over the liver is rare – this may be due to a hepatoma or acute alcoholic hepatitis.
- Rectal examination for stool color – pale in cholestatic jaundice.

Investigations

Blood tests

The following blood tests should be performed:

- **Liver enzymes** – bilirubin, alkaline phosphatase, transaminases (aspartate transaminase (AST) and alanine aminotransferase (ALT)), gamma glutamyl transferase (gamma-GT), albumin. Typical values that help distinguish different types of jaundice are shown in Table 5.4. An AST > 500 is very rare in alcoholic hepatitis and usually indicates coexistent viral infection or drug toxicity (e.g. acetaminophen/ paracetamol) or prolonged hypotension. In rare instances, ALT elevation can be seen in biliary obstruction but biliary pain is a feature. Gamma GT is an unreliable test for alcohol abuse. Gamma-GT will be

Table 5.4 Liver enzymes in different types of jaundice.

Test	Normal	Prehepatic	Hepatic	Cholestatic/obstructive
Bilirubin (μmol/L)	<17	50–150	50–400	100–900
(mg/dL)	<1	3–9	3–20	6–45
AST (IU/L)	<35	<35	300–10 000	35–400
ALP (IU/L)	<120	<120	<120–300	>300
γ-GT (IU/L)	15–40	15–40	15–200	80–1000
Albumin (g/dL)	3.5–5	3.5–5	2–5	3–5
Prothrombin time (s)	13–15	13–15	15–45	15–45

Source: Travis et al. 2005 [2]. Reproduced with permission from Wiley.

elevated in liver disease of any cause including non-alcoholic fatty liver disease. A combination of a high gamma-GT and alkaline phosphatase (ALP) is consistent with cholestasis/obstruction. Albumin is a better marker of liver function although it can be altered by redistribution of body fluids.

- **Prothrombin time** – this is a good marker of liver function.

The following blood tests should be performed depending on the type of jaundice. In *prehepatic jaundice*, the following should be performed:
- peripheral blood film;
- reticulocyte count – raised in hemolysis;
- Coomb test (direct antihuman globulin);
- serum haptoglobins – absent in hemolysis but also low in cirrhosis.

In *hepatic jaundice*, the following should be performed:
- hepatitis A, B, C serology
- monospot (Paul–Bunnell) for infectious mononucleosis, serum for cytomegalovirus, mycoplasma. If renal failure is present, check *Leptospira* titers;
- autoantibody screen – mitochondrial, smooth muscle, nuclear; (liver, kidney, microsomal);
- immunoglobulins;
- iron studies – iron, iron-binding capacity (transferrin saturation) and ferritin to look for hemochromatosis. In hemochromatosis, serum iron is high and transferrin saturation is high, often .80% although values of .55% warrant further investigations. Ferritin is markedly elevated when cirrhosis is present but may be at the upper limit of normal in earlier stages. It is an acute phase protein and is elevated in inflammatory conditions as well as in alcoholics.
- thyroid function tests
- coeliac serology.

The following blood tests should be considered if history or physical examination suggests this:
- alpha-1-antitrypsin – if deficiency is considered;
- copper and ceruloplasmin and 24-hour urinary copper – if Wilson's disease is considered, e.g., 40 years old, viral titers and autoantibodies negative;
- alpha fetoprotein – should be checked if a hepatoma is suspected;
- tests for adrenal Insufficiency if it is suspected.

Urine

Bilirubin is absent in prehepatic causes. Urobilinogen is absent in complete cholestasis/obstruction.

Ultrasound scan

This is the preferred initial screening test for evaluating biliary obstruction. It determines the caliber of the extrahepatic biliary tree and reveals mass lesions. The sensitivity of abdominal ultrasound for the detection of biliary obstruction in jaundiced patients ranges from 55% to 91% and the specificity from 82% to 95%. It can also demonstrate cholelithiasis. Common duct stones may not be seen; the negative predictive value of a dilated duct seen on scan with no stones seen is about 50% for actual common duct stones. The positive predictive value of a dilated duct with ductal stones seen on scan is about 90%. The variability in sensitivity reflects limitations from overlying bowel gas, site and size of the stones, and presence or absence of duct dilation. Ultrasound is inconsistent in determining the site of obstruction, partly because the distal duct is not well seen in 30–50% of patients. In cases of acute obstruction it may take 4 hours to 4 days for the ducts to dilate. The ducts of some patients with partial or intermittent obstruction may not dilate. Ultrasound can detect space-occupying lesions greater than 1 cm in diameter.

Computerized tomography

Computerized tomography (CT) is not as accurate as ultrasound in detecting cholelithiasis. It can detect space-occupying lesions as small as 5 mm. It provides technically superior images to ultrasound in obese patients and those in whom the biliary tree is obscured by bowel gas. Its accuracy for detecting biliary obstruction is similar to ultrasound. CT with intravenous contrast material can evaluate the etiology of biliary obstruction such as stone or stricture.

Magnetic resonance imaging (MRI)

Magnetic resonance cholangiopancreatography (MRCP) can detect bile duct stones or extrahepatic and intrahepatic strictures. MRCP is comparable to endoscopic retrograde cholangiopancreatography (ERCP) in the detection of bile duct stones (sensitivity and specificity 93% and 100%; 94% and 100% respectively). For the detection of strictures, for example in primary sclerosing cholangitis, MRCP is comparable to ERCP (sensitivity and specificity about 90%). MRI is more sensitive and specific than CT with contrast for the detection and evaluation of focal and malignant lesions. In patients with renal impairment, MRI has the advantage over

CT in avoiding the potentially nephrotoxic agents used with CT. In patients who may not require therapeutic intervention, MRCP can be performed and if a stone or stricture is identified then a therapeutic intervention can follow. In patients who are likely to require intervention such as stone extraction or stenting, ERCP may be preferable as the initial investigation rather than MRCP.

Endoscopic retrograde cholangiopancreatography

ERCP is highly accurate in the diagnosis of biliary obstruction with a sensitivity of 89–98% and specificity of 89–100% but its use is now mainly confined to therapy as the diagnosis can be made by other modalities. Biopsy specimens, brushings for cytology can be obtained. Therapeutic maneuvers to relieve the obstruction from stones or strictures such as sphincterotomy, stone extraction, dilatation, and stent placement can be performed. The risk of complications in about 5–10% (pancreatitis, hemorrhage, perforation, cholangitis). See Chapter 11 regarding ERCP complications.

Percutaneous transhepatic cholangiography

Percutaneous transhepatic cholangiography (PTC) visualizes the biliary tree in 90–100% of patients with dilated ducts. PTC requires the passage of a needle through the skin into the hepatic parenchyma and peripheral bile duct. The sensitivity and specificity are comparable to ERCP. PTC may be technically more difficult in the absence of intrahepatic duct dilatation. Therapeutic procedures such as stent placement can be performed. However, bile duct stones cannot be extracted. Minor complications occur in 30% of patients. Major complications, including sepsis, bleeding, biliary leak, pneumothorax, arteriovenous fistula, hematoma, abscess, and peritonitis occur in 1–10%. PTC is usually performed for therapeutic indications, such as biliary stenting, if ERCP is unsuccessful. In patients with bile duct stones where ERCP is unsuccessful in obtaining biliary access, a combined PTC followed by ERCP rendezvous procedure can be performed to allow biliary access with sphincterotomy and stone extraction.

Endoscopic ultrasound

Endoscopic ultrasound (EUS) is superior to ultrasound and CT for diagnosing bile duct stones. Its accuracy is comparable to MRCP and ERCP. EUS may be more accurate than MRCP or ERCP in detecting biliary sludge. It has fewer complications than ERCP. EUS should be considered for diagnosing or excluding bile duct stones when there are contraindications to MRCP or if prior ERCP was unsuccessful.

Liver biopsy

Liver biopsy provides information regarding hepatic lobular architecture and is most helpful in patients with undiagnosed persistent jaundice. It permits the diagnosis of viral hepatitis, non-alcoholic steatohepatitis, alcoholic hepatitis, Wilson disease, hemochromatosis, alpha-1-antitrypsin deficiency, fatty liver of pregnancy, primary biliary cirrhosis, granulomatous hepatitis, and neoplasms. It may provide clues to unsuspected biliary tract obstruction. There is a small complication rate (bleeding and perforation) of about 1.7% (see Chapter 13). Overall this is a safe procedure but the risk to benefit ratio needs to be carefully assessed and explained to the patient.

Management

Gilbert syndrome

Jaundice is rare, as the bilirubin level is usually 70 μmol/L, except in concomitant illness with anorexia. Bilirubin increases on fasting. Liver enzymes are normal. The diagnosis is made by a combination of elevated bilirubin, normal liver enzymes and asymptomatic. No treatment other than reassurance is necessary.

Biliary obstruction

Therapy is directed at the mechanical relief of obstruction. The options include ERCP (sphincterotomy, stone extraction, stent insertion), PTC (stent insertion) or surgery. The therapeutic strategy depends on the likely etiology and local expertise.

Hepatic jaundice

The therapy is directed towards the underlying etiology: for example, stopping alcohol, discontinuation of a drug, antiviral agents, phlebotomy for hemochromatosis, copper chelation for Wilson disease.

Drug-induced jaundice

All possible drugs that can cause jaundice should be stopped. All other possible causes of jaundice should be excluded. Severe acute liver failure is managed as for other causes (see Chapter 26, Acute Liver Failure). Liver biopsy is not necessary if the drug is well known to cause liver dysfunction. Liver biopsy is indicated if the diagnosis is uncertain or if liver enzymes have not returned to normal after 8 weeks as drug reactions may unmask pre-existing liver disease. The liver enzymes should be monitored until they return to normal, usually over several weeks. Most hepatotoxic effects resolve completely after the drug is withdrawn, unless liver dysfunction is unrecognised for several months such as with methotrexate or methyldopa. Very rarely, persistent loss of small intrahepatic bile ducts (ductopenia) can occur and is manifest by persistently elevated ALP.

Pruritus

The pruritogen is thought to be a bile acid, bile acid derivative or some other substance that undergoes enterohepatic circulation. The management of pruritus is outlined in Table 5.5 [3].

Hepatic osteodystrophy

Hepatic osteodystrophy is the metabolic bone disease encompassing osteoporosis and osteomalacia, which occurs in patients with chronic liver disease, particularly

Table 5.5 Management of pruritus.

Topical therapy
Lower bathing water temperature and use fewer or lighter clothing and bed coverings
Minimize dry skin by using moisturizing soaps and applying topical moisturizers
Anion-exchange resins
Cholestyramine or colestipol: start with 4 g (packet or scoop) twice daily, starting before and after breakfast, and increasing to six packets or scoops daily, separated from other medications by 2 hours
Bile salts
Ursodeoxycholic acid, 15 mg/kg per day
Doxepin
25–50 mg once daily
Hepatic microsomal enzyme induction
Rifampicin 300–600 mg once daily
Opioid receptor antagonists
Naltrexone, 12.5 mg once daily, increasing slowly to 50–100 mg once daily
Naloxone and nalmefene are only commonly available for parenteral use

Source: Merriman and Peters 2003 [3]. Reproduced with permission from Wiley.

cholestatic disease. Osteoporosis is usually dominant. The management of hepatic osteodystrophy involves the early identification through bone mineral density screening by dual energy X-ray absorptiometry of all patients with cholestatic liver disease. If bone density measurement confirms osteoporosis, worsens rapidly or there are symptomatic fractures, antiresorptive medication with bisphosphonates or calcitonin is indicated.

Fat-soluble vitamin deficiency

This condition is common in patients with prolonged cholestasis. Replacement will depend on the extent of deficiency and response to treatment. Table 5.6 outlines the vitamins that can be monitored and replaced if deficient. Evaluation of therapy is monitored by 24 hour urine calcium after 3 months if vitamin D was low, followed by yearly 25-OH vitamin D levels. Annual vitamins A and E levels and prothrombin time can be monitored.

Jaundice in pregnancy

Consider other coincidental causes of jaundice. The following are specific conditions related to pregnancy.

- *Hyperemesis gravidarum* – occurs in the first trimester. Jaundice occurs in 10% especially those with Gilbert syndrome. High serum transaminases are common. This is self- limiting and liver failure does not occur.
- *Intrahepatic cholestasis of pregnancy* – occurs in the third trimester. This is preceded by pruritus. The liver enzymes are cholestatic. The condition resolves within 2 weeks after pregnancy. Ursodeoxycholic acid appears to improve fetal outcome but has not been subject to a randomized controlled trial. It can recur with subsequent pregnancies. It is associated with increased fetal mortality and therefore early delivery may be necessary.

Table 5.6 Monitoring and replacement of fat-soluble vitamin deficiency in prolonged cholestasis.

Monitoring fat-soluble vitamins	Replacement
25-OH Vitamin D level	Calcium
Vitamin A level	β carotene
Vitamin E level with fasting total lipid profile	D-α–tocopherol
Vitamin K – measure prothrombin time	Vitamin K 10 mg subcutaneously daily for 3 days, then monthly if cholestatic

- *Acute fatty liver of pregnancy* – occurs in the third trimester. The features are nausea, abdominal pain and encephalopathy. AST and uric acid are elevated. Coagulopathy and acidosis are seen. There is no hemolysis. As this condition is potentially fatal, early delivery is essential and will result in resolution.
- *HELLP syndrome* – occurs in the third trimester. It is characterized by hemolysis, elevated liver enzymes, and low platelets (hence the acronym). It is associated with pre-eclampsia. It has a clinical spectrum of severity up to acute liver failure. Hence early delivery is also needed to resolve the condition.

References

1. Lidofsky S, Scharschmidt BF. Jaundice. In Sleisenger and Fordtran's Gastrointestinal and Liver Disease, 6th edition, Feldman M, Scharschmidt BF, Sleisenger MH (eds). WB Saunders & Co., Philadelphia, 1998.
2. Travis SPL, Ahmad T, Collier J, Steinhart AH. Pocket Consultant: Gastroenterology. Blackwell Publishing Ltd, Oxford, 2005.
3. Merriman RB, Peters MG. Approach to the patient with jaundice. In Textbook of Gastroenterology, 4th edition, Yamada T, Alpers DH, Kaplowitz N, Laine L, Owyang C, Powell DW (eds). Lippincott Williams & Wilkins, Philadelphia, 2003; 911–28.

CHAPTER 6

Acute severe lower gastrointestinal hemorrhage

Jennifer M. Kolb[1] and Tonya Kaltenbach[2]

[1] *Icahn School of Medicine at Mount Sinai, Internal Medicine, New York, NY, USA*
[2] *Stanford University, Palo Alto, CA, USA*

Introduction

Lower gastrointestinal bleeding (LGIB) is common, resulting in approximately 25–40 hospitalizations per 100 000 adults per year and accounting for an estimated 30% of all major gastrointestinal bleeding. It is more common in the elderly and in patients on anticoagulation, aspirin, or non-steroidal anti-inflammatory drugs (NSAIDs). Its presentation can range from trivial bleeding to massive, life-threatening hemorrhage with a reported mortality rate up to 5%.

The approach to LGIB is controversial and not standardized. Various factors, including the suspected etiology, location and rapidity of bleeding, time of admission, and center experience impact the choices for radiologic, surgical, or endoscopic diagnosis and treatment approaches.

Definition

Acute severe LGIB is of recent limited duration and associated with hemodynamic instability as measured by tachycardia, hypotension, and anemia possibly requiring transfusion. It also emanates from a source between the ligament of treitz and the anus.

Presentation and differential diagnosis

Acute severe LGIB presents as bright red blood per rectum, maroon stools, or melena. Bleeding from colonic diverticula is the most common etiology of acute lower gastrointestinal bleed, followed by hemorrhoids and malignancy (Table 6.1).

Important historical questions should be asked to help aid in making a correct diagnosis: focusing on age, comorbid conditions, recent treatment with NSAID and antiplatelet agents , radiation exposure, abdominal surgical history, and anorectal trauma. For example, in patients with LGIB over age of 65, diverticular bleeding, arteriovenous malformation, or ischemic colitis, are most common; while in younger patients, infectious or inflammatory conditions are more likely.

Evaluation

The first step in management should be stratification of risk. Seventy-five percent of lower gastrointestinal bleeding is self-limiting, therefore patients with stable vital signs, no recent bloody effluent and no syncope have a low risk of continued bleeding and elective colonoscopy is appropriate.

Urgent interventions should be targeted for patients with severe bleeding with early colonoscopy within 24 hours for severe, ongoing, or recurrent LGIB.

Independent correlates of severe bleeding

- Bleeding per rectum during the first 4 hours of evaluation
- Vital sign instability
  - Tachycardia (HR $\geq$100)
  - Hypotension (SBP $\leq$ 115 mmHg)

Gastrointestinal Emergencies, Third Edition. Edited by Tony C. K. Tham, John S. A. Collins, and Roy Soetikno.

Table 6.1 Etiology of lower gastrointestinal hemorrhage.

Condition	Cause of hemorrhage
Congenital abnormalities	Meckel diverticulum Arteriovenous malformation Telangiectasia Hemorrhoids Rectal/colonic varices Vasculitis Aortoenteric fistula
Ischemia	Ischemic colitis Mesenteric ischemia Necrotizing enterocolitis Marathon runner's colon
Dysentery	Bacterial (salmonellosis, shigellosis, *E. coli*, *Campylobacter*, *Yersinia*) Parasitic (amebiasis, giardiasis, schistosomiasis)
Neoplasia	Hemangioma Leiomyoma/leiomyosarcoma Polyps (adenoma, hyperplastic, hamartoma) Colorectal cancer
Inflammation	Ulcerative colitis/Crohn's disease Radiation enterocolitis/proctitis Henoch–Schönlein purpura
Trauma	Surgery Endoscopic polypectomy
Structural	Diverticulosis Pneumatosis coli
Collagen disorders (Ehlers–Danlos syndrome, pseudoxanthoma elasticum)	Endometriosis Dieulafoy lesion
Pharmacologic	Anticoagulants Nonsteroidal anti-inflammatory drugs Cytotoxic chemotherapy

- Syncope
- Non-tender abdominal exam
- Aspirin use
- ≥2 comorbid conditions

Investigations:
Volume status
Complete blood count
Coagulation profile

Exclude an UGI source, which can occur in up to 10% of cases. Upper endoscopy for:
- ○ Patients with a positive nasogastric aspirate
- ○ Patients where a colonic source is not identified.

Management

The patient should be resuscitated with two large-bore IVs in place, transfused if appropriate, the severity and acuity of bleeding should be assessed, and an upper gastrointestinal source of bleeding excluded. Colonoscopy is the diagnostic and therapeutic procedure of choice. Colonoscopy should be performed within 24 hours, and within 12 hours if the bleeding continues or does not respond to resuscitation. (Fig. 6.1) It is important to recognize the various stigmata of diverticular bleeding including large and small vessel, adherent clot, flat pigmented spot, and erosion (Fig. 6.2). In cases of continued bleeding not amenable to endoscopic therapy or angiography, surgery should be considered. We emphasize a multidisciplinary team approach with close collaboration between the gastroenterologist, radiologist, surgeon, and internist in the successful approach to acute severe LGIB. For further reading on bleeding from diverticular disease, see Chapter 36, Diverticular Disease.

Colonoscopy
Preparation – rapid purge with polyethylene glycol based solutions.
Administration should be achieved with a nasogastric tube or by drinking 1 L every 30–45 minutes with a goal of 4–6 L over 3–4 hours. Metoclopramide 10 mg intravenous can be given immediately prior to purge to control nausea and promote gastric emptying. The stomach should be emptied before colonoscopy with a nasogastric tube if there is concern of large residual or need for deep sedation. Purging is contraindicated in the presence of bowel obstruction or suspected gastroparesis.

Equipment and accessory selection
An adult endoscope or therapeutic enteroscope in cases of a suspected small bowel bleeding source should be used. A foot-controlled irrigation device, and an additional suction line directly locked to the working

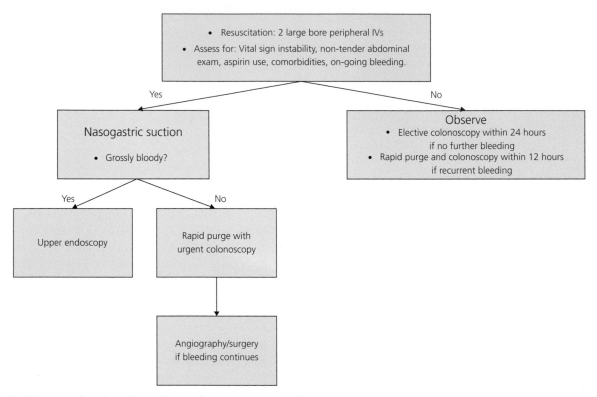

Fig. 6.1 Approach to the patient with acute lower gastrointestinal hemorrhage.

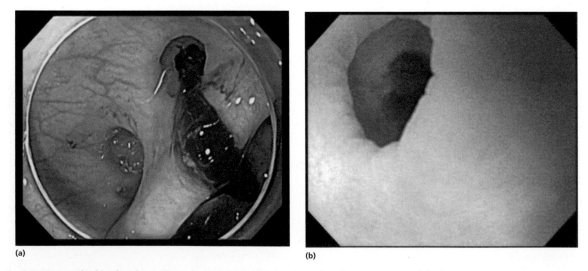

(a)

(b)

Fig. 6.2 Diverticular bleed with stigmata of an adherent clot. (*see insert for color representation of the figure.*)

channel attachment aid visualization and provide a clear field for therapeutic intervention.

The use of a translucent endoscopic mucosal resection cap or a banding cap can improve visualization behind a fold or a turn in the colon. It allows therapy of lesions hidden inside a diverticulum, or a lesion on the side. The target bleeding source should be aligned with the axis of the accessory channel with an en face view.

Direct pressure can be applied for temporary tamponade. An injection needle with epinephrine should also be available and may provide temporary hemostasis to improve visualization.

Techniques

In the treatment of LGIB, various endoscopic techniques (Table 6.2), such as clipping, looping, banding, argon plasma coagulation (APC) and thermal therapies, used alone and in combination, have been reported to be safe and efficacious. (Fig. 6.3). Familiarity with the different techniques is encouraged.

Table 6.2 Endoscopic therapies for acute bleeding.

Diagnosis	Endoscopic therapy
Diverticular	Clip, APC, thermal
Ischemic Colitis	Self-limited
Neoplasm	Clip, loop, thermal
AVM	Clip, APC, thermal
Radiation proctopathy	APC
Hemorrhoids*	Infrared coagulation, band ligation, radiofrequency ablation

APC, argon plasma coagulation.
* Contraindications to hemorrhoidal ligation: Immunocompromised state, rectal prolapse, inflammatory bowel disease, anal carcinoma, coagulopathy, thrombocytopenia, portal hypertension, pregnancy or peripartum.

Outcomes

Colonoscopy for LGIB can successfully achieve primary hemostasis in 75–100% of cases, and in up to 90% of cases when using endoscopic clips for diverticular bleed. Early (within 30 days) rebleeding and complication rates are close to 0%. Late recurrent bleeding rates approach 21% with an average time to rebleed of approximately 4 years.

- **Nuclear scan**
  Literature dating since 1990 suggests that nuclear scans are not particularly useful to confirm and localize the bleeding site in order to direct further angiographic or surgical intervention.
- **Angiography**
  Angiography can be useful if colonoscopy fails or cannot be performed. Small studies, using the coiling or gel foam embolization technique, have shown high rates (up to 96%) of successful primary hemostasis in patients with active bleeding. Short-term, less than one week, rebleeding rates were, however, high; they were found to be about 25% with a mean of 10–53%; and data on long-term rebleeding rates are lacking. Major complications occur in about 18% of cases.
- **Surgery**
  Whenever possible, it is preferable to perform surgery on an elective basis rather than emergently. Operative

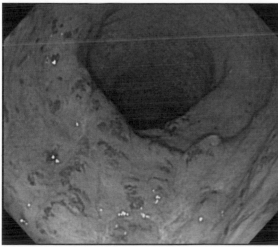
(a)

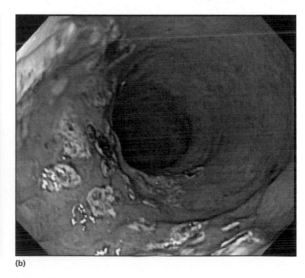
(b)

Fig. 6.3 Radiation proctopathy (a) treated with argon plasma coagulation (b).

mortality is 10% for a directed segmental colectomy and up to 27% in a subtotal colectomy.

Further reading and viewing

Bender JS, Wiencek RG, Bouwman DL. Morbidity and mortality following total abdominal colectomy for massive lower gastrointestinal bleeding. *Am. Surg.* 1991;**57**:536–40.

Elta GH. Urgent colonoscopy for acute lower-GI bleeding. *Gastrointest. Endosc.* 2004;**59**:402–8.

Gayer C, Chino A, Lucas C, et al. Acute lower gastrointestinal bleeding in 1,112 patients admitted to an urban emergency medical center. *Surgery* 2009;**146**(4):600–607.

Hreinsson JP, Gumundsson S, Kalaitzakis E, Bjornsson ES. Lower gastrointestinal bleeding: incidence, etiology, and outcomes in a population-based setting. *Eur. J. Gastroenterol. Hepatol.* 2013;**25**(1):37–43.

Jensen DM, Machicado GA, Jutabha R, et al. Urgent colonoscopy for the diagnosis and treatment of severe diverticular hemorrhage. *N. Engl. J. Med.* 2000;**342**:78–82.

Juthaba R, Kaltenbach T, Soetikno R. *Endoscopic approach to hemorrhoids – Educational DVD.* American Society of Gastrointestinal Endoscopy Endoscopic Learning Library 2006.

Kaltenbach T, Watson R, Shah J, et al. Colonoscopy with clipping is useful in the diagnosis and treatment of diverticular bleeding. *Clin. Gastroenterol. Hepatol.* 2012;**10**:131.

Khanna A, Ognibene SJ, Koniaris LG. Embolization as first-line therapy for diverticulosis-related massive lower gastrointestinal bleeding: evidence from a meta-analysis. *J. Gastrointest. Surg.* 2005;**9**:343–52.

Rockey DC. Lower gastrointestinal bleeding. *Gastroenterology* 2006; **130**:165–171.

Soetikno R, Kaltenbach T, Kelsey P, McQuaid KR. *Endoscopic interpretation and therapy of severe lower gastrointestinal bleeding – Educational DVD.* American Society of Gastrointestinal Endoscopy Endoscopic Learning Library 2007.

Strate LL, Syngal S. Predictors of utilization of early colonoscopy vs. radiography for severe lower intestinal bleeding. Gastrointest. *Endosc.* 2005;**61**:46–52.

CHAPTER 7

Approach to diarrhea

John S. A. Collins

Northern Ireland Medical and Dental Training Agency, Royal Victoria Hospital, Belfast, UK

Definition

Diarrhea is defined as a decrease in consistency or increased liquidity of the stool. Some definitions of diarrhea also include increased frequency of defecation or increased daily stool weight, but these criteria have been limited by normal variation in a patient population. Chronic diarrhea is usually defined as persistence of symptoms for at least 4 weeks.

Differential diagnosis

The normal gut receives 6–7 L of fluid daily from ingested food and liquid, plus intestinal secretions. Most of this fluid is reabsorbed by the small intestine. The colon absorbs 1.5–2.0 L and about 200 mL is excreted in the feces. Thus, a fall in small bowel absorption, increased small bowel secretion, or a fall in colonic absorptive capacity can lead to diarrhea. Acute diarrhea can be classified according to the deranged underlying physiological mechanisms (see Table 7.1).

Osmotic diarrhea results from the presence of poorly absorbed solutes, usually carbohydrates or peptides, within the gut lumen, leading to a net increase in stool water, and the passage of large volumes of liquid feces. In disaccharidase enzyme deficiency disorders such as alactasia, ingestion of lactose-rich foods such as milk can precipitate acute diarrhea due to the accumulation of high concentrations of lactose in the small bowel and loss of luminal glucose and galactose, which are the substrates for sodium-dependent sugar absorption mechanisms. The net result is an increase in stool water, leading to diarrhea.

The therapeutic use of this mechanism is employed in the use of polyethylene glycol solution or magnesium and sodium salts as bowel preparation agents or laxatives.

Osmotic diarrhea can be classified into two types:

- **Exogenous** – ingested laxatives, bowel preparations; antacids – magnesium hydroxide; dietary sugar ingestion, sorbitol, xylitol; drugs – cholestyramine, lactulose;
- **Endogenous** – disaccharidase deficiencies; abetalipoproteinemia; congenital lymphangiectasia; pancreatic insufficiency.

Secretory diarrhea is the result of disturbed transport of water and electrolytes, mainly Na, K, Cl, and HCO_3 in the presence of gut mucosal disease, toxins, or inflammatory mediators. In these conditions there is usually a stimulation of intestinal Cl and HCO_3 and inhibition of Na and Cl absorption by agents such as enterotoxins, long-chain fatty acids or ingested laxatives with a secretogog effect. Again, these can be classified as:

- **Exogenous**
  - laxatives including anthraquinones, bisacodyl, senna
  - drugs – diuretics, theophylline, prostaglandins
  - chemical toxins
  - bacterial toxins – *Clostridium difficile, Staphylococcus aureus*
  - gut allergy.
- **Endogenous**
  - congenital (rare) – microvillus inclusion disease
  - bacterial enterotoxins
  - endogenous laxatives due to build-up of dihydroxy bile acids and long-chain fatty acids
  - hormone-producing tumors – vipoma, medullary
  - carcinoma of the thyroid, mastocytosis.

Gastrointestinal Emergencies, Third Edition. Edited by Tony C. K. Tham, John S. A. Collins, and Roy Soetikno.
© 2016 John Wiley & Sons, Ltd. Published 2016 by John Wiley & Sons, Ltd.

Table 7.1 Physiological mechanisms in acute diarrhea.

Mechanism	Disorder
Osmotic	Disaccharide deficiencies
	Magnesium salts
	Short bowel
	Extensive mucosal disease
	Bile salt malabsorption
	Pancreatic insufficiency
Secretory	Stimulant laxatives
	Chemical toxins
	Bacterial toxins
	Drugs
	Allergic response
	Bacterial overgrowth
	Congenital
	Bile acids
	Long chain fatty acids
	Hormone-producing tumors
	Villous adenoma
Dysmotility	Irritable bowel syndrome
	Endocrine disorders
	Autonomic neuropathy
Inflammatory	Infection
	Inflammatory bowel disease
	Ischemic enteritis/colitis

Table 7.2 Differential diagnosis of acute onset diarrhea.

Cause	Remarks
Infections:	
Viral	Adenovirus, astrovirus, calicivirus, rotavirus
Bacterial	*Salmonella* spp, *Shigella* spp, *B. cereus*
Parasites	*Entamoeba histolytica*, *Giardia lamblia*
Toxins	*C. difficile*, *S. aureus*
Inflammatory bowel disease	Ulcerative colitis
	Crohn's disease
	Collagenous colitis
Drugs	Antibiotics
	ACE inhibitors
	Digoxin
	Chemotherapeutic agents
	Lipid-lowering drugs
	Prostaglandin analogs
	Proton pump inhibitors
	All laxatives
Ischemic colitis	
Fecal impaction with overflow	

Dysmotility diarrhea is caused by increased transit time of luminal contents and may be compounded by bacterial overgrowth due to stasis. *Inflammatory or exudative diarrhea*, as the term suggests, is the result of an acute inflammatory mucosal process, which may be idiopathic, as in ulcerative colitis or Crohn's disease, or more commonly with an infectious microorganism.

Diarrhea is often caused by several coexistent factors. For example, in ulcerative colitis, there is altered colonic permeability to water, increased prostaglandin production, and disordered motility with increased loss of blood, mucus, and water into the lumen.

The differential diagnosis of acute diarrhea is summarized in Table 7.2.

History

The onset of diarrhea is often acute and the symptoms may be of short duration.

It is important to establish that the patient is complaining of diarrhea, as defined above, and not frequent, normally formed, stools or the large-volume pale stool associated with steatorrhea. Rapid onset of symptoms with abdominal cramps and sleep disturbance usually suggests an infective or toxic etiology. The patient should be asked about recent food ingestion and its timing in relation to symptom onset. Nausea and vomiting again suggests an enteric infection. Current medications may be a factor and particular inquiry should be made about antibiotics, angiotensin-converting enzyme (ACE) inhibitors, laxatives, digoxin, proton pump inhibitors, lipid lowering agents, prostaglandin analogs, and magnesium-containing antacids.

Recent foreign travel to areas where acute enteric infections are common should raise the suspicion of infection from agents such as *Vibrio cholerae*, *Shigella*, or *Entamoeba histolytica*. The passage of bloody diarrhea may indicate an acute infective dysentery, but should always raise the suspicion of inflammatory bowel disease.

Examination

In general, the following should be assessed in all cases:
• Signs of dehydration and circulatory collapse due to water and electrolyte depletion. The patient will be pale with a rapid, low-volume pulse. The blood pressure may be low with a postural drop on standing. There will be increased skin turgor and dry mucous membranes.

- Abdominal examination is often normal but in acute onset of inflammatory bowel, the abdomen may be distended with generalized tenderness or an abdominal mass in patients with Crohn's disease.
- Rectal examination may show blood on the glove.

Investigation

Acute diarrhea is very common in the community, often occurring in isolated outbreaks associated with enteric viral infections. Most cases are diagnosed and managed by primary care physicians without resort to further investigations. However, a small proportion of cases where the symptoms are associated with dehydration, systemic illness, or rectal bleeding are referred for hospital assessment.

The following investigations are most likely to lead to a rapid diagnosis in the majority of cases.

- Fresh stool sample for ova, cysts, and parasites, culture and sensitivity as necessary, *C. difficile* enterotoxin and *Giardia* antigen. In the immunocompromised patient, it is essential to rule out the presence of cryptosporidiosis.
- Test stool for occult blood.
- Full blood count.
- Urea and electrolytes.
- Erythrocyte sedimentation rate, C-reactive protein, and alpha-1 antiglobulin as inflammatory markers.
- Tissue transglutaminase assay to rule out celiac disease.
- Blood culture if fever/rigors present.
- Visualization of the colonic mucosa by colonoscopy or flexible sigmoidoscopy, and biopsy if inflammatory bowel is suspected.
- Plain abdominal radiographs (erect and supine) in the presence of abdominal tenderness, decreased bowel sounds, and in all cases where acute inflammatory bowel disease is suspected.
- Duodenal aspirates are uncommonly required if giardiasis is suspected.

Management

The management of inflammatory bowel disease and acute infectious diarrhea will be discussed in detail in Chapters 34 and 35, respectively.

In general the management has four important components:

1 Correction of dehydration, electrolyte disturbance, anemia, and nutritional abnormalities.

2 Oral rehydration solutions, which were originally developed for fluid replacement in patients with cholera, are useful in the treatment of severe acute diarrhea provided an oral intake is tolerated. The WHO/UNICEF solution contains Na 90 mmol/L, K 20 mmol/L, Cl 80 mmol/L, HCO_3 30 mmol/L, and glucose 111 mmol/L. Dioralyte is a commercial preparation that contains Na 35 mmol/L, K 20 mmol/L, Cl 37 mmol/L, HCO_3 18 mmol/L, and glucose 200 mmol/L. Both solutions can be administered by nasogastric tube if necessary until the diarrhea has resolved.

3 Consideration of antimicrobial therapy. If an infecting agent is detected in the stool, specific antibacterial therapy is usually not indicated except in certain cases as the enteric infection is commonly self-limiting. If the patient has a severe systemic illness with fever and positive blood cultures, e.g. *Salmonella* bacteremia, then antiobiotic therapy is essential.

4 Symptomatic therapy. In milder cases of diarrhea, in the absence of fever, dehydration, and bloody stools, antimotility agents can be used to control stool frequency. Loperamide has been shown in controlled trial to be effective. The starting dose is 4 mg daily, not exceeding 16 mg daily. An alternative agent is diphenoxylate, which has also been shown to be effective in reducing stool volume and frequency in controlled trials, at a recommended dose of 4 mg given four times daily.

5 Bismuth subsalicylate has been used in some cases, but seems less effective than loperamide in trials.

It should be noted that infective causes of diarrhea can present with rectal blood loss, which can mimic inflammatory bowel disease. Stool cultures should be carried out in these patients to rule out infection before steroid therapy specific for inflammatory bowel disease is commenced.

Further reading

Camilleri M. Chronic diarrhoea: a review of pathophysiology and management for the clinical gastroenterologist. *Clin. Gastroenterol. Hepatol.* 2004;**2**:198–206.

DuPont HL. Guidelines on acute infectious diarrhea in adults The Practice Parameters Committee of the American College of Gastroenterology. *Am. J. Gastroenterol.* 1997;**92**:1962.

Powell DW. Approach to the patient with diarrhoea. In *Textbook of Gastroenterology*, Yamada T (ed.), Vol **1**. Lippincott, Philadelphia, 1991: 732–70.

Complications of gastrointestinal procedures and therapy

CHAPTER 8

Complications of upper gastrointestinal endoscopy

Daniel J. Stein and Reza Shaker

Medical College of Wisconsin, Milwaukee, WI, USA

Introduction

Complications related to diagnostic upper gastrointestinal endoscopy are rare. The American Society for Gastrointestinal Endoscopy estimated that the overall complication rate of this commonly performed diagnostic procedure was 0.13%, with an associated mortality of 0.004% [1]. The estimated average major complication rates for diagnostic and therapeutic upper endoscopic procedures range from 0.2% to 8%, with associated mortality rates of 0.01% to 1.5% [2]. Major complications include cardiopulmonary compromise, sedation-related side effects, infectious complications, perforation, and hemorrhage.

Late complications may be underestimated, primarily due to under-reporting by the patient or medical staff In a prospective study, physicians reported complications in only 2.1% of procedures; however, patients reported an 18.2% complication rate up to 30 days after the upper endoscopy [3]. Oropharyngeal or abdominal discomfort accounted for the majority of these late complications and most were minor; only 2.5% and 1.1% required a physician visit and/or hospitalization, respectively [3].

Appreciation of potential complications and the frequency of their occurrence by both physicians and patients allows for improved risk benefit analysis. The early recognition of complications permits prompt investigation and treatment, hence minimizing patient morbidity and mortality.

Complications of sedation

Intravenous medications used for moderate sedation in the majority of upper endoscopies include benzodiazepines, usually midazolam, together with a narcotic such as merperidine or fentanyl. Titrated dosing should be administered with continuous monitoring of the patient's blood pressure, cardiac rhythm and oxygen saturation. Clinical assessment of the patient's pulmonary status should be continuously observed during sedation. End-tidal CO_2 monitoring is not currently recommended for routine upper endoscopy, but may be indicated for more complicated patients [4].

Cardiopulmonary complications account for approximately half of the morbidity and mortality related to diagnostic endoscopic procedures [5,6]. Serious cardiopulmonary events may complicate as many as 0.5% of upper endoscopic procedures and more than 50% of deaths are related to cardiopulmonary complications [7,8]. Complications related to over-sedation include: acute myocardial infarction, cardiac arrhythmias, hypoventilation, hypotension, vasovagal episodes, aspiration, respiratory depression, and shock. Hence, full resuscitation equipment should be readily available in the endoscopy area. Use of a combination of medications, such as midazolam and fentanyl, for moderate sedation increases the incidence of respiratory depression significantly [9].

Gastrointestinal Emergencies, Third Edition. Edited by Tony C. K. Tham, John S. A. Collins, and Roy Soetikno.
© 2016 John Wiley & Sons, Ltd. Published 2016 by John Wiley & Sons, Ltd.

Cardiopulmonary complications

Oxygen desaturation may occur in up to 70% of patients undergoing various endoscopic evaluations [10]. Factors contributing to oxygen desaturation include difficulty with intubation of the esophagus, advanced patient age and a history of cardiopulmonary disease [9]. Difficult esophageal intubation, over-insufflation of the stomach or small bowel with air and the use of larger-diameter endoscopes are risk factors for vasovagal episodes. Cardiac rhythm abnormalities during upper endoscopy are most frequently seen in patients with underlying chronic heart or lung disease [11]. Furthermore, American Society of Anesthesiologists (ASA) class III or greater or an increased modified Goldman score have been associated with an increased frequency of unplanned cardiopulmonary events [6,12].

Other adverse events related to medications include drug allergy, paradoxical excitement with benzodiazepines, and benzocaine-induced methemoglobinemia in genetically predisposed individuals. Aspiration may occur in only 0.08% of cases but the mortality rate of this complication may reach 10%. Sedation, supine positioning and pharyngeal anesthesia utilized for upper endoscopy contribute to the development of pulmonary aspiration. Hence, aspiration precautions and readily available suctioning apparatus are integral to performing upper endoscopic procedures safely.

Management of sedation-related complications

Naloxone reverses the respiratory depression, sedation and hypotensive effects of narcotics in 1–2 minutes. Flumazenil, a benzodiazepine antagonist, significantly reduces patient recovery time following moderate sedation. Recurrent doses of both may be required in view of the relatively short half-life of these medications. Both naloxone and flumazenil should be readily available in the endoscopy room and staff should be familiar with dosage.

Infectious complications

Infectious complications may be related to the procedure itself, or the equipment used during the procedure. The incidence of bacteremia is low and the rate of subacute bacterial endocarditis (SBE) in patients not at risk for SBE is extremely low; it has been estimated to be 1 in 5–10 million [13]. Bacteremia is highest following esophageal dilation and esophageal variceal sclerotherapy, with a mean incidence of 45% and 18%, respectively. By contrast, bacteremia in diagnostic upper endoscopy is extremely low, less than 5% [14,15]. However, bacteremia is also associated with activities of daily life such as teeth brushing (20–68%) and chewing food (7–51%), so the exposure during endoscopy is likely trivial when compared to daily activities [16]. For this reason, the American Society of Gastrointestinal Endoscopy and the American Heart Association do not recommend SBE antibiotic prophylaxis for any upper endoscopy [16,17].

Other infectious complications include retropharyngeal and retroesophageal abscesses. These are related to trauma or unrecognized perforations at the time of the procedure.

Infectious complications related to equipment are very rare and are estimated to be 1 per 1.8 million procedures. Transmissions of bacteria such as *Helicobacter pylori* and viruses such as hepatitis B virus (HBV) and hepatitis C virus (HCV) have been reported and are fortunately very rare. Transmission of human immunodeficiency virus (HIV) has not been reported.

Perforation

The rate of perforation in upper endoscopy is relatively low, and has been reported in 1 in 2500 to 1 in 11 000 [18,19]. Factors predisposing to perforation include blind passage of the endoscope, anterior cervical osteophytes, presence of a Zenker diverticulum, esophageal strictures, and esophageal malignancy. Perforation occurs more frequently in the esophagus than the stomach and is associated with a relatively high mortality rate approximating 2% to 25% [20–22]. Pain is the most common symptom related to perforation. Other symptoms include shortness of breath, pleuritic chest pain, fever, and crepitus of the neck (subcutaneous emphysema). Early recognition of this complication, confirmation of perforation radiographically, and collaboration with cardiothoracic surgery have been shown to decrease mortality [21]. The main risk of endoscopic mucosal resection (EMR) is perforation, ranging from 0.7% to 2.5% in esophageal cancer and 0.06% to 2.4% for gastric cancers [23,24].

Bleeding

Bleeding from diagnostic upper endoscopy is very rare, estimated to occur in 0.03% of cases, and is usually gastric in origin [25]. A Mallory–Weiss tear may occur during upper endoscopy secondary to patient retching. These arise in less than 0.1% of diagnostic endoscopies and are usually not associated with significant bleeding. Overall therapeutic procedures cause bleeding more frequently than diagnostic evaluations. Generally, this rare complication occurs primarily in patients with thrombocytopenia and/or coagulopathy. Upper endoscopy without biopsy has been determined to be safe in patients with platelet counts greater than 20 000 [25]. Platelet counts of greater than 50 000 are likely required to safely perform biopsies [26].

Use of dual antiplatelet therapy (DAT), aspirin and clopidogrel, has become more common, particularly in the care of patients with a vascular stent, acute coronary syndrome (ACS), and cerebrovascular disease [28]. For routine upper endoscopy in this patient population, with and without biopsy, it is recommended that at least aspirin be continued and both aspirin and clopidogrel should be continued in those patients with a recent coronary stent [29]. Patients undergoing procedures that are at higher risk for bleeding such as polypectomy, endoscopic mucosal resection or percutaneous gastrostomy tube placement consideration for delaying the procedure should be made [29].

Patients on antithrombotic therapy with warfarin, unfractionated heparin, or low-molecular-weight heparin likely can safely continue their anticoagulation for low risk upper endoscopy with and without biopsy [30]. Patients at low risk for thrombotic events should consider having their anticoagulation held or bridged prior to the procedure; however, those at high risk for thrombotic event should not [30]. Timing of post-procedure resumption of anticoagulation or antiplatelet therapy is not clearly defined at this time. Delaying non-urgent elective procedures in the setting of temporary anticoagulation or antiplatelet therapy should always be considered. Consulting with the patient's cardiologist, hematologist, or primary doctor is recommended in individual cases [29].

Complications of common endoscopic procedures

Dilation

Major complications may occur in 0.5% of esophageal dilations and death in 0.01% [31]. The complication rate for esophageal dilation with mercury dilators has been reported to be 0.4% [1]. Through-the-scope balloon dilation and wire-guide bougie dilation have similar rates of complications and success when dilating benign esophageal strictures and may be safer than blindly passed dilators [32,33]. Other complications of esophageal dilation include abdominal pain, aspiration, bleeding, and bacteremia.

Balloon dilation of benign esophageal strictures is complicated by perforation in 0.4% of cases. In pyloric stenosis the risk of perforation is 0.5%, whereas with gastroenterostomy (anastomotic) stricture and gastric staple line dilation, the risk is 2.2% and 0.8%, respectively [34]. Caustic strictures are at higher risk of perforation due to the length of the lesion and luminal compromise. Perforation rates up to 17% have been reported [35].

In achalasia the rate of perforation with pneumatic balloon dilation is approximately 5% [36,37]. This risk may be reduced to 2% if a gradual dilation is performed and inflation pressures of greater than 11 psi are avoided [36,37].

With regard to malignant strictures, the rate of perforation is approximately 10% [2,38]. Post-radiation strictures have the same risk of perforation as a malignant stricture, ranging from 2% to 6.5% [39]. It has been established that relatively safe dilation of malignant strictures can be performed up to a diameter of 15 mm.

Dilation of malignant and benign gastric outlet obstruction strictures carry a perforation risk of 6.7% and 7.4%, respectively [2,37,41]. Dilation greater than 15 mm and active ulceration are risk factors to perforation, for this reason a stepwise approach to dilation is preferred [37,42].

Variceal sclerotherapy and banding

(See also Chapter 10.) The overall complication rate for variceal sclerotherapy (EVS) is between 35% and 78%. Major complications occur in 8.0% of cases and the mortality rate is in the range of 1% to 5% [43,44]. Esophageal ulcers occur in 50% to 78% of cases. Treatment with proton pump inhibitors does not prevent occurrence, but may allow healing [45]. Significant bleeding occurs in up to 6% of patients [46,47]. The retreatment interval should be greater than 1 week, as the only factor relating to multiple ulcerations is a treatment interval shorter than 1 week. The perforation rate ranges from 2% to 5% [48]. Chest pain after EVS occurs in up to 50% of patients but rarely lasts longer than 48 hours. Strictures can occur weeks to months after variceal sclerotherapy sessions in 2% to 20% of cases. Other complications of this emergent procedure include aspiration (5%), pneumonitis, pleural effusions and bacteremia [49].

Esophageal band ligation (EBL) is fortunately associated with a lower complication rate of 2% to 3% [50,5]). The overall mortality attributed to an acute complication of EBL is 1%. Hence, EBL is the endoscopic intervention of choice in the management of esophageal varices. Esophageal ulcers are reported in 5% to 15% of patients after EBL with a low tendency for bleeding [49]. Perforation had been reported in 0.7% of cases when band ligation was performed with a facilitating overtube [51]. The introduction of multiple band devices has resulted in the discontinuance of the use of overtubes for this procedure. Formation of strictures has been limited to case reports and was not seen in clinical trials [49–52].

Endoscopic non-variceal hemostasis

Overall, the incidence of major complications in the setting of non-variceal hemostasis is less than 0.5% [52]. Randomized controlled trials using MPEC (multipolar electrocoagulation) have reported rates of perforation of 0% to 2%. Induction of bleeding by electrocoagulation occurs in up to 5% of cases [54]. Repeated therapy with electrocoagulation within 24 to 48 hours is associated with an up to 4% risk of perforation [55].

Epinephrine, the most commonly used injection agent to achieve initial hemostasis, may cause mucosal ulceration but has not been associated with perforation [56]. Clinical trials into the use of endoscopic clips did not demonstrate a significantly increased rate procedure related complications [57].

Foreign body removal

(See also Chapter 20 on Foreign Body Impaction.) Adverse events that are caused by the object itself or by its removal can often be difficult to discern. Complications of endoscopic foreign body removal and meat disimpaction

have been reported in up to 8% of cases [58]. Complications include mucosal laceration, aspiration of the foreign body, GI bleeding and perforation [58]. The risks of aspiration and perforation may be decreased by the use of an overtube [59]. The use of overtubes has been associated with complications such as bleeding and perforation, and requires judicious use by an experienced operator [10,50].

Summary

Upper gastrointestinal endoscopy, a very commonly performed procedure, is fortunately relatively safe with few complications and extremely low mortality. Careful preprocedure evaluation of the patient can help avoid unnecessary risks and careful intraprocedural monitoring can help avoid unwanted complications. Lastly, early recognition of complications and prompt investigation, diagnosis and treatment can minimize patient morbidity and mortality.

References

1. Silvis SE, Nebel O, Rogers G, Sugawa C, Mandelstam P. Endoscopic complications. Results of the 1974 American Society of Gastrointestinal Endoscopy Survey. *JAMA* 1976; **235**(9):928–30.
2. Newcomer MK, Brazer SR. Complications of upper gastrointestinal endoscopy and their management. *Gastrointest. Endosc. Clin. N. Am.* 1994;**4**(3):551–70.
3. Zubarik R, Eisen G, Mastropietro C, et al. Prospective analysis of complications 30 days after outpatient upper endoscopy. *Am. J. Gastroenterol.* 1999;**94**(6):1539–45.
4. Lichtenstein D.R., Jagannath S., Baron T.H., et al. Sedation and anesthesia in GI endoscopy. *Gastrointest. Endosc.* 2008;**68**: 815–26.
5. Hart R, Classen M. Complications of diagnostic gastrointestinal endoscopy. *Endoscopy* 1990;**22**(5):229–33.
6. Sharma VK, Nguyen CC, Crowell MD, Lieberman DA, de Garmo P, Fleischer DE. A national study of cardiopulmonary unplanned events after GI endoscopy. *Gastrointest. Endosc.* 2007;**66**(1):27–34.
7. Arrowsmith JB, Gerstman BB, Fleischer DE, Benjamin SB. Results from the American Society for Gastrointestinal Endoscopy/US Food and Drug Administration collaborative study on complication rates and drug use during gastrointestinal endoscopy. *Gastrointest. Endosc.* 1991;**37**(4):421–7.
8. Bell GD. Review article: Premedication and intravenous sedation for upper gastrointestinal endoscopy. *Aliment. Pharmacol. Ther.* 1990;**4**(2):103–22.

9. Fleischer D. Monitoring the patient receiving conscious sedation for gastrointestinal endoscopy: issues and guidelines. *Gastrointest. Endosc.* 1989;**35**(3):262–6.

10. Dark DS, Campbell DR, Wesselius LJ. Arterial oxygen desaturation during gastrointestinal endoscopy. *Am. J. Gastroenterol.* 1990;**85**(10):1317–21.

11. Lee JG, Leung JW, Cotton PB. Acute cardiovascular complications of endoscopy: prevalence and clinical characteristics. *Dig. Dis.* 1995;**13**(2):130–5.

12. Clarke GA, Jacobson BC, Hammett RJ, et al. The indications, utilization and safety of gastrointestinal endoscopy in an extremely elderly patient cohort. *Endoscopy* **33**. 580–584.2001;

13. Mogadam M, Malhotra SK, Jackson RA. Pre-endoscopic antibiotics for the prevention of bacterial endocarditis: do we use them appropriately? *Am. J. Gastroenterol.* 1994;**89**(6):832–4.

14. Botoman VA, Surawicz CM. Bacteremia with gastrointestinal endoscopic procedures. *Gastrointest. Endosc.* 1986;**32**(5): 342–6.

15. Neu HC, Fleischer D. Controversies, dilemmas, and dialogues. Recommendations for antibiotic prophyaxis before endoscopy. *Am. J. Gastroenterol.* 1989;**84**(12):1488–91.

16. Hirota WK, Petersen K, Baron TH, et al.; Standards of Practice Committee of the American Society for Gastrointestinal Endoscopy. Guidelines for antibiotic prophylaxis for GI endoscopy. Gastrointest. *Endosc.* 2003;**58**(4):475–82.

17. Wilson W, Taubert KA, Gewitz M, et al. Prevention of infective endocarditis: guidelines from the American Heart Association. *Circulation* 2007;**116**:1736–54.

18. Quine MA, Bell GD, McCloy RF, et al. Prospective audit of perforation rates following upper gastrointestinal endoscopy in two regions of England. *Br. J. Surg.* 1995;**82**:530–3.

19. Sieg A, Hachmoeller-Eisenbach U, Eisenbach T. Prospective evaluation of complications in outpatient GI endoscopy: a survey among German gastroenterologists. *Gastrointest. Endosc.* 2001;**53**:620–7.

20. Pettersson G, Larsson S, Gatzinsky P, Sudow G. Differentiated treatment of intrathoracic oesophageal perforations. *Scand. J. Thorac. Cardiovasc. Surg.* 1981;**15**(3):321–4.

21. Abbas G, Schuchert MJ, Pettiford BL, et al. Contemporaneous management of esophageal perforation. *Surgery* 2009; **146**:749–55.

22. Eroglu A, Turkyilmaz A, Aydin Y, et al. Current management of esophageal perforation: 20 years experience. *Dis. Esophagus* 2009;**22**:374–80.

23. Inoue H, Tani M, Nagai K, et al. Treatment of esophageal and gastric tumors. *Endoscopy* 1999;**31**(1):47–55.

24. Makuuchi H, Kise Y, Shimada H, Chino O, Tanaka H. Endoscopic mucosal resection for early gastric cancer. *Semin. Surg. Oncol.* 1999;**17**(2):108–16.

25. Montalvo RD, Lee M. Retrospective analysis of iatrogenic Mallory–Weiss tears occurring during upper gastrointestinal endoscopy. *Hepatogastroenterology* 1996;**43**:174–7.

26. Chu DZ, Shivshanker K, Stroehlein JR, et al. Thrombocytopenia and gastrointestinal hemorrhage in the cancer patient: prevalence of unmasked lesions. *Gastrointest. Endosc.* 1983;**29**: 269–72.

27. Van Os EC, Kamath PS, Gostout CJ, et al. Gastroenterological procedures among patients with disorders of hemostasis: evaluation and management recommendations. *Gastrointest. Endosc.* 1999;**50**:536–43.

28. King 3rd, SB, Smith Jr, SC, Hirshfeld Jr, JW, et al. 2007 focused update of the ACC/AHA/SCAI 2005 guideline update for percutaneous coronary intervention: a report of the American College of Cardiology/American Heart Association Task Force on Practice guidelines. *J. Am. Coll. Cardiol.* 2008;**51**:172–209.

29. Anderson MA, Ben-Menachem T, Gan SI, et al. ASGE Standards of Practice Committee, Management of antithrombotic agents for endoscopic procedures. *Gastrointest. Endosc.* 2009;**70**(6):1060–70.

30. Gerson LB, Gage BF, Owens DK, et al. Effect and outcomes of the ASGE guidelines on the periendoscopic management of patients who take anticoagulants. *Am. J. Gastroenterol.* 2000;**95**:1717–24.

31. Mandelstam P, Sugawa C, Silvis SE, et al. Complications associated with esophagogastroduodenoscopy and with esophageal dilation. *Gastrointest. Endosc.* 1976;**23**(1):16–19.

32. Saeed ZA, Winchester CB, Ferro PS, Michaletz PA, Schwartz JT, Graham DY. Prospective randomized comparison of polyvinyl bougies and through-the-scope balloon for dilation of peptic strictures of the esophagus. *Gastrointest. Endosc.* 1995;**41**(3):189–95.

33. Scolapio JS, Pasha TM, Gostout CJ, et al. A randomized prospective study comparing rigid to balloon dilators for benign esophageal strictures and rings. *Gastrointest. Endosc.* 1999;**50**:13–17.

34. Kozarek RA. Hydrostatic balloon dilation of gastrointestinal stenoses: a national survey. *Gastrointest. Endosc.* 1986;**32**(1):15–19.

35. Karnak I, Tanyel FC, Buyukpamukcu N, Hicsonmez A. Esophageal perforations encountered during dilation of caustic esophageal strictures. *J. Cardiovasc. Surg.* 1998;**39** (3):373–7.

36. Nair LA, Reynolds JC, Parkman HP, et al. Complications during pneumatic dilation for achalasia or diffuse esophageal spasm. Analysis of risk factors, early clinical characteristics, and outcome. *Dig. Dis. Sci.* 1993;**38**(10):1893–904.

37. Lau JY, Chung SC, Sung JJ, et al. Through-the-scope balloon dilation for pyloric stenosis: long-term results. *Gastrointest. Endosc.* 1996;**43**:98–101.

38. Neuhaus H, Hoffman W, Dittler HJ, Neidermeyer HP, Classen M. Implantation of self-expanding esophageal metal stents for palliation of malignant dysphagia. *Endoscopy* 1992;**24**(5):405–10.

39. Ng TM, Spencer GM, Sargeant IR, Thorpe SM, Brown SG. Management of strictures after radiotherapy for esophageal cancer. *Gastrointest. Endosc.* 1996;**43**(6):584–90.

40. Fukami N, Anderson MA, Khan K, et al. The role of endoscopy in gastroduodenal obstruction and gastroparesis. *Gastrointest. Endosc.* 2011;**74**:13–21.

41. Disario JA, Fennerty MB, Tietze CC, Hutson WR, Burt RW. Endoscopic balloon dilation for ulcer-induced gastric outlet obstruction. *Am. J. Gastroenterol.* 1994;**89**(6):868–71.

42. Boeckxstaens GE, Annese V, des Varannes SB, et al. The European Achalasia Trial: a randomized multi-centre trial comparing endoscopic pneumodilation and laparoscopic myotomy as primary treatment of idiopathic achalasia. *Gastroenterology* 2010;**138**:S-53.

43. Schuman BM, Beckman JW, Tedesco FJ, Griffin JW, Assad RT. Complications of endoscopic injection sclerotherapy: a review. *Am. J. Gastroenterol.* 1987;**82**(9):823–30.

44. Zambelli A, Arcidiacano PG, Arcidiacano R et al. Complications of endoscopic variceal sclerotherapy (EVS): a multicenter study of 1192 patients. *Gastroenterology* 1993;**104**:1023.

45. Shephard H, Barkin JS. Omeprazole heals mucosal ulcers associated with endoscopic injection sclerotherapy. *Gastrointest. Endosc.* 1993;**39**:474–5.

46. Piai G, Cipolleta L, Claar M, et al. Prophylactic sclerotherapy of high risk esophageal varices: results of a multicentric prospective controlled trial. *Hepatology* 1988; **8**(6):1495–500.

47. Gimson A, Polson R, Westaby D, Williams R. Omeprazole in the management of intractable esophageal ulcerations following injection sclerotherapy. *Gastroenterology* 1990;**99**(6):1829–31.

48. The Copenhagen Esophageal Varices Sclerotherapy Project. Sclerotherapy after first variceal hemorrhage in cirrhosis. *N. Engl. J. Med.* 1984;**311**(25):1594–600.

49. Stiegmann GV, Goff JS, Michaletz-Onody PA, et al. Endoscopic sclerotherapy as compared with endoscopic ligation for bleeding esophageal varices. *N. Engl. J. Med.* 1992;**326**(23):1527–32.

50. Laine L, Cook D. Endoscopic ligation compared with sclerotherapy for treatment of esophageal variceal bleeding. A meta-analysis Ann. Intern. *Med.* 1995;**123**:280–7.

51. Lo GH, Lai KH, Cheng JS, et al. A prospective, randomized trial of sclerotherapy versus ligation in the management of bleeding esophageal varices. *Hepatology* 1995;**22**:466–71.

52. Rai RR, Nijhawan S, Singh G. Post-ligation stricture: a rare complication. *Endoscopy* 1996;**28**:406.

53. Sung JJ, Tsoi KK, Ma TK, et al. Causes of mortality in patients with peptic ulcer bleeding: a prospective cohort study of 10,428 cases. *Am. J. Gastroenterol.* 2010;**105**: 84–9.

54. Jensen DM. Endoscopic control of nonvariceal upper gastrintestinal hemorrhage. In Textbook of Gastroenterology, Yamada T, Alpers DH, Laine L, Owyang C, Powell DW (eds). Lippincott Williams & Wilkins, Philadelphia, 1999;2857–79.

55. Lau JY, Sung JJ, Lam YH, et al. Endoscopic retreatment compared with surgery in patients with recurrent bleeding after initial endoscopic control of bleeding ulcers. *N. Engl. J. Med.* 1999;**340**(10):751–6.

56. Lin HJ, Tseng GY, Perng CL, Lee FY, Chang FY, Lee SD. Comparison of adrenaline injection and bipolar electrocoagulation for the arrest of peptic ulcer bleeding. *Gut* 1999;**44**(5):715–19.

57. Sung JJ, Tsoi KK, Lai LH, et al. Endoscopic clipping versus injection and thermo-coagulation in the treatment of nonvariceal upper gastrointestinal bleeding: a meta-analysis. *Gut* 2007;**56**:1364–73.

58. Berggreen PJ, Harrison E, Sanowski RA, Ingebo K, Noland B, Zierer S. Techniques and complications of esophageal foreign body extraction in children and adults. *Gastrointest. Endosc.* 1993;**39**(5):626–30.

59. Ginsberg GG. Management of ingested foreign objects and food bolus impactions. *Gastrointest. Endosc.* 1995; **41**(1):33–8.

CHAPTER 9

Complications of percutaneous endoscopic gastrostomy

Barbara Willandt[1] and Jo Vandervoort[2]

[1] KU Leuven, Netherlands
[2] Onze-Lieve-Vrouw Ziekenhuis, Aalst, Belgium

Introduction

Since the introduction of percutaneous endoscopic gastrostomy (PEG) in 1980 by Gauderer et al., it has become a popular technique for enteral feeding [1]. PEG has proven, in controlled trials, to be a relatively safe and effective method to provide long-term enteral feeding in patients with an intact, functional gastrointestinal tract, but who are unable to maintain their nutrition status orally.

The most frequent indications for PEG placement are neurologic or general debilitating disorders and oropharyngeal or esophageal obstruction caused by benign or neoplastic lesions [2]. PEG placement is considered to be an easy procedure, with a high success rate of 95–98% [3,4]. The procedure-related mortality is less than 1% [2,4,5]. The frequency of complications observed in the various reports depends upon the definitions used and the population under study. The overall complication rate ranges from 4.9–10.8% (incidence of major complications varies from 1–4%) [3,4].

Minor complications are infection of insertion site, peristomal leakage, tube dislodgement, pneumoperitoneum, and gastric ileus, and can mostly be treated conservatively. Major complications such as hemorrhage, necrotizing fasciitis (NF), perforation, fistulization, and buried bumper syndrome often require further endoscopic procedure or surgical intervention [5–7].

Minor complications

Pneumoperitoneum

Pneumoperitoneum after PEG placement is frequent, but mostly benign and self-limiting. Its true incidence is subject to debate (variable from 12–56%) [5,8,9]. It originates from air insufflations at endoscopy and by introducing air through the puncture needle. It can be present for a few days, but may persist up to 4 weeks [8,10]. In the absence of signs of peritonitis it is of no clinical significance. It is seen on plain abdominal radiography and CT scan can rule out other complications [10–12].

Infectious complications

The most common complication is PEG site infection [3,5]. Patients undergoing PEG tube placement are often vulnerable to infection because of advanced age, poor nutritional state, immunosuppression or underlying disease such as malignancy and diabetes [13].

Serious infections are extremely rare, occurring in less than 1.6% [5]. Prophylactic administration of a single dose of systemic broad-spectrum antibiotics, 30 min before insertion of PEG tube, significantly reduces the number of post-PEG infections and should be routinely administered [3,13,14]. Type of antibiotics used in different trials depend on the origin of the study. Similar rates of wound infections occur with either penicillin

Gastrointestinal Emergencies, Third Edition. Edited by Tony C. K. Tham, John S. A. Collins, and Roy Soetikno.
© 2016 John Wiley & Sons, Ltd. Published 2016 by John Wiley & Sons, Ltd.

based antibiotics or cephalosporin based antibiotics [13,15]. A meta-analysis by Jafri et al. [15] showed that the number needed to treat (NNT) for cephalosporin was 10 compared with six for penicillin, but this was not statistically significant. Some studies also support nasopharyngeal decolonization for methicillin-resistant *Staphylococcus aureus* (MRSA) prior to PEG placement, because of the emergence of MRSA as a common pathogen in peristomal infections [15–17].

Treatment consists of good local wound care and intravenous antibiotic therapy. Progression to peritonitis is only seen in 0.4–1.6% of cases and should be treated with intravenous antibiotics and surgical exploration [5].

Peristomal leakage

Although the reported incidence of peristomal leakage is 1–2%, it is probably much more common. It's precipitated by the use of corrosive agents (ascorbic acid, hydrogen peroxide use for cleansing), peristomal infection, granulation tissue, torsion on the tube, absence of an external bolster, or by complications such as buried bumper. Diagnosis and subsequent treatment should be directed against the specific exacerbating factor; relieve excessive torsion, start proton pump inhibitors, stop the use of hydrogen peroxide and ascorbic acid, and apply zinc oxide or an antifungal paste on the PEG-site. Replacing the tube with a larger size should be avoided, because it will distend the tract even more and cause further leakage [5,7].

Ileus and gastroparesis

Post-procedural gastroparesis occasionally occurs, especially in patients with a history of diabetes. Metoclopramide, or even erythromycin, can be useful in stimulating gastrointestinal motility. Prolonged ileus occurs in 1–2% of cases after PEG placement. Supportive measures are indicated and sometimes discontinuing enteral nutrition is necessary [5,7].

Major complications

Aspiration

Procedure-related aspiration is only reported in 0.3–1% of cases, but most aspiration events occur at a later time, unrelated to the PEG procedure [5,7]. Advanced age, supine position, neurologic impairment, and level of sedation are considered risk factors for aspiration.

Symptoms are high temperature and respiratory distress. Oxygen desaturation during the procedure usually occurs. Aiming for a short procedure time, avoiding excessive sedation, controlled air-insufflation and maximal aspiration of gastric contents can reduce the risk of aspiration. Treatment with IV antibiotics is indicated [5,7,18].

Hemorrhage

Gastrointestinal hemorrhage following PEG is rare, with an incidence of 0.2–2.5% [5,19]. It may be due to direct puncture of a blood vessel in the abdominal wall, but mostly it is caused by ulceration of the mucosa underneath the internal bumper. Another mechanism of ulcer formation after PEG-insertion, is friction of the tip of the PEG against the posterior gastric wall [20]. Unrelated peptic ulcer disease is less frequent.

The risk of puncturing a large abdominal wall vessel is increased in patients with portal hypertension. Careful transillumination of the abdominal wall should prevent this complication [20]. Inability to obtain good transillumination whatever the cause (obesity, prior surgery, ascites) should always be a contraindication for PEG placement [2,19].

Management of a post-PEG haemorrhage is similar to other gastrointestinal bleeding with upper endoscopy, anti-ulcer therapy. If there is deep ulceration underneath the internal bumper, which may be at risk of perforation, the PEG-tube should be removed [19].

PEG placement is considered a high-risk procedure for bleeding. Anticoagulation and antiplatelet therapies should be discontinued in accordance with current guidelines published. A recent study by Richter et al. concluded that use of serotonin reuptake inhibitors 24 hours before the procedure was associated with an increased risk of bleeding, rather than use of aspirin or clopidogrel [21].

Necrotizing fasciitis

NF, first described by Wilson in 1952, is a rapid and progressive soft-tissue infection leading to necrosis of the fascia, subcutaneous tissue and overlying skin. It is a rare complication after PEG tube placement that constitutes a surgical emergency with high morbidity and mortality [22,23].

Predisposing factors are diabetes, wound infections, malnutrition, and impaired immunity [23–25]. Traction and pressure on the PEG tube can also predispose to development of NF. Some authors suggest that a skin incision of at least 1 cm can avoid infectious complications; however, there is some controversy with this practice. A controlled trial by Sedlack et al. found no difference in wound healing between two patient groups with or without skin incision [26].

Symptoms of NF can be very subtle and a high index of suspicion is necessary. Patients usually present with pain, localized edema, erythema, and fever progressing to formation of bullae (with subcutaneous crepitus), and eventually septic shock. NF is usually seen within 72 hours after placement, though longer intervals have been described [23–28].

A plain abdominal X-ray shows signs of subcutaneous emphysema, a pathognomonic sign for NF. Computerized tomography (CT) scan or magnetic resonance imaging (MRI) of the abdomen are useful to evaluate the extension of the infection. It may allow the surgeon to avoid opening the visceral fascia if there's no evidence of peritoneal spread [24].

The treatment of NF requires immediate intervention with a rapid and extensive surgical debridement, broad-spectrum antibiotics and, according to certain authors, hyperbaric oxygen [22]. Mortality varies between 35–70% and there is a correlation with the delay to surgical intervention. Repeated surgery until all non-viable tissue has been resected is necessary for the wound to heal and healthy granulation tissue to form [23–25,27,28].

Most common organisms are group A haemolytic *Streptococcus*, often together with *Staphylococcus* species, *Enterococcus*, *Escherichia coli*, *Proteus*, and *Bacteroides*. In post-traumatic NF *Clostridium* is usually present, in association with other aerobic or anaerobic bacteria [22].

Provision of adequate nutrition is an important factor for these patients. Placement of nasoenteric feeding tubes or even surgical gastrostomy or jejunostomy are preferable, given the known limitations of long-term parenteral nutrition.

Perforation and gastroenteric fistula

Perforation of other intra-abdominal organs like colon, small bowel, and liver during PEG placement have been described, but are rare complications that can be difficult to diagnose.

Larson et al. [3] described gastric or esophageal perforation in 4 of the 314 cases during or after PEG placement, often with progression to peritonitis. It occurs when the mushroom-shaped head of the PEG is pulled through the tighter gastroesophageal junction or, more likely, through a (benign or malignant) stricture. In such cases dilatation of the stricture to at least 36 F is necessary prior to PEG insertion [3].

As the result of interposition of bowel – usually the splenic flexure – between the anterior abdominal wall and the gastric wall during PEG placement colonic perforation can occur with formation of a gastrocolocutaneous fistula, by placing the tube directly through the bowel into the stomach [7]. This complication occurs more frequently in pediatric population, with a 2–3% incidence [29,30]. Gastroenteric fistulae are often asymptomatic for a long time; the problem is usually discovered several months after PEG procedure, when the tube is removed or manipulated. Sometimes fistulae are diagnosed when the patient develops watery diarrhea, unexplained weight loss, or if fecaloid output appears around the PEG tube. Persistent peristomal leakage and inflammation or bowel obstruction can also indicate fistula formation [4,7,31].

Management of gastrocolocutaneous fistula consists of removing the PEG tube and allowing spontaneous closure of the fistula. In rare cases surgery is required if there is evidence of peritonitis, abscess or the fistula fails to close spontaneously [4,7]. As a precaution, Quadri et al. [32] propose elevating the head end of the bed 30° during PEG insertion to displace the bowel caudally. Careful transillumination and finger pressure as guide to point out the puncture site are also very important during placement. By using a syringe with saline solution attached to a needle, one can more easily determine a "safe tract", determined by simultaneous air return and endoscopic visualization of the needle. Abnormal posture of the patient, spinal deformations, and previous abdominal surgery with adhesions are risk factors and are considered relative contraindications for PEG placement [31,33].

Buried bumper

Migration of the internal bolster of the PEG into the gastric mucosa, is a rare complication, referred to as the "buried bumper syndrome" (Fig. 9.1). It was first described by Klein et al[34] in 1988. In a series of 115 patients, Gençosmanoglu et al. [35] found two cases of buried bumper (1.7%), which corresponds with the incidence of 1.5–1.9% reported in the literature [5]. Intramucosal migration of the rigid bumper of a PEG

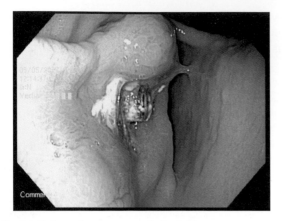

Fig. 9.1 Endoscopic appearance of a buried bumper at endoscopy. (*see insert for color representation of the figure.*)

tube is caused by ischemic pressure necrosis from the underlying gastric mucosa. Following re-epithelialization, the bumper is completely embedded in the gastric wall. Pressure necrosis is a result of either too strong a tension on the bolster causing hypoperfusion of the stomach wall, or because patients apply aggressive traction on the external portion of the tube. This is a long-term complication after PEG. Often it is only noticed on endoscopy during PEG replacement [34].

The depth of the intramucosal migration defines the clinical presentation. Symptoms may vary from pain at the insertion place with edema and erythema, more difficult tube mobilization, or difficulties at infusion of the feeding solution. Patients can also present with melena from bleeding ischemic ulcers at the site of the buried bumper [36]. Most often patients complain of sudden pain at infusion or have abdominal bloating, indicative of gastric dysmotility [34]. Although the clinical presentation of buried bumper is frequently asymptomatic, it may evolve to gastric perforation, diffuse peritonitis with acute abdomen, and even death of the patient.

Diagnosis can be made from the clinical examination, where the PEG is immoveable at a point where you can no longer push it inward. Gastroscopy is the most accurate way of diagnosing a buried bumper. Supplementary diagnostic work-up often comprises a plain abdominal X-ray, contrast radiography through the PEG, and an abdominal CT scan or MRI to facilitate the localization of the bumper and decide whether surgical or endoscopic approach is necessary to remove the tube [7,34].

Whatever the presentation, it is imperative that the PEG-tube is removed to prevent further migration through the stomach wall and gastric perforation. One technique uses the needle knife to cut the overlying mucosa, so the bumper can be pushed into the stomach, cut near the tip and endoscopically removed. The remaining part of the tube is removed externally. In another technique a guide wire is pushed through the PEG-tube. Next a skin incision is made up to the imbedded bumper, which can then be removed without opening the peritoneum, reducing infectious complications.

As a precaution, nursing staff are best advised to push the tube inward 1 cm and rotating it a few times, every time they clean the tube, thus preventing intramucosal migration [36,37].

PEG replacement

Replacement of a gastrostomy tube is considered as a safe and simple procedure, but can sometimes result in serious complications such as gastrocutaneous tract disruption and intraperitoneal tube placement, leading to chemical peritonitis with significant morbidity and even mortality. The tract of a percutaneous gastrostomy begins to mature in 7–10 days and is well formed in 4–6 weeks. However, in malnourished or immunosuppressed patients this process can take much longer. When a PEG tube needs to be replaced within the first 4 weeks after initial placement (either because of occlusion or breakage of the tube, or by inadvertent PEG tube removal – a common complication in confused and agitated patients), this should not be done blindly at the bedside, because the gastric and abdominal walls may have separated, resulting in an intraperitoneal tube placement. If intraperitoneal placement of the tube is suspected, a water-soluble contrast study through the gastrostomy should be performed to confirm the position of the tube. In the absence of peritonitis conservative treatment with removal of the tube, nasogastric tube decompression, and intravenous broad-spectrum antibiotics may be sufficient. However, a surgical intervention will normally be necessary [5,38,39].

References

1. Gauderer MWL, Ponsky JL, Izant RJ Jr. Gastrostomy without laparotomy: a percutaneous endoscopic technique. *J. Pediatr. Surg.* 1980;**15**(6):872–5.
2. Nicholson FB, Korman MG, Richardson MA. Percutaneous endoscopic gastrostomy: a review of indications, complications and outcome. *J. Gastroenterol. Hepatol.* 2000;**15**:21–5.

3. Larson DE, Burton DD, Schroeder KW, DiMagno EP. Percutaneous endoscopic gastrostomy: indications, success, complications and mortality in 314 consecutive patients. *Gastroenterology* 1987;**93**:48–52.

4. Verhoef MJ, Van Rosendaal GM. Patient outcomes related to percutaneous endoscopic gastrostomy placement. *J. Clin. Gastroenterol.* 2001;**32**:49–53.

5. McClave A, Chang W-K. Complications of enteral access. *Gastrointest. Endosc.* 2003;**58**(5):739–51.

6. Mathus-Vliegen EMH, Koning H, Taminiau JAJM, Moorman-Voestermans CGM. Percutaneous endoscopic gastrostomy and gastrojejunostomy in psychomotor retarded subjects: a follow-up covering 106 patient years. *J. Pediatr. Gastroenterol. Nutr.* 2001;**33**:488–94.

7. Schrag SP, Sharma R, Jaik NP, et al. Complications related to percutaneous endoscopic gastrostomy (PEG) tubes. A comprehensive clinical review. *J. Gastrointest. Liver Dis.* 2007; **16**(4):407–18.

8. Wiesen AJ, Sideridis K, Fernandes A, et al. True incidence and clinical significance of pneumoperitoneum after PEG placement: a prospective study. *Gastrointest. Endosc.* 2006; **64**:886–9.

9. Blum CA, Selander C, Ruddy JM, Leon S. The incidence and clinical significance of pneumoperitoneum after percutaneous endoscopic gastrostomy: a review of 722 cases. *Am. Surg.* 2009;**75**(1):39–43.

10. Dulabon GR, Abrams JE, Rutherford EJ. The incidence and significance of free air after percutaneous endoscopic gastrostomy. *Am. Surg.* 2002;**68**(6):590–3.

11. Roberts PA, Wrenn K, Lundquist S. Pneumoperitoneum after percutaneous endoscopic gastrostomy : a case report en review. *J. Emerg. Med.* 2005;**28**(1):45–8.

12. Faias S, Buck G, DeLegge M. Peritonitis after percutaneous endoscopic gastrostomy and jejunostomy : where there is smoke, there may not be fire. *Endoscopy* 2006;**38**(7):745–8.

13. Lipp A, Lusardi G. Systematic antimicrobial prophylaxis for percutaneous endoscopic gastrostomy (Review). Cochrane Database Syst Rev. 2006 Oct 18;(4):CD005571.

14. Miller RE, Castlemain B, Lacqua FJ, Kotler DP. Percutaneous endoscopic gastrostomy. Results in 316 patients and review of the literature. Surg. *Endosc.* 1989;**3**:186–90.

15. Jafri NS, Mahid SS, Minor KS, Idstein SR, Hornung CA, Galandiuk S. Meta-analysis: antibiotic prophylaxis to prevent peristomal infection following percutaneous endoscopic gastrostomy. *Alim. Pharm. Ther.* 2007;**25**:647–56.

16. Horiuchi A, Nakayama Y, Kajiyama M, Fujii H, Tanaka N. Nasopharyngeal decolonization of methicillin-resistant *Staphylococcus aureus* can reduce PEG peristomal wound infection. *Am. J. Gastroenterol.* 2006;**101**(2):274–7.

17. Thomas S, Cantrill S, Waghorn DJ, McIntyre A. The role of screening and antibiotic prophylaxis in the prevention of percutaneous gastrostomy site infection caused by methicillin-resistant Staphylococcus aureus. *Aliment. Pharmacol. Ther.* 2007;**25**(5):593–7.

18. Kadakia S, O'Sullivan H, Starnes E. Percutaneous endoscopic gastrostomy or jejunostomy and the incidence of aspiration in 79 patients. *Am. J. Surg.* 1992;**164**:114–18.

19. Cappell MS, Abdullah M. Management of gastrointestinal bleeding induced by gastrointestinal endoscopy. *Gastroenterol. Clin. N. Am.* 2000;**29**(1):125–67.

20. Kanie J, Akatsu H, Suzuki Y, Shimokata H, Iguchi A. Mechanism of the development of gastric ulcer after percutaneous endoscopic gastrostomy. *Endoscopy* 2002;**34**(6):480–2.

21. Richter JA, Patrie JT, Richter RP, et al. Bleeding after percutaneous endoscopic gastrostomy is linked to serotonin reuptake inhibitors, not aspirin or clopidogrel. *Gastrointest. Endosc.* 2011;**74**:22–34.

22. Catena F, La Donna M, Ansaloni L, Agrusti S, Taffurelli M. Necrotizing fasciitis: a dramatical surgical emergency. *Eur. J. Emerg. Med.* 2004;**11**(1):44–8.

23. Haas D, Dharmaraja P, Morrison JG, Pots III Jr. Necrotizing fasciitis following percutaneous endoscopic gastrostomy. *Gastrointest. Endosc.* 1988;**34**(6):487–8.

24. Maclean AA, Miller G, Bamboat ZM, Hiotis K. Abdominal wall necrotizing fasciitis from dislodged percutaneous endoscopic gastrostomy tubes: a case series. *Am. Surg.* 2004;**70**(9):827–31.

25. Martindale R, Witte M, Hodges G, Kelley J, Harris S, Andersen C. Necrotizing fasciitis as a complication of percutaneous endoscopic gastrostomy. *J. Parent. Enteral Nutr.* 1987;**11**(6):583–585.

26. Sedlack RE, Pochron NL, Baron TH. Percutaneous endoscopic gastrostomy placement without skin incision: results of a randomized trial. *J. Parent. Enteral Nutr.* 2006;**30**:240–5.

27. Cave DR, Robinson WR, Brotschi EA. Necrotizing fasciitis following percutaneous endoscopic gastrostomy. *Gastrointest. Endosc.* 1986;**32**(4):294–6.

28. Greif JM, Ragland JJ, Ochsner MG, Riding R. Fatal necrotizing fasciitis complicating percutaneous endoscopic gastrostomy. *Gastrointest. Endosc.* 1986;**32**(4):292–294.

29. Patwardhan N, McHugh K, Drake D, Spitz L. Gastroenteric fistula complicating percutaneous endoscopic gastrostomy. *J. Pediatr. Surg.* 2004;**39**:561–4.

30. Khatak IU, Kimber C, Kiely EM, et al. Percutaneous endoscopic gastrostomy in paediatric practice : complications and outcome. *J. Pediatr. Surg.* 1998;**33**:67–72.

31. Friedmann R, Feldman H, Sonnenblick M. Misplacement of percutaneously inserted gastrostomy tube into the colon: report of 6 cases and review of the literature. *J. Parent. Enteral Nutr.* 2007;**31**:469–76.

32. Quadri AHA, Puetz TR, Dindzans V, Canga C, Sincaban M. Enterocutaneous fistula: a rare complication of PEG tube placement. *Gastrointest. Endosc.* 2001; **53**(4):529–31.

33. Yamazaki T, Sakai Y, Hatakeyama K, Hoshiyama Y. Colocutaneous fistula after percutaneous endoscopic gastrostomy in a remnant stomach. *Surg. Endosc.* 1999;**13**:280–2.

34. Klein S, Heare BR, Soloway RD. The "Buried bumper syndrome": a complication of percutaneous endoscopic gastrostomy. *Am. J. Gastroenterol.* 1990;**85**(4):448–51.

35. Gençosmanoglu R, Koç D, Tözün N. The buried bumper syndrome : migration of internal bumper of percutaneous endoscopic gastrostomy tube into the abdominal wall. *J. Gastroenterol.* 2003;**38**:1077–80.

36. Anagnostopoulos GK, Kostopoulos P, Arvanitidis DM. Buried bumper syndrome with a fatal outcome, presenting early as gastrointestinal bleeding after percutaneous endoscopic gastrostomy placement. *J. Postgrad. Med.* 2003; **49**:325–7.

37. Rino Y, Tokunaga M, Morinaga S, et al. The buried bumper syndrome: an early complication of percutaneous endoscopic gastrostomy. *Hepato-Gastroenterology* 2002;**49**:1183–4.

38. Lohsiriwat V. Percutaneous endoscopic gastrostomy tube replacement: A simple procedure? World J. *Gastrointest. Endosc.* 2013;**5**(1):14–18.

39. Taheri M, Singh H, Duerksen DR. Peritonitis after gastrostomy tube replacement: a case series and review of literature. *J. Parent. Enteral Nutr.* 2011;**35**:56–60.

CHAPTER 10

Complications of endoscopic variceal ligation, sclerotherapy, and balloon tamponade

Aarti K. Rao[1] and Roy Soetikno[2,3]

[1] Department of Internal Medicine, Stanford University, Stanford, CA, USA
[2] Stanford University, Stanford, CA, USA
[3] Veterans Affairs Palo Alto Health Care System, Palo Alto, CA, USA

Endoscopic variceal ligation (EVL), endoscopic variceal sclerotherapy (EVS), and balloon tamponade are commonly performed to treat esophageal variceal bleeding, and all of these modalities carry risks of complications. The risks, however, are much lower compared to the significant risk of mortality from esophageal bleeding. While EVL and EVS can be used in both acute and prophylactic settings, balloon tamponade is typically reserved for severe acute bleeding that cannot otherwise be controlled by EVL or EVS. In addition to risks inherent to the procedures themselves, patients with upper gastrointestinal bleeding are at increased risk of infection, namely aspiration pneumonia and spontaneous bacterial peritonitis (SBP). EVL is the preferred method of endoscopic treatment in acute variceal bleeding, both in terms of safety and efficacy, combined with vasoactive medication, such as somatostatin [1].

EVL has a lower risk of complications than EVS. Major risks include bleeding from treatment-induced ulcers, esophageal perforation and strictures [1–10]. Minor complications such as dysphagia and chest pain are common and resolve within a few days. Esophageal ulcer is reported in between 2.7 and 20% of patients undergoing EVL [3,4,6,9,10]. Proton pump inhibitor treatment is recommended post-EVL [11,12]. Perforation has been reported in the past when an overtube was more commonly used to allow repeated intubation of the esophagus because the banding accessory was "single shot" [13,14]. However, the introduction of "multiple-shot" ligation devices has helped reduce this risk since it has six to ten bands and no overtube. Stricture formation

is very rare [2,3]. It occurs as a result of multiple bands being applied to the same area of the esophageal wall. Aspiration pneumonia has been reported in between 1.5 and 5.3% of patients and spontaneous bacterial peritonitis has been reported in between 2.7 and 15.9% of patients undergoing EVL [1,5–7,9,15]. Frequent suctioning of the oropharynx can reduce the risk of aspiration of secretions. The risk of aspiration and subsequent pneumonia is highest in patients with massive bleeding. It may even be higher during the introduction of the instrument when the stomach is filled with blood or food, particularly in patients with altered consciousness. In such circumstances, endoscopy should best be performed under general anesthesia after securing the circulatory and respiratory status. In conscious patients, endoscopy may be carried out without any sedation or pharyngeal anesthesia. The use of a therapeutic upper gastrointestinal endoscope with a working channel of 6.0 mm is strongly recommended, because it enables rapid evacuation of the gastric contents and simultaneously compresses the bleeding site at the esophagus. An additional suction pump is needed to clear the oropharyngeal cavity.

Antibiotic prophylaxis is recommended for patients with ascites. Typically, ceftriaxone is given intravenously for 7 days. Once the patient stops bleeding and has resumed oral intake, the remainder of the 7 day course can be completed with twice daily norfloxacin [16].

It is important to perform EVL in the most distal portion of the esophagus, typically up to 5 cm from the squamocolumnar junction (SCJ). Esophageal varices develop from the esophageal palisade vessels. Bleeding

Gastrointestinal Emergencies, Third Edition. Edited by Tony C. K. Tham, John S. A. Collins, and Roy Soetikno.
© 2016 John Wiley & Sons, Ltd. Published 2016 by John Wiley & Sons, Ltd.

occurs from the engorged mucosal vessels, but is less likely from vessels as they become submucosal at 5 cm proximal to the SCJ. EVL of the submucosal vessels is thus unnecessary. It has been reported to cause fatal bleeding as the band captures only a portion of the varix. If a band falls off, bleeding from the remnant vessels may occur. Bleeding may rarely occur during a banding procedure if the varix ruptures while being sucked into the barrel of the ligator. However, this kind of bleeding is easily stopped by immediately releasing the band. Early rebleeding may occur after initial band ligation sessions as long as varices are not completely thrombosed.

EVS has been reported to be associated with a higher rate of ulcer formation than EVL – up to 78% [17]. EVS-induced ulcers penetrate deeper while EVL-induced ulcers cover more surface area. Proton pump inhibitors may be effective in healing these ulcers. Dysphagia from irritation of the esophagus after sclerotherapy can be alleviated with the use of a soft diet after treatment until symptoms subside. Up to 24% of patients develop recurrent bleeding [1]. This can be from treatment-induced ulcers eroding persistently patent varices after an unsuccessful sclerotherapy attempt. Patients treated with EVS can also develop portal hypertensive gastropathy, which can take months to recover. EVS is associated with a high rate of stricture formation (20%) [17]. Mechanisms include tissue reaction to sclerosant, acid reflux and EVS-induced changes in motility [3]. The rate of stricture formation may also correlate with the number of EVS sessions, the volume of sclerosant used and the amount of excessive or inadvertent paravariceal injections. Fewer complications, including strictures, may occur with the use of ethanolamine and polidocanol instead of tetradecyl sulfate as the sclerosing agent of choice [10]. Treatment-induced strictures can be successfully dilated with a TTS balloon or Savory dilators [3].

Perforations have also been reported in up to 2.2% of patients undergoing EVS [3,10]. EVS-induced ulcers are deeper than those seen after EVL, which may account for the higher risk of perforation associated with EVS. Respiratory or renal failure can result from intravariceal injection of sclerosants, such as sodium morrhuate or ethanolamine oleate. Injections should be submucosal and either paravariceal or perivariceal. Transmural injection can cause mediastinitis, suggested by persistent fever and chest pain, which should resolve on its own. Pleural and mediastinal changes following sclerotherapy in the form of minor pleural effusion and atelectasis are frequently seen radiologically. If fever does not subside within 2–3 days and massive pleural effusion occurs, a perforation should be considered. Prophylactic antibiotics are also recommended for actively bleeding cirrhotic patients [18].

Esophageal rupture following treatment with the Sengstaken–Blakemore tube is a known and dreadful complication. This complication is mainly caused by the overinflation and prolonged use of the esophageal balloon. Inflation of the esophageal balloon with 80 mL air or water exerts a pressure of around 40 mmHg, which is sufficient to control the bleeding. The use of balloon tamponade should not exceed 24 hours, in order to prevent pressure necrosis of the esophageal wall. Within this time span, endoscopy should be performed to achieve definitive haemostasis.

Rupture is often a result of iatrogenic misplacement of the tube and inflation of the gastric balloon in the esophagus. Relying solely on auscultation to confirm balloon placement is insufficient, and chest radiographs should be performed both before and after balloon inflation.

Esophageal perforation can also be a result of technical difficulty in tube placement, removal of the tube prior to complete balloon deflation, vomiting or recent sclerotherapy, which can weaken the esophageal wall [19–21]. Other major complications include: aspiration pneumonia, pressure necrosis of the mucosa, airway obstruction, and cardiac inflow obstruction. Minor complications include: mucosal tears, chest pain, agitation, gastric erosion, and nasal mucosa or cartilage injury [22–26]. Treatment of this severe complication is usually conservative, since patients are usually unfit for surgery. Apart from parenteral nutrition and administration of broad-spectrum antibiotics, thoracic drainage is the mainstay of therapy.

Chylothorax due to perforation of the thoracic duct and bronchoesophageal fistula are very rare complications of sclerotherapy that may be related to the use of excess amounts of sclerosant and a long injection needle.

Aspiration is the most frequent complication once the balloon is in place and has been reported in 10–20% of cases. Oral and nasogastric suction should be performed prior to insertion of the tube. Aspiration risk is reduced with the four-lumen tube, which, in addition to the gastric and esophageal balloon lumens, includes a lumen in the stomach and above the esophageal balloon for decompression and excess secretion management [26]. Intubation decreases the aspiration risk but is not always necessary prior to tube insertion as long as the patient will be under close surveillance in an intensive care setting. To prevent pressure necrosis of the nares from the tube, a Preston helmet is sometimes placed on the patient to keep tension on the tube [24].

Airway obstruction may result from proximal migration of the balloon. In this situation, the tube should be cut to enable balloon deflation and subsequent immediate removal. The Sengstaken–Blakemore tube is rarely used because of its known high complication rate. Rebleeding is common, likely since balloon tamponade is used in cases initially unmanageable by endoscopy. If placement is necessary as a temporizing measure before definitive endoscopic management, it should be done in the intensive care setting. Minimizing the amount of time that the tube is left in also reduces the risk of complications. Typically the Sengstaken–Blakemore tube is in place from 24 to 48 hours, after which point the balloon is deflated and cessation of bleeding is confirmed prior to its removal.

Acknowledgements

We would like to acknowledge the contribution of the authors of this chapter in the second edition of this book; Drs Yan Zhong, Stefan Seewald and Nib Soehendra. We have utilized some of their previous sections for this chapter.

References

1. Villanueva C, Piqueras M, Aracil C, et al. A randomized controlled trial comparing ligation and sclerotherapy as emergency endoscopic treatment added to somatostatin in acute variceal bleeding. *J. Hepatol.* 2006;**45**:560–7.
2. Sarin SK, Govil A, Jain AK, et al. Prospective randomized trial of endoscopic sclerotherapy versus variceal band ligation for esophageal varices: influence on gastropathy, gastric varices and variceal recurrence. *J. Hepatol.* 1997;**26**:826–32.
3. Schmitz RJ, Sharma P, Badr AS, Qamar MT, Weston AP. Incidence and management of esophageal stricture formation, ulcer bleeding, perforation, and massive hematoma formation from sclerotherapy versus band ligation. *Am. J. Gastroenterol.* 2001;**96**:437–41.
4. Saeed ZA, Stiegmann GV, Ramirez FC, et al. Endoscopic variceal ligation is superior to combined ligation and sclerotherapy for esophageal varices: a multicenter prospective randomized trial. *Hepatology* 1997;**25**:71–4.
5. Laine L, Cook D. Endoscopic ligation compared with sclerotherapy for treatment of esophageal variceal bleeding: a meta-analysis. *Ann. Intern. Med.* 1995;**123**:280–7.
6. Hou MC, Lin HC, Kuo BIT, Chen CH, Lee FY, Lee SD. Comparison of endoscopic variceal injection sclerotherapy and ligation for the treatment of esophageal variceal hemorrhage: a prospective randomized trial. *Hepatology* 1995;**21**:1517–22.
7. Stiegmann GV, Goff JS, Michaletz-Onody PA, et al. Endoscopic sclerotherapy as compared with endoscopic ligation for bleeding esophageal varices. *N. Engl. J. Med.* 1992;**326**:1527–32.
8. Young MF, Sanowski RA, Rasche R. Comparison and characterization of ulcerations induced by endoscopic ligation of esophageal varices versus endoscopic sclerotherapy. *Gastrointest. Endosc.* 1993;**39**:119–22.
9. Lo G, Lai K, Cheng J, et al. Emergency banding ligation versus sclerotherapy for the control of active bleeding from esophageal varices. *Hepatology* 1997;**25**:1101–4.
10. de la Peña J, Rivero M, Sanchez E, Fábrega E, Crespo J, Pons-Romero F. Variceal ligation compared with endoscopic sclerotherapy for variceal hemorrhage: prospective randomized trial. *Gastrointest. Endosc.* 1999;**49**:417–23.
11. Garcia-Tsao G, Sanyal AJ, Grace ND, Carey W. Prevention and management of gastroesophageal varices and variceal hemorrhage in cirrhosis. *Hepatology* 2007;**46**:922–38.
12. Shaheen NJ, Stuart E, Schmitz SM, et al. Pantoprazole reduces the size of postbanding ulcers after variceal band ligation: a randomized, controlled trial. *Hepatology* 2005;**41**:588–94.
13. Holderman WH, Ftzkorn KP, Patel SA, Harig JM, Watkins JL. Endoscopic findings and overtube-related complications associated with esophageal variceal ligation. *J. Clin. Gastroenterol.* 1995;**21**:91–4.
14. Dinning JP, Jaffe PE. Delayed presentation of esophageal perforation as a result of overtube placement. *J. Clin. Gastroenterol.* 1997;**24**:250–2.
15. Lo GII, Lai KH, Cheng JS, et al. Endoscopic variceal ligation plus nadolol and sucralfate compared with ligation alone for the prevention of variceal rebleeding: a prospective, randomized trial. *Hepatology* 2000;**32**:461–5.
16. Runyon BA. Management of adult patients with ascites due to cirrhosis: an update. *Hepatology* 2009;**49**:2087–107.
17. Sarles Jr HE, Sanowski RA, Talbert G. Course and complications of endoscopic variceal sclerotherapy: a prospective study of 50 patients. *Am. J. Gastroenterol.* 1985;**80**:595–9.

18. Lee YY, Tee H-P, Mahadeva S. Role of prophylactic antibiotics in cirrhotic patients with variceal bleeding. *World J. Gastroenterol.* 2014;**20**:1790.

19. Chong C-F. Esophageal rupture due to Sengstaken–Blakemore tube misplacement. *World J. Gastroenterol.* 2005;**11**:6563.

20. Nielsen TS, Charles AV. Lethal esophageal rupture following treatment with Sengstaken–Blakemore Tube in management of variceal bleeding: A 10-year autopsy study. *Forens. Sci. Int.* 2012;**222**:e19–e22.

21. Crerar-Gilbert A. Oesophageal rupture in the course of conservative treatment of bleeding oesophageal varices. *J. Accident Emerg. Med.* 1996;**13**:225–7.

22. Collyer TC, Dawson SET, Earl D. Acute upper airway obstruction due to displacement of a Sengstaken–Blakemore tube. *Eur. J. Anaesthesiol.* 2008;**25**:341–2.

23. Panes J, Teres J, Bosch J, Rodes J. Efficacy of balloon tamponade in treatment of bleeding gastric and esophageal varices. *Dig. Dis. Sci.* 1988;**33**:454–9.

24. Cook D, Laine L. Indications, technique, and complications of balloon tamponade for variceal gastrointestinal bleeding. *J. Intens. Care Med.* 1992;**7**:212–8.

25. De Cock D, Monballyu P, Voigt J-U, Wauters J. Extra-cardiac compression and left ventricular inflow obstruction as a complication of a Sengstaken–Blakemore tube. *Eur. Heart J.-Cardiovasc. Imag.* 2011:jer170.

26. Avgerinos A, Armonis A. Balloon tamponade technique and efficacy in variceal haemorrhage. *Scand. J. Gastroenterol.* 1994;**29**:11–6.

CHAPTER 11

ERCP complications

Constantinos P. Anastassiades[1,2] and Richard C. K. Wong[2,3]

[1] Khoo Teck Puat Hospital, Singapore
[2] Case Western Reserve University School of Medicine, Cleveland, OH, USA
[3] University Hospitals Case Medical Cente, Cleveland, OH, USA

Introduction

Endoscopic retrograde cholangiopancreatography (ERCP) was first introduced 45 years ago. It has since evolved to become a common and minimally invasive therapeutic tool for the management of pancreatobiliary disorders [1]. The recent, parallel evolution of less invasive imaging modalities that allow dedicated and detailed imaging of the pancreatobiliary tree (e.g. endoscopic ultrasound (EUS) and magnetic resonance cholangiopancreatography (MRCP)), have limited the diagnostic applications of ERCP. ERCP has, therefore, become primarily therapeutic. ERCP is generally considered safe and effective in trained hands but, as any therapeutic procedure, it is associated with an inherent risk of complications. The mechanism of some complications (such as cholangitis, post-sphincterotomy bleeding, post-ERCP pancreatitis) is specific to ERCP, whereas other complications are applicable to any endoscopic procedure: for example, cardiopulmonary complications, aspiration, risk of sedation, or anesthesia.

The ways to minimize, avoid and manage these complications are discussed.

Post-ERCP pancreatitis

Pancreatitis is the most common serious complication related to ERCP [2]. Asymptomatic elevation in the serum pancreatic enzymes is prevalent and of no clinical significance. Routinely checking enzyme values post-ERCP in patients who need to have blood drawn for other reasons (e.g., hospitalized patients) should, therefore, not be ordered unless there is clinical concern for pancreatitis. Debate as to what truly constitutes post-ERCP pancreatitis (PEP) as well as over-diagnosis of PEP has led to a consensus definition, which requires three criteria to be satisfied: new or worsening abdominal pain; serum amylase elevation to three times or more the upper limit of normal when measured at least 24 hours post-procedure; and new or prolonged hospitalization for at least 2 days [3]. The incidence of clinically significant post-ERCP pancreatitis ranges between 2% and 16% [4,5].

Risk factors for PEP have been widely studied and several risk factors have been identified. In multivariate analysis, risk factors for PEP include: female gender; young age; absence of chronic pancreatitis; suspected sphincter of Oddi dysfynction; previous history of PEP; pancreatic duct injection; pancreatic sphincterotomy; and balloon dilation of the biliary sphincter [6,7]. Precut (needle knife) sphincterotomy has also been shown to be a risk factor but this is considered by some to be controversial [2].

Awareness of these risk factors can help guide careful patient selection and permit close attention to endoscopic technique in order to minimize the risk of PEP. For instance, imaging modalities may need to be considered in patients at high-risk for PEP and in whom a therapeutic intervention is unlikely. Similarly, wire-guided cannulation is increasingly being used in preference to contrast-guided cannulation, as this has been shown in meta-analyses to lower the risk of PEP [8,9].

Gastrointestinal Emergencies, Third Edition. Edited by Tony C. K. Tham, John S. A. Collins, and Roy Soetikno.
© 2016 John Wiley & Sons, Ltd. Published 2016 by John Wiley & Sons, Ltd.

Methods to reduce PEP risk have attracted significant attention and are likely to continue to do so in view of the magnitude of the problem. Prophylaxis is mainly divided into pharmacologic and mechanical means. Placement of a temporary pancreatic duct stent has been shown in meta-analyses and several prospective studies to be effective [10–12]. It has gained acceptance as an established intervention to prevent PEP and is now commonly utilized for patient populations who are considered to be at high-risk for PEP (Fig. 11.1). Potential issues with pancreatic duct stent placement relate to the comfort level and expertise of gastroenterologists to endoscopically manipulate and perform interventions in the pancreatic duct. For this reason, it is generally recommended for such procedures to be performed at centers where expertise and training in ERCP is available. Another issue is the need to ensure that the pancreatic duct stent is either removed by repeat endoscopy, or that it has spontaneously passed as shown by X-ray imaging, to avoid the potential risk of complications such as stent occlusion and stent-induced injury to the pancreatic duct. Despite these issues, pancreatic duct stent placement has been shown to be cost-effective in a relevant analysis [13]. The electrocautery settings used for biliary sphincterotomy do not appear to have an impact on the risk of PEP; a meta-analysis showed no statistically significant difference when four studies were pooled, which compared blended

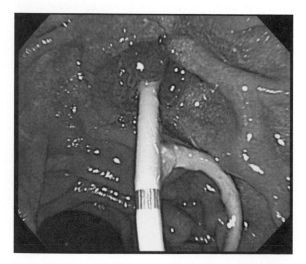

Fig. 11.1 Temporary pancreatic duct stent with single external pigtail, inserted for post-ERCP pancreatitis prophylaxis in a high-risk patient. (*see insert for color representation of the figure.*)

current to pure-cut current [14]. As previously mentioned, wire-guided cannulation is now preferred as this can lower the risk of PEP.

Based on pathways thought to mediate the process of pancreatic inflammation, many pharmacologic agents have been studied over many decades. Such pharmacologic agents have included octreotide, ulinastatin, corticosteroids, nitroglycerin, and allopurinol [15]. Until recently, these studies have yielded negative and/or inconclusive results. Following an initial meta-analysis showing a statistically significant benefit with rectal indomethacin [16], new high-quality data from a recently published, multicenter, prospective randomized controlled study have demonstrated significant benefit in the reduction of PEP with administration of rectal indomethacin at a dose of 100 mg [17]. Many patients in this study additionally underwent pancreatic duct stent placement, the benefit of which was not directly studied. Furthermore, many patients in this prospective randomized study had sphincter of Oddi dysfunction. Despite these potential limitations, the ease, cost, and benefit of this intervention have already led to popular use and it is likely that new studies will shed more light on issues such as the benefit of administration of rectal indomethacin, with or without pancreatic duct stent placement, a direct comparison between rectal indomethacin alone versus pancreatic duct stent placement alone, universal versus selective use, etc. A subsequent meta-analysis published in 2013 concluded that rectal indomethacin administered around the time of ERCP significantly reduced the risk of PEP in both low-risk and high-risk populations. The meta-analysis advocated routine administration for all patients undergoing ERCP [18], which is the protocol we now follow at our institution.

The management of pancreatitis is discussed in Chapter 23, Acute Pancreatitis.

Post-sphincterotomy bleeding (PSB)

Bleeding as a result of ERCP almost always occurs as a result of sphincterotomy (Fig 11.2). The incidence of PSB is approximately 2% [19,20]. Most bleeding is mild and occurs immediately or soon after sphincterotomy. However, delayed (within 2 weeks) bleeding can also occur [21]. Severe bleeding is observed in 0.1% or less of sphincterotomy cases, characterized by the requirement for transfusion of multiple (5 or more) units of blood and/or need for angiography and/or surgery [19,20].

Immediate bleeding can occur at the time of sphincterotomy in 10 to 30% of patients, but most cases are minor and not clinically significant [22], and can be controlled at the time of initial ERCP. Delayed post-sphincterotomy bleeding can occur up to 2 weeks in about half the cases. The risk of clinically significant, severe hemorrhage requiring blood transfusions and/or angiographic or surgical intervention is uncommon at 0.1 to 0.5% [23].

Other than sphincterotomy itself, risk factors that have been shown in multivariate analysis to be associated with PSB include coagulopathy and the use of anticoagulants within 72 hours of the procedure, concomitant ampullary stenosis or cholangitis, use of access (precut) sphincterotomy, and low endoscopic volume by the endoscopist (defined as 1 sphincterotomy per week or less) [19,20,24]. Factors previously suspected but shown not to be associated with bleeding include incision length and the use of aspirin and other non-steroidal anti-inflammatory drugs (NSAIDs) [19]. Immediate bleeding may be a factor associated with delayed bleeding [19]. The choice of

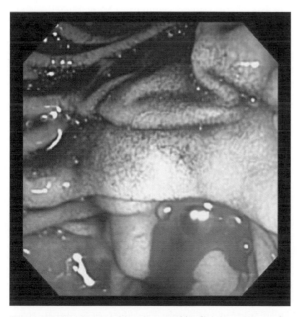

Fig. 11.2 Delayed post-sphincterotomy bleeding in a patient who had to start full anticoagulation therapy soon after ERCP with sphincterotomy. (*see insert for color representation of the figure.*)

electrosurgical current for biliary sphincterotomy is controversial as it relates to PSB [25]. It is not known if the participation of a trainee in the performance of a biliary sphincterotomy, particularly when this involves pre-cut techniques, is associated with an increased risk of PSB, but in view of the data on low-volume endoscopists, this may be a subject of study and point of interest in the ERCP training curriculum issued by professional societies [26].

In the performance of a biliary sphincterotomy, the 11 to 1 o'clock position is preferred, as this is believed to be the axis of the least concentration of arterial supply; incision along this axis is thought to minimize the risk of bleeding [27]. In the endoscopic management of PSB, the apex of the previously performed sphincterotomy is often the preferred target of endoscopic therapy, particularly when an alternative bleeding site cannot be identified. Extension of a biliary sphincterotomy is also sometimes performed to address possible partial severing of blood vessels in order to completely sever the artery and cause vasospasm, thereby limiting further PSB.

PSB can sometimes be prevented with careful preprocedural preparation and assessment of the patient and their comorbidities, their medication list and laboratory studies. The endoscopist should seek the results of a complete blood count, platelet count and basic coagulation studies (prothrombin time, International Normalized Ratio, and partial thromboplastin time) prior to a planned sphincterotomy, and any abnormalities should be corrected whenever possible. For anticoagulant medications, these should be adjusted accordingly based on the patient's risks of thromboembolism weighed against the risks of post-sphincterotomy bleeding [28]. It is also important that the endoscopist carefully review, on a case-by-case basis, the indications for endoscopic sphincterotomy and whether it is essential. This is especially critical in high-risk patients. For example, in a critically ill patient with ascending cholangitis and coagulopathy from sepsis, decompression of an obstructed bile duct by placement of a temporary biliary stent is usually adequate. Delayed biliary sphincterotomy and stone extraction can then be performed after the patient's clinical status has improved and coagulopathy resolved.

Medical management of PSB is similar to that of upper gastrointestinal bleed with fluid resuscitation and hemodynamic support, blood transfusion, and correction of coagulopathy and thrombocytopenia. The use of proton pump inhibitor therapy has not been specifically studied in the context of PSB, but is often recommended and utilized. Endoscopic intervention is usually effective. Injection of dilute epinephrine at the apex of the sphincterotomy site, or directly at the bleeding site, is the most common effective method of hemostasis [14,29]. Endoscopic therapy can be delivered either through a sclerotherapy needle or a submucosal injection through a tapered-tip ERCP catheter. Other options include standard endoscopic thermal therapy and endoscopic clip placement [21,30], which are often employed when there is failure of hemostasis with initial epinephrine injection. Balloon tamponade is also sometimes used. Caution should be exercised with the application of endoscopic thermal therapy to avoid targeting the orifice of the pancreatic duct, which can lead to resultant pancreatitis and pancreatic injury. It should be noted that while endoscopic clip placement is possible, deployment of endoscopic clips using a duodenoscope can be technically challenging due to possible distortion of the clip delivery system by the elevator of the duodenoscope during passage.

The use of a fully covered self-expandable metal stent has been shown in some studies to be effective in refractory bleeding cases [31]. However, such stents are very expensive and this approach may not be cost effective. Rescue therapy for failed endoscopic hemostasis includes angiography with selective embolization and, more rarely, surgery [21].

Finally, endoscopists should be aware that PSB can occasionally lead to superimposed biliary obstruction and/or cholangitis due to the presence of blood clots obstructing the bile duct. In addition to endoscopic hemostasis, the occurrence of bile duct obstruction due to intraductal blood clots necessitates biliary cannulation, clearing of the bile duct and possible temporary biliary stent placement. When there is a high clinical suspicion for PSB, it is prudent for endoscopists with training in ERCP and familiarity with the use of a side-viewing duodenoscope, to be the ones performing the upper endoscopy rather than gastroenterologists without ERCP training.

Infectious complications

Cholangitis is one of the most serious ERCP complications. It occurs in up to 1% of cases, although transient bacteremia has been reported in up to 27% of therapeutic ERCP procedures [19,24,32]. While the incidence of infection is low (1%), a large retrospective study showed that the mortality rate from infection is relatively high (8%) [22]. Risk factors for cholangitis include combined percutaneous and endoscopic procedures (e.g. rendez-vous procedures), jaundice, low case volume for the endoscopist, stent placement in malignant strictures and failed or incomplete biliary drainage [19]. The immunocompromised patient population is at higher risk of an infectious complication following ERCP [33]. It should also be noted that pancreatitis, including PEP, also carries a risk of superimposed infection, which is usually delayed and can manifest as infected parenchymal necrosis of the pancreas or infected pancreatic pseudocysts [34].

Securing complete biliary drainage is of paramount importance in the prevention of cholangitis. Malignant hilar obstruction (i.e. cholangiocarcinoma) can be particularly challenging and the preferred drainage strategy remains controversial. However, data show that unilateral endoscopic bile duct stent placement can be equally effective for palliation of jaundice compared to bilateral stent placement and may carry less risk of cholangitis [35,36]. Pre-procedural guidance by MRCP is helpful in targeting the desired obstructed biliary segment [37]. Limiting the amount of injected contrast can help reduce the risk of undrained segments of the biliary system [36]. Air cholangiography has been shown to be associated with a lower risk of post-ERCP cholangitis compared to traditional contrast injection before placement of a stent in patients with unresectable malignant hilar obstruction [38].

Routine use of prophylactic antibiotics in all ERCP cases has not been shown to be beneficial [39,40]. Current guidelines by the American Society for Gastrointestinal Endoscopy (ASGE) recommend the use of antibiotic prophylaxis for ERCP in patients with known or suspected mechanical biliary obstruction that may not be completely alleviated at ERCP (e.g. incomplete or failed biliary decompression, in patients with primary sclerosing cholangitis [PSC] or a hilar obstruction) [41]. Antibiotic prophylaxis is also recommended when performing ERCP with a pre-existing sterile pancreatic fluid collection (e.g. a pseudocyst in communication with the pancreatic duct) and for endoscopic transpapillary or transmural drainage procedures of sterile pancreatic fluid collections [41]. If biliary drainage is thought to be complete at the end of ERCP, post-procedure antibiotics is not necessary except in patients with PSC and those with post-liver transplantation biliary strictures, for whom oral antibiotics are administered 3–5 days post-procedure [2]. As previously mentioned, antibiotics should also be continued in patient in whom biliary drainage is thought to be incomplete; such patients should be promptly evaluated on a case-by-case basis for an early repeat attempt at ERCP drainage versus expedited biliary drainage by alternative means such as a percutaneous transhepatic approach by interventional radiology versus antegrade EUS-guided access to the obstructed bile duct by an endoscopist experienced in this technique. These considerations would be dependent on local institutional expertise and may require prompt referral to a tertiary care medical center with a high-volume ERCP practice. In terms of antimicrobial coverage, medications should cover biliary flora including enteric Gram-negative organisms and enterococci. Ciprofloxacin and other fluoroquinolones are generally effective against the most common organisms [42,43].

Cholecystitis can also be seen as a complication in up to 0.5% cases of ERCP [19,24]. It is associated with cholelithiasis and possibly with filling of the gallbladder with contrast during the ERCP procedure [19]. The risk of cholecystitis is thought to be increased by the placement of a fully covered self-expandable metal stent that may obstruct the cystic duct [44,45].

It should be noted that in terms of antibiotic administration for prophylaxis against infective endocarditis, new guidelines include significant deviations from previously issued recommendations. A landmark change is that the use of prophylactic antibiotics solely to prevent infective endocarditis is not recommended for patients who undergo endoscopy, even in subjects with high-risk cardiac conditions such as prosthetic valves. It is recommended that patients with high-risk cardiac conditions and *concomitant* gastrointestinal tract infection, such as cholangitis, who undergo ERCP be administered periprocedural antibiotics that cover enterocci [41]. However, such a recommendation is arguably redundant, as such antibiotics should routinely be administered for patients with known or suspected cholangitis undergoing ERCP, irrespective of their cardiac condition.

For patients who experience cholangitis as a complication of ERCP, the management principles for cholangitis are the same. If sepsis is present, broad-spectrum intravenous antibiotics should be administered and appropriate management should be instituted with fluid resuscitation and close hemodynamic monitoring and support. The latter may require admission of the patient to an intensive care unit (ICU). Biliary drainage should also be quickly established (Fig. 11.3). This can include repeat ERCP with clearing of the bile duct and placement of a large-caliber (e.g. 10-French) temporary bile duct stent to ensure adequate biliary drainage. If bile duct obstruction is present (e.g. presence of a stricture, stone, mass, etc.), the bile duct stent has to be of sufficient length to bridge the obstructed area and allow complete decompression and drainage of the biliary system. If repeat ERCP with stent placement is thought to be unlikely to achieve drainage, or if such a procedure fails or drainage is thought to be incomplete in a patient with ongoing sepsis, urgent rescue therapy through a percutaneous transhepatic approach by interventional radiology is recommended.

Perforation

Perforation is rare and occurs in 1% or less of ERCP cases [46–48]. It can transmurally involve the bowel lumen (i.e. duodenum), as is the risk with all upper endoscopy. It can also affect the bile duct and the pancreatic duct [49]. It is important to appreciate that small amounts of incidental free air on abdominal

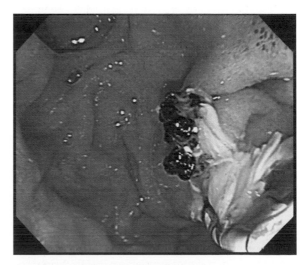

Fig. 11.3 Cholangitis with immediate release of intraductal stones and pus from the bile duct after biliary sphincterotomy. (*see insert for color representation of the figure.*)

imaging may be observed in up to 30% of asymptomatic patients after ERCP and this alone is not a reason for additional medical, endoscopic or surgical management [50,51]. Careful correlation of imaging findings with the clinical picture is therefore always required.

Perforation of the ducts can be caused by guide wire manipulation, sphincterotome manipulation, or from dilation. Perforation of the bile duct can result in a bile leak and the intra-abdominal collection of bile, which is referred to as a biloma. Similarly, perforation of the pancreatic duct can lead to a pancreatic duct leak and the formation of peri-pancreatic fluid collections. Perforation of the duodenum during ERCP can be intraperitoneal or retroperitoneal. The former (intra-peritoneal) is usually related to endoscopic trauma and the latter (retroperitoneal) is usually related to sphinc-terotomy or guide wire manipulation. Sometimes, the exact cause is unknown [48].

Factors associated with an increased risk of perforation may include suspected sphincter of Oddi dysfunction, the presence of dilated bile ducts and biliary strictures, and the performance of a biliary sphincterotomy [46]. Post-Billroth II partial gastrectomy is notoriously associ-ated with an increased risk of complications, including jejunal loop perforation when using a side-viewing endoscope compared with a forward-viewing endoscope [52,53] (Fig. 11.4).

If the patient's clinical and hemodynamic status allows, and advanced endoscopic expertise is available, luminal perforations nowadays can often be closed immediately and effectively with endoscopic clips or larger over-the-scope closure devices, followed by imaging studies with oral contrast to look for extravasa-tion. Bile and pancreatic duct perforations and leaks are usually managed by stent placement with the stent ideally bridging the disrupted duct. The development of a biloma often requires percutaneous drainage by inter-ventional radiology and the administration of broad-spectrum intravenous antibiotics in addition to endoscopic bile duct stent placement. In general, retro-peritoneal perforations with little or no evidence of contrast extravasation, can be managed conservatively without need for surgery (Fig. 11.5). Intraperitoneal perforation with significant extravasation of free air usually requires prompt surgical intervention [46]. Rapid clinical assessment, computerized tomography (CT) imaging, emergent surgical consultation, and close clinical monitoring in an ICU are crucial in the effective

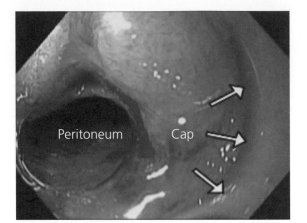

Fig. 11.4 Perforation of the afferent enteral limb with a duodenoscope in a patient with Billroth II anatomy. After obtaining an emergent surgical consultation in the endoscopy unit, the defect was immediately managed endoscopically with a cap-fitted, forward-viewing gastroscope with complete clip-closure of the perforation. The ERCP was then able to be completed in the same session with the cap-fitted, forward-viewing instrument [53]. (*see insert for color representation of the figure.*)

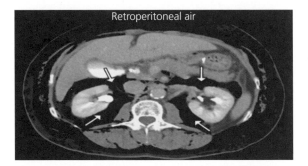

Fig. 11.5 Retroperitoneal air (white arrows) on computerized tomography (CT) of the abdomen and pelvis in a patient with retroperitoneal perforation during ERCP. Despite the CT findings and subcutaneous air leading to clinical crepitus and periorbital edema, the patient was successfully managed conservatively after obtaining an emergent surgical consultation in the endoscopy unit.

management of ERCP-associated perforations. It is essential that the endoscopist work very closely with a surgeon to jointly manage these types of complications.

Cardiopulmonary complications

Cardiopulmonary complications can occur during any endoscopic procedure and are not specific to ERCP. In general, however, ERCP requires higher doses of sedatives than colonoscopy or upper endoscopy. Cardiopulmonary complications are rarely encountered and may occur in 1% of ERCP cases [22]. Cardiac arrhythmias, hypoventilation, or aspiration can occur. Most cardiopulmonary injury has been shown to be associated with prolonged (longer than 30 minutes) procedures [54]. Patients with severe cholangitis may be very ill, with hemodynamic changes and altered mental status. In such patients, it is important to have an anesthesiologist assess the patient and to provide monitored anesthesia care or more commonly general anesthesia, as appropriate, during ERCP [55]. Furthermore, patients who undergo ERCP for suspected pancreatic malignancy tend to be older and have more co-morbidities. "Over-sedation" in the setting of acute illness and pre-existing co-morbidities contribute to most cardiopulmonary complications from ERCP, many of which respond rapidly to intravenous reversal agents (flumazenil and/or naloxone), close monitoring, and supportive care. Some endoscopists advocate the routine use of deep sedation with propofol for ERCP, due to similar efficacy and safety as conventional moderate sedation, but with fewer associated hypoxemic events [56–59]. Capnography monitoring in one study was shown to be associated with fewer episodes of hypoxemia and apnea in ERCP compared with conventional monitoring [60]. Capnography is used routinely for ERCP at our institution.

Contrast media-related reactions

As part of the pre-procedural assessment for ERCP, any allergy history to intravenous contrast media used in CT studies or an allergy to shellfish should be established. Such patients are at increased risk for adverse reactions from the contrast used in ERCP and should receive appropriate allergy prophylaxis.

Water-soluble, iodine-based contrast media are used to opacify the biliary and/or pancreatic ducts during ERCP [61]. Practice standards are based primarily on radiological recommendations for intravenous contrast. The actual risk of systemic, contrast-related reactions from ERCP is much less than with intravenous contrast administration because of limited systemic absorption. Nonetheless, idiosyncratic non-IgE-mediated anaphylactic reactions can occur immediately and non-idiosyncratic reactions can occur from 1 hour

to 7 days after contrast injection, but these reactions are usually mild and self-limited.

Patients at increased risk for adverse reactions, such as those with prior history of allergy to CT contrast media or shellfish, should receive *non-ionic* contrast agents. For high-risk patients, appropriate allergy prophylaxis should be administered at several scheduled time points before the ERCP, as a single dose of corticosteroid given before the procedure is inadequate. This often involves the use of corticosteroid and antihistamine-type medications given at scheduled timed intervals before the ERCP. Recommendations from the American College of Radiology for intravenous contrast-related reactions are often extrapolated for use in ERCP [61].

Conclusions

ERCP is expected to continue to play an important therapeutic role in the management of patients with pancreatic and biliary diseases. Adverse events are inherent to ERCP practice. The risk of complications, their avoidance and their successful management once they happen can be addressed by adequate and formal ERCP training on the endoscopist's part; a thorough knowledge of the indications and alternatives of the procedure, as well as the management principles of any complications that may arise from it; ongoing close collaboration with and the availability of resources such as interventional radiology and surgical services; tertiary care referral institutions in close proximity, and the endoscopist's commitment to be up-to-date with his or her ongoing experience, education and ERCP volume.

References

1. McCune WS, Shorb PE, Moscovitz H. Endoscopic cannulation of the ampulla of vater: a preliminary report. *Ann. Surg.* 1968;**167**:752–6.
2. Anderson MA, Fisher L, Jain R, et al. Complications of ERCP. *Gastrointest. Endosc.* 2012;**75**:467–73.
3. Cotton PB, Lehman G, Vennes J, et al. Endoscopic sphincterotomy complications and their management: an attempt at consensus. *Gastrointest. Endosc.* 1991;**37**:383–93.
4. Cotton PB, Garrow DA, Gallagher J, Romagnuolo J. Risk factors for complications after ERCP: a multivariate analysis of 11 497 procedures over 12 years. *Gastrointest. Endosc.* 2009;**70**:80–8.

5. Barthet M, Lesavre N, Desjeux A, et al. Complications of endoscopic sphincterotomy: results from a single tertiary referral center. *Endoscopy* 2002;**34**:991–7.

6. Freeman ML. Adverse outcomes of ERCP. *Gastrointest. Endosc.* 2002;**56**:S273–82.

7. Cheon YK, Cho KB, Watkins JL, et al. Frequency and severity of post-ERCP pancreatitis correlated with extent of pancreatic ductal opacification. *Gastrointest. Endosc.* 2007;**65**: 385–93.

8. Cennamo V, Fuccio L, Zagari RM, et al. Can a wire-guided cannulation technique increase bile duct cannulation rate and prevent post-ERCP pancreatitis?: A meta-analysis of randomized controlled trials. *Am. J. Gastroenterol.* 2009;**104**:2343–50.

9. Shao LM, Chen QY, Chen MY, Cai JT. Can wire-guided cannulation reduce the risk of post-endoscopic retrograde cholangiopancreatography pancreatitis? A meta-analysis of randomized controlled trials. *J. Gastroenterol. Hepatol.* 2009;**24**:1710–5.

10. Freeman ML. Pancreatic stents for prevention of post-endoscopic retrograde cholangiopancreatography pancreatitis. *Clin. Gastroenterol. Hepatol.* 2007;**5**:1354–65.

11. Ito K, Fujita N, Noda Y, et al. Can pancreatic duct stenting prevent post-ERCP pancreatitis in patients who undergo pancreatic duct guidewire placement for achieving selective biliary cannulation? A prospective randomized controlled trial. *J. Gastroenterol.* 2010;**45**:1183–91.

12. Mazaki T, Masuda H, Takayama T. Prophylactic pancreatic stent placement and post-ERCP pancreatitis: a systematic review and meta-analysis. *Endoscopy* 2010;**42**:842–53.

13. Das A, Singh P, Sivak MV, Jr., Chak A. Pancreatic-stent placement for prevention of post-ERCP pancreatitis: a cost-effectiveness analysis. *Gastrointest. Endosc.* 2007;**65**:960–8.

14. Verma D, Kapadia A, Adler DG. Pure versus mixed electro-surgical current for endoscopic biliary sphincterotomy: a meta-analysis of adverse outcomes. *Gastrointest. Endosc.* 2007;**66**:283–90.

15. Woods KE, Willingham FF. Endoscopic retrograde cholangiopancreatography associated pancreatitis: A 15-year review. *World J. Gastrointest. Endosc.* 2010;**2**:165–78.

16. Elmunzer BJ, Waljee AK, Elta GH, Taylor JR, Fehmi SM, Higgins PD. A meta-analysis of rectal NSAIDs in the prevention of post-ERCP pancreatitis. *Gut* 2008;**57**:1262–7.

17. Elmunzer BJ, Scheiman JM, Lehman GA, et al. A randomized trial of rectal indomethacin to prevent post-ERCP pancreatitis. *N. Engl. J. Med.* 2012;**366**:1414–22.

18. Yaghoobi M, Rolland S, Waschke KA, et al. Meta-analysis: rectal indomethacin for the prevention of post-ERCP pancreatitis. *Aliment. Pharmacol. Ther.* 2013;**38**:995–1001.

19. Freeman ML, Nelson DB, Sherman S, et al. Complications of endoscopic biliary sphincterotomy. *N. Engl. J. Med.* 1996;**335**:909–18.

20. Loperfido S, Angelini G, Benedetti G, et al. Major early complications from diagnostic and therapeutic ERCP: a prospective multicenter study. *Gastrointest. Endosc.* 1998;**48**:1–10.

21. Ferreira LE, Baron TH. Post-sphincterotomy bleeding: who, what, when, and how. *Am. J. Gastroenterol.* 2007;**102**: 2850–8.

22. Andriulli A, Loperfido S, Napolitano G, et al. Incidence rates of post-ERCP complications: a systematic survey of prospective studies. *Am. J. Gastroenterol.* 2007;**102**: 1781–8.

23. Freeman ML. Adverse outcomes of endoscopic retrograde cholangiopancreatography: avoidance and management. *Gastrointest. Endosc. Clin. N. Am.* 2003;**13**:775–98, xi.

24. Masci E, Toti G, Mariani A, et al. Complications of diagnostic and therapeutic ERCP: a prospective multicenter study. *Am. J. Gastroenterol.* 2001;**96**:417–23.

25. Perini RF, Sadurski R, Cotton PB, Patel RS, Hawes RH, Cunningham JT. Post-sphincterotomy bleeding after the introduction of microprocessor-controlled electrosurgery: does the new technology make the difference? *Gastrointest. Endosc.* 2005;**61**:53–7.

26. Anastassiades CP, Saxena A. Precut needle-knife sphincterotomy in advanced endoscopy fellowship. *Gastrointest. Endosc.* 2013;**77**:637–40.

27. Mirjalili SA, Stringer MD. The arterial supply of the major duodenal papilla and its relevance to endoscopic sphincterotomy. *Endoscopy* 2011;**43**:307–11.

28. Anderson MA, Ben-Menachem T, Gan SI, et al. Management of antithrombotic agents for endoscopic procedures. *Gastrointest. Endosc.* 2009;**70**:1060–70.

29. Leung JW, Chan FK, Sung JJ, Chung S. Endoscopic sphincterotomy-induced hemorrhage: a study of risk factors and the role of epinephrine injection. *Gastrointest. Endosc.* 1995;**42**:550–4.

30. Katsinelos P, Paroutoglou G, Kountouras J, et al. Partially covered vs uncovered sphincterotome and post-endoscopic sphincterotomy bleeding. *World J. Gastroenterol.* 2010;**16**: 5077–83.

31. Shah JN, Marson F, Binmoeller KF. Temporary self-expandable metal stent placement for treatment of post-sphincterotomy bleeding. *Gastrointest. Endosc.* 2010;**72**:1274–8.

32. Kullman E, Borch K, Lindstrom E, Ansehn S, Ihse I, Anderberg B. Bacteremia following diagnostic and therapeutic ERCP. *Gastrointest. Endosc.* 1992;**38**:444–9.

33. Subhani JM, Kibbler C, Dooley JS. Review article: antibiotic prophylaxis for endoscopic retrograde cholangiopancreatography (ERCP). *Aliment. Pharmacol. Ther.* 1999;**13**: 103–16.

34. Beger HG, Rau B, Mayer J, Pralle U. Natural course of acute pancreatitis. *World J. Surg.* 1997;**21**:130–5.

35. De Palma GD, Galloro G, Siciliano S, Iovino P, Catanzano C. Unilateral versus bilateral endoscopic hepatic duct drainage in patients with malignant hilar biliary obstruction: results of a prospective, randomized, and controlled study. *Gastrointest. Endosc.* 2001;**53**:547–53.

36. Sherman S. Endoscopic drainage of malignant hilar obstruction: is one biliary stent enough or should we work to place two? *Gastrointest. Endosc.* 2001;**53**:681–4.

37. Hintze RE, Abou-Rebyeh H, Adler A, Veltzke-Schlieker W, Felix R, Wiedenmann B. Magnetic resonance cholangiopancreatography-guided unilateral endoscopic stent placement for Klatskin tumors. *Gastrointest. Endosc.* 2001;**53**:40–6.

38. Pisello F, Geraci G, Modica G, Sciume C. Cholangitis prevention in endoscopic Klatskin tumor palliation: air cholangiography technique. *Langenbecks Arch. Surg.* 2009;**394**: 1109–14.

39. Harris A, Chan AC, Torres-Viera C, Hammett R, Carr-Locke D. Meta-analysis of antibiotic prophylaxis in endoscopic retrograde cholangiopancreatography (ERCP). *Endoscopy* 1999;**31**:718–24.

40. Bai Y, Gao F, Gao J, Zou DW, Li ZS. Prophylactic antibiotics cannot prevent endoscopic retrograde cholangiopancreatography-induced cholangitis: a meta-analysis. *Pancreas* 2009;**38**:126–30.

41. Banerjee S, Shen B, Baron TH, et al. Antibiotic prophylaxis for GI endoscopy. *Gastrointest. Endosc.* 2008;**67**:791–8.

42. Alveyn CG, Robertson DA, Wright R, Lowes JA, Tillotson G. Prevention of sepsis following endoscopic retrograde cholangiopancreatography. *J. Hosp. Infect.* 1991;**19** Suppl C:65–70.

43. Mehal WZ, Culshaw KD, Tillotson GS, Chapman RW. Antibiotic prophylaxis for ERCP: a randomized clinical trial comparing ciprofloxacin and cefuroxime in 200 patients at high risk of cholangitis. *Eur. J. Gastroenterol. Hepatol.* 1995;**7**:841–5.

44. Suk KT, Kim HS, Kim JW, et al. Risk factors for cholecystitis after metal stent placement in malignant biliary obstruction. *Gastrointest. Endosc.* 2006;**64**:522–9.

45. Fumex F, Coumaros D, Napoleon B, et al. Similar performance but higher cholecystitis rate with covered biliary stents: results from a prospective multicenter evaluation. *Endoscopy* 2006;**38**:787–92.

46. Enns R, Eloubeidi MA, Mergener K, et al. ERCP-related perforations: risk factors and management. *Endoscopy* 2002;**34**:293–8.

47. Vandervoort J, Soetikno RM, Tham TC, et al. Risk factors for complications after performance of ERCP. *Gastrointest. Endosc.* 2002;**56**:652–6.

48. Fatima J, Baron TH, Topazian MD, et al. Pancreaticobiliary and duodenal perforations after periampullary endoscopic procedures: diagnosis and management. *Arch. Surg.* 2007;**142**:448–54; discussion 54–5.

49. Howard TJ, Tan T, Lehman GA, et al. Classification and management of perforations complicating endoscopic sphincterotomy. *Surgery* 1999;**126**:658–63; discussion 64–5.

50. de Vries JH, Duijm LE, Dekker W, Guit GL, Ferwerda J, Scholten ET. CT before and after ERCP: detection of pancreatic pseudotumor, asymptomatic retroperitoneal perforation, and duodenal diverticulum. *Gastrointest. Endosc.* 1997;**45**:231–5.

51. Wu HM, Dixon E, May GR, Sutherland FR. Management of perforation after endoscopic retrograde cholangiopancreatography (ERCP): a population-based review. *HPB (Oxford)* 2006;**8**:393–9.

52. Kim MH, Lee SK, Lee MH, et al. Endoscopic retrograde cholangiopancreatography and needle-knife sphincterotomy in patients with Billroth II gastrectomy: a comparative study of the forward-viewing endoscope and the side-viewing duodenoscope. *Endoscopy* 1997;**29**:82–5.

53. Anastassiades CP, Salah W, Pauli EM, Marks JM, Chak A. Cap-assisted ERCP with a forward-viewing gastroscope as a rescue endoscopic intervention in patients with Billroth II anatomy. *Surg. Endosc.* 2013;**27**:2237.

54. Fisher L, Fisher A, Thomson A. Cardiopulmonary complications of ERCP in older patients. *Gastrointest. Endosc.* 2006;**63**:948–55.

55. Lichtenstein DR, Jagannath S, Baron TH, et al. Sedation and anesthesia in GI endoscopy. *Gastrointest. Endosc.* 2008;**68**:815–26.

56. Wehrmann T, Kokabpick S, Lembcke B, Caspary WF, Seifert H. Efficacy and safety of intravenous propofol sedation during routine ERCP: a prospective, controlled study. *Gastrointest. Endosc.* 1999;**49**:677–83.

57. Vargo JJ, Zuccaro G, Jr., Dumot JA, et al. Gastroenterologist-administered propofol versus meperidine and midazolam for advanced upper endoscopy: a prospective, randomized trial. *Gastroenterology* 2002;**123**:8–16.

58. Riphaus A, Stergiou N, Wehrmann T. Sedation with propofol for routine ERCP in high-risk octogenarians: a randomized, controlled study. *Am. J. Gastroenterol.* 2005;**100**:1957–63.

59. Kongkam P, Rerknimitr R, Punyathavorn S, et al. Propofol infusion versus intermittent meperidine and midazolam injection for conscious sedation in ERCP. *J. Gastrointest. Liver Dis.* 2008;**17**:291–7.

60. Qadeer MA, Vargo JJ, Dumot JA, et al. Capnographic monitoring of respiratory activity improves safety of sedation for endoscopic cholangiopancreatography and ultrasonography. *Gastroenterology* 2009;**136**:1568–76; quiz 819–20.

61. Mishkin D, Carpenter S, Croffie J, et al. ASGE Technology Status Evaluation Report: radiographic contrast media used in ERCP. *Gastrointest. Endosc.* 2005;**62**:480–4.

CHAPTER 12

Complications of laparoscopic surgery

Stephen Attwood[1] and Khalid Osman[2]

[1] *Durham University, Durham, UK*

[2] *North Tyneside General Hospital, Tyne & Wear, UK*

Introduction

The advantages of laparoscopy are numerous and it is important to emphasize at the beginning of this chapter on complications that the advantages of laparoscopy outweigh the disadvantages and potential complications.

In general, compared to the equivalent open surgical procedure, laparoscopic procedures result in reduced pain, earlier return to mobility, reduced incidence of chest infections, reduced Incidence of deep venous thrombosis and pulmonary embolus, earlier return to normal gut function (less ileus), reduced wound infections, earlier discharge from hospital, and earlier return to work and sporting activity. Long-term outcomes show that with laparoscopy there is a reduced rate of incisional hernia, reduced rate of peritoneal adhesions, and improved cosmetic appearance. Laparoscopy often allows for a more accurate diagnosis, especially in acute abdominal pain and malignancy. It also allows a useful alternative access, for example in recurrent inguinal hernia where the previous scar tissue from open surgery can be avoided, and it allows multiple operations through the same access – for example bilateral inguinal hernia.

While bleeding can be a difficult problem to control if it occurs during laparoscopy, in general there is reduced blood loss, less transfusion and less cost of blood replacement. Laparoscopy allows an improved opportunity for teaching, an operative field visible to all personnel and facilitates telemedicine or even telepresence operating.

The best way of avoiding complications is to know about them. This chapter will highlight as many of the known complications of laparoscopic surgery as possible.

Many will be the same as for the equivalent open operation. Some will be unique and some will be commoner because of the laparoscopic approach (see Table 12.1). An interesting feature of complications after laparoscopy is that the skin incisions may give little clue as to what has been done internally. From a periumbilical access point the laparoscopist may have been operating anywhere from the mid mediastinum down to the lowest part of the pelvis. Therefore accurate, contemporaneous notes are an essential part of laparoscopic practice and reading these is an essential part of assessing a patient with complications after laparoscopic surgery.

Many of the complications of laparoscopy have been associated with the learning curve of taking a new approach to an old problem. Despite the large number of potential pitfalls the balance of benefit (by avoiding other complications from open surgery, or improving overall outcomes) is still in favor of laparoscopy.

Assessment, investigation, and management of laparoscopic complications

Assessment

- Understand the underlying operation: read the operation notes.

Gastrointestinal Emergencies, Third Edition. Edited by Tony C. K. Tham, John S. A. Collins, and Roy Soetikno.
© 2016 John Wiley & Sons, Ltd. Published 2016 by John Wiley & Sons, Ltd.

Table 12.1 Categorization of specific risks of complications in laparoscopic versus open operations.

Operations that have a specific risk of complication when done laparoscopically

Gastric bypass for obesity: anastomotic leaks
Resection of the stomach or esophagus: anastomotic leaks
Pancreatic resection: anastomotic leaks
Colectomy: anastomotic leaks
Nissen fundoplication: bougie perforation of the cardia
Incisional hernia repair: enterotomy, seroma
Adrenalectomy: renal arterial injury

Operations where there is significant debate on the relative risks of open versus laparoscopic approach

Appendicectomy: deep pelvic abscess
Cholecystectomy: relative risk of common bile duct injury

Operations where the complications of laparoscopic surgery seem little different in nature, and no more frequent than open surgery

Inguinal hernia repair
Heller's myotomy
Splenectomy
Rectopexy
Nephrectomy (live related donor)
Liver resection (for disease)
Ovarian tubal surgery

- Look for methods of access to the peritoneum (Veress needle/open cut down).
- Consider the underlying primary pathology.
- Consider any secondary pathology in the operative field (adhesions).
- Does the patient have co-morbidity such as obesity, cardiac failure, or respiratory failure?
- Use a multidisciplinary approach (radiology, gastroenterology, anesthesiology, and surgical teams).
- Examine the patient comprehensively:
  - Area of surgery – abdomen or chest;
  - Outside the area – head, neck, limbs, and cardiorespiratory system.

Investigation

- Radiography – within 24 hours note that the free air may be due to pneumoperitoneum.
- Ultrasound is not often helpful initially because of gas.
- Blood tests: check for anemia, blood gases, and liver function tests after cholecystectomy.

Management

- Discuss the case with the operating surgeon and anesthetist.
- Inform the patient of the concerns.
- Do not delay with reoperation if the need arises.
- Reoperation usually is by laparoscopy.
- There is no gain in laparoscopy if open surgery is safer in the hands of the local team.
- Involve specialist referral for specific complications such as bile duct injury.
- Collect data for subsequent audit.

Types of complication

Cardiorespiratory system

Gas in the wrong cavity

Extraperitoneal insufflation may result in surgical emphysema, palpable anywhere on the neck, chest, or abdomen.

Pneumothorax or carbothorax (since the gas is CO_2) occurs by accidental pleural puncture, when dissecting the mediastinum or diaphragm. As long as positive pressure ventilation is maintained, an underwater seal drain is not required at the end of the procedure. Gas can also escape through a congenital foramen such as Morgagni or Bochdalek into the chest without any instrumental injury. A needle placed into the suspected chest cavity and CO_2 analysis may reveal a 100% concentration and confirm the diagnosis. This is treated by leaving in a wide-bore needle during the operation to allow gas to escape and remove the needle after ceasing the insufflation of CO_2 at the end of the procedure.

Gas embolism is a possibility but is rarely reported. It results in acute hypotension, cyanosis, hypoxia and a characteristic "millwheel" murmur on cardiac auscultation. Treat by releasing the pneumoperitoneum. Place the patient in a steep Trendelenburg, left lateral decubitus position and aspirate gas using a central line.

Hypercarbia may occur with underlying lung disease such as emphysema and chronic obstructive airway disease causing premature ventricular contraction and arrhythmias. The anesthetist should be aware of the risk and monitor the exhaled CO_2 concentration. Increasing ventilation volume and frequency at an early stage will prevent this becoming a substantial problem.

Postoperative shoulder tip pain (Kehr sign) is common and may be due to carbonic acid irritating the diaphragm; overstretch of the diaphragm muscle fibers, or chemical irritating effects of blood in the peritoneal cavity. This is treated with reassurance, simple analgesia, and mobilization of the patient. It almost always resolves within 24 hours.

Complications in the systemic circulation

Reduced venous return due to compression of the inferior vena cava (IVC) is a theoretical risk that is rarely a clinical problem. In obese patients the upright position actually makes ventilation easier and venous return is usually good in practice. Bradycardia can occur with vasovagal activity induced by the rapid insufflation of CO_2 during the establishment of the pneumoperitoneum. Treat by reduction of the CO_2 insufflation and administration of intravenous atropine. Respiratory gas exchange increases during laparoscopy and core temperature rises but there is no scientific evidence that this effect is beneficial or detrimental [1].

Deep venous thrombosis is relatively rare after laparoscopic surgery due to improved mobilization postoperatively and the often shorter operative time than open surgery for cholecystectomy and hernia repair.

Complications of access
Enterotomy, vascular injury, and bladder injury

More than 50% of complications of laparoscopic surgery occur during obtaining access. A review of 25 67 gynaecological procedures, found that 57% of complications occurred while obtaining access [2]. When a vascular injury occurs during laparoscopic access it is usually after the use of a Veress needle (spring-mounted ball on the tip of a safety needle) to introduce the CO_2 into the peritoneum and may occur from the needle itself or the blind introduction of a sharp port. When it occurs, it is catastrophic and so it has received much attention, but it is rare, at 1 in 1333 cases, and the associated mortality is 1 in 33 333 [3]. All of the complications of access are reduced by the use of a direct cut down (Hasson's) technique. While some experienced operators (particularly gynecologists) continue to safely use a Veress needle it is easier and safer to teach the open cut down method. A meta-analysis of 760 890 cases of closed laparoscopic surgery (Veress technique and 22 465 cases of the open technique) reported that the incidence of vascular injury is very rare in the closed technique 0.44% and 0% in the open technique, $p = 0.003$[4].

An alternative is a translucent plastic port (optical port) with a 0° lens to allow direct view of the inserted port, useful for obese patients, for bariatric surgery, or for placing the first port laterally when starting a laparoscopic incisional hernia repair. However, visceral and vascular Injuries have been reported with this technique.

No method of port insertion is perfectly safe in the presence of dense adhesions but being aware of the possibility, taking specific steps to avoid the problem and carefully assessing any areas of potential damage will limit these events to a minimum [3, 5].

Port site hernia

Port site hernia is important; however, it is under-recognized complication of laparoscopic surgery. It carries a high risk of obstruction and strangulation due to the small defect. In systematic review of 11,699 patients undergoing gastrointestinal operations, the incidence of port site herniae was 0.74% with a mean follow up of 24 months [6]. It is much less common than incisional hernias for midline laparotomy (10%). They usually occur within 3–6 weeks of the operation, and occur at 10–12 mm port sites, often one that has been extended to remove a large gallbladder. The lowest incidence of port site hernia was in bariatric surgery 0.57% in 2644 patient after a follow up of approximately 6 years, the highest incidence was in laparoscopic colorectal surgery 1.4% in 477 patient followed up for 6 years [6]. To prevent the port site herniae from occurring in first instance all fascial defects larger than 10 mm should be closed. The herniae are best repaired laparoscopically using mesh (Fig. 12.1).

Complications of operative injury during laparoscopy

Enterotomy

Inadvertent injury of an abdominal organ can occur during the removal and replacement of surgical instruments. If this happens out of view of the camera then the injury may go unnoticed until there is a significant leakage of intestinal content and possible established peritoneal sepsis. The incidence of bowel Injury is 0.7% when using Veress needle compared with 0.5% when using the open technique [4].

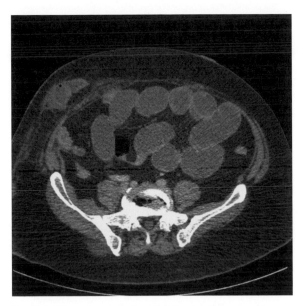

Fig. 12.1 CT scan: port site hernia following laparoscopic Incisional hernia repair.

Enterotomy may occur during the dissection of adhesions of intestinal loops. In many circumstances adhesions may be left alone but in patients with adhesion obstruction, or patients with incisional hernia, there is a need to clear the operative field of adhesions. During laparoscopy the detection of such an injury may be hampered by limitations of the field of view of the laparoscopic camera. Recognition is critically important because immediate repair is simple either laparoscopically or by externalizing the bowel through a small incision.

Diathermy
Diathermy injury may occur as in open surgery, with the additional risk of capacitance coupling, which occurs if a conductor is placed inside an insulator (such as a plastic sheath around a metal port) and this can randomly discharge electricity out of view of the operator.

Adhesions
Laparoscopy greatly reduces the incidence of adhesions compared to equivalent open operations, resulting in fewer early and late postoperative complications of pain and obstruction. The long-term comparative figures are not well reported but clinical experience indicates a dramatic reduction in scar tissue compared to the effects of open intra-abdominal surgery.

Hemorrhage
The problem of bleeding during laparoscopy has required the design of special tools. The Harmonic scalpel, a vibrating blunt blade device that coagulates with minimal heat and can seal arteries up to 7 mm in diameter, is useful for Nissen's fundoplication. The Ligasure™ is a form of multipolar electrocoagulation, useful for large arteries and popular in colectomy or splenectomy. For liver resection compression collars, microwave application and argon beam plasma coagulation (a form of spray diathermy) all have a role to play in dealing with potential major hemorrhage. Injury to inferior epigastric arteries (IEAs) can be avoided by knowing the surface landmarks for IEAs. Injury to IEA results in a large haematoma. To prevent this from occurring, a large Foley catheter should be inserted in the port site over the bleeding and inflated with 30 mL of saline. This will cause a tamponade and stop the bleeding.

Conversion to open surgery

Whether conversion to open surgery can be defined as a complication is debatable. From the perspective of consent and education, the patient must be aware of the possibility but it may not be appropriate to term it a complication. When applied to large numbers conversion rates do give an indication of the quality of outcome from laparoscopic surgery and they may be audited in departments of surgery. For some operations such as Nissen's fundoplication conversion to open surgery is so rare (1% in expert institutions) that a high rate signifies potential problems with surgical standards. In contrast, for colectomy, conversion rates still vary from 11% to 29% and it will take some time before we understand whether such conversion is required to achieve adequate cancer clearance or whether the underlying issue is a lack of appropriate laparoscopic technique to achieve the same result [5, 7].

Complications specific to procedures

Cholecystectomy, exploration of common bile duct
The complications of bile duct injury were frequent during the introduction of laparoscopiccholecystectomy (see Table 12.2) but are now much less frequent due to

Table 12.2 Complications of laparoscopic cholecystectomy.

Injury to common bile duct or other biliary anatomy
Strictures, bile leaks, obstructive jaundice
Injury to duodenum
Leak from closure of cholecystoduodenal fistula
Retained gallstones in peritoneum
Retained common bile duct stones
Postoperative hemorrhage

improved training. The risk of a major duct injury (incision, transaction, ischemic stricture) of a major bile duct is now less than 1:500 [8]. Cholecystectomy is relatively common, and in a unit such as ours where we perform up to 1000 cholecystectomies per annum, such a risk may produce two injuries each year. The risk of minor injuries (bile leaks requiring stenting or suture) is approximately 1:200 (see also Chapter 24 – Biliary Tract Emergencies). All of these are reduced by careful technique with good exposure of Calot's triangle and assurance of the anatomy of the cystic duct and cystic artery before clipping or division. The mobilization of the Hartmann pouch and extending this along the body of the gallbladder can greatly help in defining any potential aberrant anatomy. In patients with very inflamed, thickened tissues it is safer to steer clear of Calot's triangle and perform a fundus-first dissection. This requires the ability to deal with hemorrhage from the liver bed, and having an argon beam plasma coagulator is a great asset in this circumstance.

When in doubt about the anatomy an intraoperative cholangiogram is useful. Referral centers seeing common bile duct injuries tend to advise routine cholangiography. This is a subject about which there has been controversy since before the days of laparoscopy.

Spilt gallstones may cause the rare complication of infection from actinomycosis and reports of this are unique to laparoscopy. To reduce the risk of stones being left behind use a tissue retrieval bag whenever the gallbladder wall is opened and place any loose stones in the bag before attempts are made to remove it from the abdomen.

Hernia repair: inguinal, femoral, incisional

Retention of urine after hernia repair is common (10% after bilateral repair). Bruising in the scrotum is common but significant hematoma in the scrotum is rare. Small bowel obstruction may occur due to adhesion or internal hernia through peritoneal repair. Nerve entrapment from a staple or tack can cause significant groin pain, but overall chronic groin pain is less common after laparoscopy than open surgery. After incisional hernia repair the sac may fill with blood-stained fluid (seroma) and be palpable as a persistent lump. These nearly always resolve after 6 months.

Enterotomy is likely when extensive adhesions require division during incisional hernia repair. This occurs in 2–5% of complex incisional hernias. Enough postoperative observation (2–3 days) is needed to ensure that peritonitis is not developing. In our experience we have seen delayed perforation at 7–10 days postoperatively and patients need to be educated to return and given easy access to the surgical team if significant postoperative symptoms develop.

Nissen fundoplication

The only complication of fundoplication that is specific to the laparoscopic approach is perforation of the esophagogastric junction. It is related to the use of a bougie. The incidence is 1–2%. Most observers advise careful use of the bougie with the anesthesiologist in direct view of the laparoscopic image during its introduction. The author believes that there is no need to subject the patient to the risk of a bougie perforation and the wrap can be calibrated using instruments that are 10 mm in diameter (such as a 10 mm Babcock introduced between the completed wrap and the esophagus.

Wrap migration may occur into the chest but is reduced by closing the diaphragmatic hiatus even when a hernia is not present. A slipped Nissen wrap occurs when the fundoplication moves down onto the proximal stomach and is prevented by fixing the wrap to the esophagus and retaining the hepatic branch of the vagus nerve. Dysphagia may occur regardless of the approach. There is no difference between preserving, or dividing, the short gastric arteries, in randomized trials. These trials compare one blanket policy versus another. In some patients a tight fundus might benefit from mobilization of the short gastric arteries, whereas some loose fundi, especially after mobilizing a large hiatus hernia, become excessively mobile (and therefore liable to tort) if the short gastric arteries are mobilized as well. Therefore the author believes that the right technique is to be selective and choose mobilization of the short gastric arteries when there is an operative feeling of tension in the wrap (20%).

Splenectomy

Residual splenunculi may be more common after laparoscopic splenectomy as they occur along the surface of the pancreas, within and behind the greater omentum, areas not easily seen at laparoscopy.

Major operative hemorrhage is a worry during laparoscopic splenectomy but measures to handle it are well established. Having a swab available to place laparoscopically directly on arterial bleeding while suction, irrigation and proximal control is achieved allows laparoscopic control of such a surgical mishap.

Operations for morbid obesity: gastric bands/stapling/bypass

These are frequently performed laparoscopically. For laparoscopic bands, slippage may occur in 0.7–3% [9, 10], erosion in 0.7% and band obstruction in 1.5%. All these require revision surgery. For bypass operations anastomotic leaks are the gravest of problems and the incidence of these after laparoscopic operations may be higher than after open ones (2.3% vs. 4.2%) [9, 11].

Colectomy

The complications of laparoscopic colorectal surgery are summarized in Table 12.3. Conversion to open surgery is frequent (11–29% in recent series) [12] and current thinking accepts the need to convert to achieve cancer clearance. In a meta-analysis of 10 randomized controlled trials (RCTs) of 4055 patients (2059 in laparoscopic group and 1896 in open group) there was a higher rate of intraoperative complications (OR 1.37, $p = 0.010$) and a higher rate of bowel injury in the laparoscopic group (OR 1.88, $p = 0.020$) [13]. In this meta-analysis of 20 out of 30 RCTs, some of them were relatively large, and were excluded as they did not report intraoperative complications; also, there was a lack of standardized

Table 12.3 Complications of laparoscopic colorectal surgery

Small and large bowel injury
Conversion to open
Port site hernia 1.4%
Port site metastasis (no difference between open and laparoscopic)
Lower limb compartment syndrome
Brachial plexus injury: associated with abduction of the arm and lengthy procedure

definitions of postoperative complications, which may have caused heterogeneity in the result. Furthermore a Cochrane meta-analysis in 2005 demonstrated a lower rate of postoperative complications after laparoscopic colorectal resections [14]. Since this meta-analysis was published three major RCTs have reported equivalent postoperative complications rates for open and laparoscopic techniques. Additionally, the American College of surgeon Quality Improvement Program (ACS NSQIP) demonstrated lower postoperative complications rates after laparoscopic colorectal surgery [15].

Specific early fears about the high incidence of metastatic deposits along the track of the ports used for laparoscopic access, especially among UK observers, have not proved to be a real issue. Randomized trials show comparative figures for port site or incisional metastases (0.5–0.9% vs. 0.2% laparoscopic vs. open) [7, 16] and these differences are not clinically significant in the overall context of survival.

During colectomy, swelling and dependent edema of head, neck, and upper limbs may occur from prolonged positioning in steep Trendelenburg. A sensible precaution is to provide the patient and the surgeons some respite from the positional effects by reversing the head-down position after each hour. These can be very long procedures – median operating times 275 minutes. Injury to brachial plexus is very rare and has been reported in only 10 cases in the literature. It is due to arm abduction and prolonged procedure [17].

Appendicectomy

Specific complications after appendicectomy performed by the laparoscopic route are rare but pelvic abscesses are commoner in some series. A thorough cleansing by irrigation and aspiration and the use of drains for patients with significant peritoneal soiling after perforation will minimize this problem. A very rare event is the reinfection of the stump of appendix and this will be minimized by careful dissection of the appendix down onto the cecum at the time of the first operation.

Upper gastrointestinal cancer resections

Pancreatic, esophageal, and gastric resection are probably not done in sufficient numbers to be regarded as routine and the risks of complication are not well described. Anastomotic leak rates for esophageal resections are 12% but, so far, only small series have been reported [18].

Adrenalectomy

For laparoscopic adrenalectomy there is the potential for rare complications such as renal arterial injury, not reported with open adrenalectomy [19]. In the largest study to date of 3100 patients (644 undergoing open versus 2456 patients undergoing laparoscopic adrenalectomy. Patients undergoing laparoscopic adrenalectomy had significantly lower postoperative morbidity and shorter length of stay compared to patients undergoing open adrenalectomy [20].

Solid organ resection

Nephrectomy, common for live related donor, or for disease, and liver resection have a greater challenge for the surgeon in control of major blood vessels and techniques are evolving to deal with these issues using specific new technologies. Radical prostatectomy performed laparoscopically has the same range of operative complications as the open operation.

Gynecology

Tubal surgery, ectopic pregnancy, ovarian cyst, and endometriosis treatment are all achievable by laparoscopy and the main issue in dealing with operative complications is the potential lack of the necessary skills of the gynecologist to deal with them. For instance, bowel injury may occur from dissection or from laser/argon beam and so it is good practice to ensure that there is a suitably qualified general surgeon available to handle these (or prevent them) by laparoscopic techniques.

References

1. McHoney MC, Corizia L, Eaton S, et al. Laparoscopic surgery in children is associated with an intraoperative hypermetabolic response. *Surg. Endosc.* 2006;**20**:452–7.
2. Jansen F W, Kapiteyn K, Trimbos-Kemper T, Hermans J, Trimbos JB. Complications of laparoscopy: a prospective multicentre observational study. Br. *J. Obstet. Gynecol.* 1997;**104**:595–600.
3. Bonjer HJ, Hazebrook EJ, Kezemier G, Giuffrida MC, Meijer WS, Lange JF. Open versus closed establishment of pneumoperitoneum in laparoscopic surgery. *Br. J. Surg.* 1997;**84**: 599–602.
4. Larobina M, Nottle P. Complete evidence regarding major vascular injuries during laparoscopic access. *Surg. Laparosc. Endosc. Percutan. Tech.* 2005;**15**(3):119–23.
5. Pickersgill A, Slade RJ, Falconer GF, Attwood S. Open laparoscopy: the way forward. *Br. J. Obs. Gynaecol.* 1999;**106**: 1116–19.
6. Owens M, Barry M, Janjua AZ, Winter DC. A systematic review of laparoscopic port site hernias in gastrointestinal surgery. *Surgeon* 2011;**9**(4):218–24.
7. Lacy Am, Garcia-Valdecasas JC, Delgado S, et al. Laparoscopically assisted colon resection for treatment of non-metastatic colon cancer: a randomised trial. *Lancet* 2002;**359**:2224–9.
8. Gentileschi P, DiPaola M, Catarci M, et al. Bile duct injuries during laparoscopic cholecystectomy: a 1994–2001 audit on 13,718 operations in the Rome area. *Surg. Endosc.* 2004;**18**:232–6.
9. Nguyen NT, Morton JM, Wolfe BM, Schirmer B, Ali M, Traverson LW. The Sages Bariatric Surgery Outcome Initiative. *Surg. Endosc.* 2005;**19**:1429–38.
10. Parikh MS, Fielding GA, Ren CJ. US experience with 749 laparoscopic adjustable gastric bands: intermediate outcomes. *Surg. Endosc.* 2005; **19**:1631–5.
11. Fernandez AZ, DeMaria EJ, Tichansky DS, et al. Experience with over 3,000 open and laparoscopic bariatric procedures: multivariate analysis of factors related to leak and resultant mortality. *Surg. Endosc.* 2004;**18**:193–7.
12. Reza MM, Blasco JA, Andradas E, Cantero R, Mayol J. Systematic review of laparoscopic versus open surgery for colorectal cancer. *Br. J. Surg.* 2006;**93**:921–8.
13. Sammour T, Kahokehr A, Srinivasa S, Bissett IP, Hill AG. Laparoscopic colorectal surgery is associated with a higher intraoperative complication rate than open surgery. *Ann. Surg.* 2011;**253**(1):35–43.
14. Schwenk W, Haase O, Neudecker J, Müller JM. Short term benefits for laparoscopic colorectal resection. *Cochrane Database Syst Rev.* 2005;(**3**):CD003145.
15. Kennedy GD, Heise C, Rajamanickam V, Harms B, Foley EF. Laparoscopy decreases postoperative complication rates after abdominal colectomy: results from the national surgical quality improvement program. *Ann. Surg.* 2009;**249**(4): 596–601.
16. Clinical Outcomes of Surgical Therapy Study Group. A comparison of laparoscopically assisted and open colectomy for colon cancer. *N. Engl. J. Med.* 2004;**350**:2050–9.
17. Codd RJ, Evans MD, Sagar PM, Williams GL. A systematic review of peripheral nerve injury following laparoscopic colorectal surgery.*Colorectal Dis.* 2013;**15**(3):278–82.
18. 18.Collins G, Johnson E, Korshus T, et al. Experience with minimally invasive esophagectomy. *Surg. Endosc.* 2006;**20**: 298–301.
19. Brunt LM. Minimal access adrenal surgery. *Surg. Endosc.* 2006;**20**:351–61.
20. Elfenbein DM, Scarborough JE, Speicher PJ, Scheri RP. Comparison of laparoscopic versus open adrenalectomy: results from American College of Surgeons-National Surgery Quality Improvement Project. *J. Surg. Res.* 2013;**184**(1): 216–20.

CHAPTER 13

Complications of liver biopsy

Robert J. Wong and Aijaz Ahmed

Stanford University School of Medicine, Stanford, CA, USA

Introduction

Liver biopsy has traditionally been considered the gold standard in the evaluation of chronic liver diseases, including the assessment of hepatic inflammation and fibrosis. The importance of liver biopsy reflects its role both as a diagnostic and prognostic tool. However, significant advances in non-invasive techniques to assess severity of hepatic inflammation and fibrosis may avoid the need for liver biopsy in certain clinical situations. Nevertheless, there remain several clinical situations (e.g. evaluating for allograft rejection post-liver transplantation, making a definitive diagnosis of clinical conundrums) that rely on the important histopathological information provided by liver biopsy, and a thorough understanding of the potential complications of liver biopsy is critical to the care of patients with liver disease.

Liver biopsy can be performed with three different techniques: percutaneous, transjugular, or laparoscopic. Percutaneous liver biopsy can be safely performed in the outpatient setting or at the patient's bedside using percussion and/or imaging guided localization. Transjugular liver biopsy is most commonly performed via a fluoroscopy-guided catheter that is directed from the right internal jugular vein to the hepatic vein. Laparoscopy-guided liver biopsy has the additional advantage of allowing inspection of the liver surface while a tissue sample is collected. Percutaneous liver biopsy is the most common technique utilized worldwide and this approach will be the focus of this chapter.

Complications

Despite being a highly vascular organ, major complications following liver biopsy are rare, with the most common complication being hemorrhage. Overall, the reported complication rate ranges from 0.6–3.7% and the mortality rate ranges from 0.01–0.3%. Over 95% of complications are encountered within the first 24 hours, and 60% within 2 hours following liver biopsy. Rates of hospitalization following liver biopsy, primarily for management of pain or hemodynamic derangements, are reported to be 1.4–3.2%. The complication rate increases with factors such as number of passes, presence of hepatic malignancy and advanced liver disease. Some studies also found the complication rate to be related to the type of biopsy needle and operator experience. Table 13.1 details the major complications associated with liver biopsy.

Pain
Clinical features
Approximate 30% of patients report some degree of pain in the right upper quadrant and/or right shoulder following liver biopsy. While the pain is commonly mild and dull, demonstrating relief with analgesic treatment, pain that is persistent, more severe, or demonstrates alarming features (e.g. pleuritic pain, pain associated with hypotension, tachypnea, or impaired oxygen saturation) should prompt urgent evaluation for other complications such as hemorrhage or peritonitis.

Gastrointestinal Emergencies, Third Edition. Edited by Tony C. K. Tham, John S. A. Collins, and Roy Soetikno.
© 2016 John Wiley & Sons, Ltd. Published 2016 by John Wiley & Sons, Ltd.

Table 13.1 Complications of percutaneous liver biopsy.

Complication	Incidence (%)
Pain	0.06–33
Intraperitoneal hemorrhage	0.03–0.7
Intra-/extrahepatic hematoma	0.06–2.7*
Biliary	
Perforation of gallbladder	0.012
Hemobilia	0.06–1
Bile peritonitis	0.03–0.22
Pulmonary complications	0.01–0.35
Pneumothorax	0.08–0.8
Hemothorax	0.18–0.49
Sepsis	0.09
Seeding of malignant lesion	0.003–0.009
Biopsy of other organs	0.004–0.12
Rare complications	
Subphrenic abscess	
Bile embolism	
Air embolism	
Biloma from bile leak	
Hemobilia-related obstructive jaundice, acute cholecystitis, acute pancreatitis	

*Up to 23% if post-biopsy ultrasound is performed on all patients.

Management points

- Mild pain should be treated with analgesics, depending on the severity. Moderately severe pain should be treated with an opiate analgesic intravenously for rapid onset of action.
- Severe pain or pain associated with alarm features (e.g. pleuritic pain, hypotension or tachypnea, oxygen desaturation) should prompt urgent evaluation for bleeding or peritonitis.
- Patients demonstrating alarm features that raise suspicion for bleeding or peritonitis, must be admitted to the hospital with close monitoring of vital signs, serial hemoglobin, and pertinent radiographic imaging (e.g. chest X-ray if concern for hemothorax).

Hemorrhage

Risk of hemorrhage is higher in the presence of cirrhosis, intrahepatic malignancy, use of True-cut needle, and the need for multiple passes. There is also an increased risk in the presence of coagulopathy, and platelet count >60 000/mm³ and International Normalized Ratio (INR) > 1.5 has been recommended prior to performing percutaneous liver biopsy. Aspirin or other antiplatelet agents should be avoided for 5–7 days and non-steroidal anti-inflammatory drugs (NSAIDs) for 1–3 days prior to biopsy to reduce the risk of significant hemorrhage. Patients on anticoagulant therapy should cease the medication for at least 3 days prior to the procedure, although the decision to hold anticoagulants depends on the underlying etiology for which the anticoagulant was prescribed and must take into account the risks of benefits of holding this therapy for liver biopsy. Furthermore, significant hemorrhage following liver biopsy is 10-fold higher in patients with malignancy as compared to those without underlying malignancy.

Clinical features

Significant hemorrhage following liver biopsy is rare, and while the majority of significant bleeding manifests soon after the biopsy is performed, it is important to recognize that bleeding complications can present up to 3 weeks later. Delayed bleeding carries a greater risk of morbidity and mortality given delayed diagnosis and the development of bleeding outside of an acute care setting.

Hemorrhage following liver biopsy may be intraperitoneal, intrahepatic, subcapsular, or into the bilary tract (hemobilia). Although rare (one study of 68 276 liver biopsies reported a rate of 0.32%), intraperitoneal hemorrhage is the most serious bleeding complication and usually manifests within 3 hours following biopsy. Clinical symptoms include abdominal pain and hemodynamic derangements including hypotension and/or tachycardia. Diagnostic imaging with ultrasonography or computerized tomography (CT) can help confirm the diagnosis. More common, but less serious of a complication, intrahepatic or subcapsular hemorrhage has been observed in up to 23% of patients undergoing liver biopsy. Intrahepatic or subscapular hematomas are usually asymptomatic, although large hemotomas following liver biopsy can cause significant pain secondary to capsular distension, hypotension, tachycardia, and blood loss anemia. In addition, depending on the locations and severity of bleeding, it is a rare possibility that intrahepatic or subcapsular hemorrhage may evolve into intraperitoneal hemorrhage. Conservative measures with pain-level directed analgesia are usually sufficient.

Management points

- Hemorrhage should be considered in a patient with severe abdominal pain who responses poorly to analgesics, accompanied by a drop in serum hemo-globin, tachycardia, and hypotension.

- When bleeding is suspected, patients should be admitted to the hospital for frequent vital signs including serial hemoglobin.
- Diagnostic imaging with abdominal ultrasound or CT scan can be utilized to confirm the diagnosis of hemorrhage.
- Pseudoaneurysms and arteriovenous fistulae, which are the causes of delayed hemorrhage following liver biopsy, are detected by ultrasound with Doppler and biphasic CT scan.
- If diagnostic imaging fails to identify hemorrhage, but suspicion for clinically significant bleeding remains, an interventional radiologist should be consulted for selective diagnostic +/– therapeutic angiography.
- Type- and-cross-packed red blood cells should be performed.
- If bleeding is suspected or confirmed, volume resuscitation with intravenous fluids and correction of any underlying coagulopathy with appropriate blood product transfusion should be initiated (e.g. platelets, fresh frozen plasma).
- If signs/symptoms of shock or significant bleeding are present (i.e. persistent hypotension despite intravenous fluid resuscitation, persistent severe anemia despite blood product transfusion) consult a surgeon or interventional radiologist depending on local expertise, for immediate intervention after the patient is stabilized.
- Bleeding secondary to pseudoaneurysms should be managed initially with angiographic embolization, and if it fails then surgery will be required (hepatic lobectomy or debridement followed by ligation of the pseudoaneurysm).

Hemobilia
Clinical features
Hemobilia occurs secondary to injury and bleeding into the biliary system, and presents with signs of gastrointestinal bleeding, biliary colic, and jaundice (Quincke's triad). Hemobilia following liver biopsy is rare, with one large study of 68,276 biopsies reporting four cases of hemobilia. While the predominant clinical feature of hemobilia is upper gastrointestinal bleeding via the ampulla of Vater, the onset of bleeding is usually delayed, with a mean interval of 5 days following percutaneous liver biopsy. Endoscopic evaluation can demonstrate hemorrhage

from the ampulla of Vater, and endoscopic retrograde cholangiopancreatography (ERCP) may visualize irregular densities in the biliary tract that represent blood. Hemorrhage into the biliary tree contributes to obstructive cholangiopathy and increases the risk for cholangitis. ERCP (i.e. sphincterotomy, balloon extraction of the clot, or placing a nasobiliary tube or biliary stent for drainage) can aid with decompression and removal of blood clots if there is evidence of obstruction. However, interventional radiology consultation should be considered for angiography and selective embolization therapy.

Management points
- Hemobilia can present with signs of gastrointestinal bleeding, biliary colic, and jaundice (Quincke's triad).
- Correction of any underlying coagulopathy with appropriate blood product transfusion should be initiated when there is concern for hemobilia.
- Diagnosis can be confirmed with endoscopic evaluation demonstrating bleeding from the ampulla of Vater.
- ERCP can confirm the diagnosis of hemobilia and techniques such as sphincterotomy, balloon extraction of blood clots in the biliary system, or placement of a nasobiliary tube or biliary stent for drainage can be utilized in the management.
- Diagnostic imaging with abdominal ultrasonography or CT scan can be helpful for excluding other etiologies of biliary obstruction.
- Interventional radiology should be consulted for selective angiography with embolization if significant bleeding persists despite endoscopic treatment.

Infectious considerations
Clinical features
While clinically significant infections secondary to percutaneous liver biopsy is rare, transient bacteremia has been reported in 5.8–13.5% of patients. Routine prophylactic antibiotics, however, are not currently recommended. Rarely, the development of bile peritonitis is a serious complication that must be closely evaluated and treated.

Bile peritonitis is commonly caused by puncture of the gallbladder during liver biopsy, which can be detected with evidence of bile aspiration into the biopsy syringe. Clinical features of bile peritonitis include the sudden onset of severe abdominal pain and right shoulder pain within minutes of the biopsy. Severe persistent right upper quadrant tenderness, peritoneal signs, ileus, fever, leucocytosis, hypotension, and tachycardia are signs/symptoms concerning for the development of peritonitis and septic shock. The risk of bile peritonitis is increased if there is evidence of concurrent biliary obstruction. Diagnostic imaging with abdominal ultrasonography or CT scan may help identify bile fluid collection in the abdominal cavity. Endoscopic evaluation with ERCP may help with the diagnosis and treatment of bile leak.

Management points

- Routine prophylactic antibiotics are not recommended following liver biopsy.
- Signs of clinically significant infection (e.g. fever, leukocytosis, hypotension, tachycardia) should prompt a more thorough evaluation for peritonitis.
- Severe abdominal pain, peritoneal signs, or signs/symptoms of septic shock should prompt urgent evaluation for peritonitis.
- Diagnostic imaging with abdominal ultrasonography or CT scan can aid in detection bile fluid collections.
- Technetium-99m dimethyl iminodiacetic acid (HIDA) scan and ERCP can further aid in the detection and treatment of biliary leaks.
- When bile peritonitis is suspected, intravenous fluid resuscitation and broad-spectrum antibiotics to cover enteric organisms should be promptly initiated.
- Percutaneous drainage and cholecystostomy can be utilized for the management of biliary leak if endoscopic management is not available.
- Peritoneal signs or evidence of shock should prompt urgent surgical consultation.

Pulmonary considerations
Clinical features

Pulmonary complications following liver biopsy include right-sided chest wall pain, pneumothorax, and hemothorax. Chest wall pain is not uncommon, and can additionally manifest as mild pleuritic chest pain 2–3 hours following liver biopsy. Mild discomfort can be managed with oral or intravenous analgesia. More severe pain, or symptoms associated with hypotension, tachycardia, dyspnea, cough, or hemoptysis must prompt urgent evaluation. Diagnostic imaging with chest X-ray will help evaluate for pneumothorax,

hemothorax, or development of pleural effusion. Large, symptomatic pneumothorax require chest tube placement for decompression.

Management points

- Chest wall pain following liver biopsy can be managed with oral or intravenous analgesia.
- Severe or persistent pain associated with alarm features (e.g. hypotension, tachycardia, dyspnea, cough, oxygen desaturation) should prompt urgent evaluation for hemo/pneumothorax.
- Diagnostic imaging with chest radiography (posteroanterior and lateral) should be performed immediately.
- Hospital admission with close monitoring of vital signs and serial haemoglobin is recommended if hemothorax is suspected.
- Chest tube placement is needed if there is evidence of large or symptomatic pneumothorax.

Acknowledgments

We would like to thank Ramsey Cheung, MD, who wrote this chapter in the previous edition of this book that served as the basis for this updated revision.

Further reading

Bravo AA, Sheth SG, Chopra S. Liver biopsy. N. Engl. J. Med 2001;**344**:495–500.

Campbell MS, Jeffers LJ, Reddy KR. Liver biopsy and laparoscopy. In *Diseases of the Liver*, 10th edition, Schiff ER, Sorrell MF, *Maddrey WC (eds)*. Wiley-Blackwell, Oxford, 2007: 61–81.

Campbell MS, Reddy KR. Review article: the evolving role of liver biopsy. Aliment. Pharmacol. Ther. 2004;**20**:249–59.

McGill DB, Rakela J, Zinsmeister AR, Ott BJ. A 21-year experience with major hemorrhage after percutaneous liver biopsy. Gastroenterology 1990;**99**:1396–1400.

Piccino T, Sagnelli E, Pasquale G, Giusti G. Complications following percutaneous liver biopsy: a multicenter retrospective study on 68,276 biopsies. J. Hepatol. 1986;**2**:165–73.

Sheela H, Seela S, Caldwell C, Boyer JL, Jain D. Liver biopsy: evolving role in the new millennium. J. Clin. Gastroenterol. 2005;**39**:603–10.

CHAPTER 14

Complications of colonoscopy

Matthias Steverlynck[1] and Jo Vandervoort[2]

[1] Centre Hospitalier de Mouscron, Belgium
[2] Onze-Lieve-Vrouw Ziekenhuis, Aalst, Belgium

Introduction

Colonoscopy, introduced in the late 1960s, allows diagnosis and treatment of a wide range of conditions and symptoms and is the "gold standard" for early detection and removal of colorectal cancer and its precursors.

Up to 1.9 % of more than 500 000 colonoscopies performed in the US each year result in significant complications. The major complications of colonoscopy are bleeding from biopsy and polypectomy sites, colonic perforation and post-polypectomy syndrome [1, 2].

Complications

Hemorrhage

Hemorrhage is the most common polypectomy complication, occurring in 1 to 6 per 1000 colonoscopies (0.1–0.6%) [3]. Early (<24 h) and late (>24 h to 30 days) bleeding may occur. The risk for gastrointestinal bleeding is more than four times higher for those undergoing polypectomy (8.7 per 1000) compared to screening procedures without polypectomy (2.1 per 1000) [4]. The severity of bleeding ranges from slight ooze to arterial pumping.

The risk is related to the type and size of the polyp, the number of polyps removed, the technique of polypectomy, proximal location, and anticoagulation use [2, 5–10].

Colonoscopy is commonly performed in patients on medication affecting their coagulation status. The American Society for Gastrointestinal Endoscopy (ASGE)

guidelines recommend that thienopyridines (e.g. clopidogrel) should be discontinued 7–10 days before a high bleeding risk procedure, low-molecular-weight heparin and warfarin should be discontinued 8 hours and 3–5 days, respectively, before the procedure. Aspirin and non-steroidal anti-inflammatory drugs need not be discontinued, but discontinuation may be considered in high-risk procedures. There is no consensus for the optimal timing of reinitiating anticoagulant therapy after endoscopic interventions. Decisions are likely to depend on procedure-specific circumstances as well as the indications for anticoagulation. Benefits of immediate anticoagulant therapy in preventing thromboembolic events have to be weighed against the risk of hemorrhage and determined on a case-by-case basis [11].

Management of hemorrhage

Most bleeding occurring can be controlled by the endoscopist [12]. The technique depends upon the severity of bleeding, the type of polyp, and individual preference. A combination of techniques is frequently required.

Immediate bleeding after resection of a pedunculated polyp can usually be stopped by regrasping the pedicle with a snare and holding pressure on the pedicle to stop blood flow, permitting the hemostatic cascade to occur. Retransection of the pedicle can be performed, but is not the preferred approach since there may be too little of the pedicle remaining to regrasp if bleeding recommences. Another technique is epinephrine (a dilution of 1:10 000) injection directly into the bleeding site. A thermal probe, BICAP or heater probe can be used

Gastrointestinal Emergencies, Third Edition. Edited by Tony C. K. Tham, John S. A. Collins, and Roy Soetikno.
© 2016 John Wiley & Sons, Ltd. Published 2016 by John Wiley & Sons, Ltd.

for coagulation. Since the colon wall is very thin, the current delivered should be decreased by approximately 50 %. Argon plasma coagulation is effective for oozing from a superficial vessel. Hemoclips are used for bleeding from flat polypectomy sites or to stop arterial pulsatile bleeding from the stalk of pedunculated polyps. Endoloops are used to ligate the stalk to stop bleeding.

If bleeding persists, a mesenteric angiogram will help to localize the bleeding vessel, followed by embolization of this vessel. Also vasopressin can be infused locally to vasoconstrict the mucosal feeding arterioles. If the bleeding stays uncontrollable, surgery should be performed.

Prevention of hemorrhage

Measures to prevent postpolypectomy hemorrhage are epinephrine injection, use of a detachable snare, and prophylactic clip application.

The existence of a large artery in the stalk of a pedunculated polyp increases the risk of arterial bleeding after resection. In large pedunculated polyps resected without any preventive technique, the bleeding rate is between 10 and 15.1% [13–15]. In a randomized controlled trial of 488 patients with pedunculated colorectal polyps (>1 cm), post-polypectomy bleeding was reported in 4.3% of cases: 1.8% (3 of 163) in patients undergoing ligation before snare polypectomy, 3.1% (5 of 161) in patients undergoing epinephrine injection before snare polypectomy, and 7.9% (13 of 164) in patients undergoing snare polypectomy alone. In larger polyps (>2 cm), post-polypectomy bleeding occurred in 2.7% in the detachable snare group, 2.9% in the epinephrine injection group, and 15.1% in the control group [15].

Delayed bleeding does not seem to be reduced by preventive epinephrine injection [15]. Prophylactic clipping after endoscopic removal of large (≥2 cm sessile and flat) colorectal lesions reduced the risk of delayed post-polypectomy hemorrhage. In this retrospective study, the delayed hemorrhage rate was 9.7% (24/247 patients) in the not clipped group versus 1.8% (4/225 patients) in the fully clipped group [16]. In contrast, no decrease in delayed bleeding was observed after clip placement on resection sites in an earlier study, in which the mean polyp size was 7.8 mm and there were few hemorrhages in either the clipped group or the control group (two in each group) [17].

Colonic perforation

Colonic perforation is a major complication, occurring in 0.1% to 0.3% for diagnostic colonoscopy and from 0.4% to 1.0% for therapeutic colonoscopy [18–22]. The sigmoid colon and the recto-sigmoid junction is the area at greatest risk for perforation during diagnostic procedures.

Risk factors for colonic perforation include old age, female sex, diverticulosis, history of abdominal surgery, colonic obstruction, inflammatory bowel disease, colonic stricture, radiation colitis, and multiple comorbidities [23].

There are three possible mechanisms leading to perforation [24]: mechanical perforation, pneumatic perforation, and therapeutic perforation. Mechanical perforation results from excessive pressure of the tip of the colonoscope against the colonic wall. Pneumatic perforation occurs because of the over-distention of the colon by excessive air insufflation. Finally, therapeutic perforation is associated with therapeutic interventions, like dilatation, stenting and polypectomy with transmural damage. With regard to the peritoneum, colonic perforation is classified into two subgroups: intraperitoneal and extraperitoneal perforation [25]. Extraperitoneal perforation is most likely to occur in the lower rectum (usually below the middle valve of Houston), which is retroperitoneal.

Perforation from diagnostic colonoscopy requires surgical intervention more frequently than that from therapeutic colonoscopy [26], because these perforations result from mechanical and pneumatic perforation during insertion. Perforations after therapeutic procedures are more frequent.

The clinical presentation is quite variable. Early symptoms include persistent abdominal pain and abdominal distention. Later on, patients may develop peritonitis with fever, tachycardia, absent bowel sounds, and subcutaneous emphysema. The onset of pain usually occurs during or soon after completion of the procedure, but it may be delayed or even non-existent in some instances [27]. Signs can be masked for hours or days by omental plugging. In the most severe cases of perforation, spilling of bowel contents leads to peritonitis, sepsis, and circulatory collapse.

Plain radiography of the diaphragm and abdomen often reveals pneumoperitoneum, but lack of this finding does not exclude peritonitis. Abdominal computerized tomography (CT) scan is superior to plain radiography [28].

Management

The management of colon perforation secondary to colonoscopy remains controversial. It can be effectively managed by operative or non-operative measures. Surgical consultation should be obtained in all cases.

Several large studies have reported that many patients with colonic perforations may be successfully treated without surgery [29]. Non-operative treatment involves hospitalization, intestinal rest, intravenous fluids, and antibiotics to contain peritonitis and allow the perforation to seal. If the perforation is immediately seen after polypectomy and it is small and localized, it can be managed endoscopically. At that time, the colon is clean and hemoclips can be placed. Close observation is mandatory and surgical intervention is needed if the patient's condition deteriorates or there is no improvement in 72 hours. On the other hand, operative treatment is indicated for patients with diffuse peritonitis, failure of medical treatment, large colonic injuries, ongoing sepsis and those with underlying pathology (i.e. cancer, unremitting colitis, and distal obstruction). Surgical procedures range from primary repair, resection and anastomosis or defunctioning colostomy.

The ability to close the defect endoscopically will depend on four main factors: (a) localization and size of perforation, (b) stool contamination, (c) availability of instruments to close the defect, and (d) the endoscopist's expertise and skills [30–34]. Perforations larger than 10 mm, which occur during diagnostic colonoscopy, are considered contraindications to endoscopic repair [35]. However, we expect that more endoscopic closures will be possible, especially in patients with larger defects with the advent of new clipping devices and the advancement of natural orifice transluminal endoscopic surgery (NOTES).

Post-polypectomy electrocoagulation syndrome

Post-polypectomy electrocoagulation syndrome occurs in 0.003–0.1% of polypectomies [3]. It occurs also most often after the removal of large (>2 cm) sessile polyps, which usually require large amounts and long duration of thermal energy [2, 12, 19].

Post-polypectomy electrocoagulation syndrome is the result of electrocoagulation injury to the bowel wall that induces a transmural burn and localized peritonitis without evidence of perforation on abdominal radiograph or CT scan. It usually presents within 12 hours, but may occur up to 5 days after the procedure with complaints of fever, localized abdominal pain, localized peritoneal signs and leukocytosis. Recognition is important to avoid unnecessary exploratory laparotomy since it resolves with conservative treatment (IV hydration, broad-spectrum IV antibiotics, nil by mouth, and analgesia) in the majority of patients.

Prevention of post-polypectomy perforation and post-polypectomy electrocoagulation syndrome

These complications can be prevented by the use of submucosal saline elevation of large polyps prior to transection, because it prevents transmural thermal injury by increasing the degree of separation of the mucosal layers.

Cardiopulmonary complications

Intraprocedural cardiopulmonary complications range from minor fluctuations in oxygen saturation or heart rate, to significant complications like respiratory arrest, cardiac arrhythmias, myocardial infarction, and shock [36].

It is known that the risk of cardiopulmonary events associated with colonoscopy is increased with advanced age [4], higher American Society of Anesthesiologists Physical Status Classification Scores [37, 38] and the presence of comorbidities [4]. Unstable patients should have non-emergent colonoscopy delayed. In addition, continuing aspirin and other antiplatelet agents in the periendoscopic period may reduce the risk of cardiovascular events.

In addition to acute complications, colonoscopy is associated with an increased incidence of cardiovascular events in the 30-day post-procedure period. In a prospective study of patients undergoing colonoscopy, the event rate at 30 days was 1.4 per 1000 for angina, myocardial infarction, stroke, and transient ischemic attack [39].

Gas explosion

Gas explosion can occur when combustible levels of hydrogen or methane gas are present in the colonic lumen, oxygen is present, and electrosurgical energy is used (e.g. electrocautery and argon plasma coagulation). Risk factors are use of non-absorbable or incompletely absorbable carbohydrate preparations, such as mannitol, lactulose or sorbitol [40, 41] and incomplete colonic cleansing either because a sigmoidoscopy preparation was used (e.g. enemas) or because the result of a colonoscopic purge preparation was inadequate [42]. This complication is rare, but has serious consequences.

Rare complications of colonoscopy

These include splenic trauma or rupture [43–45], acute appendicitis [46], diverticulitis [3], or tearing of mesenteric vessels with intra-abdominal hemorrhage. Chemical colitis may occur if glutaraldehyde, used during disinfection, has not been adequately rinsed from the endoscope [47]. Other rare complications are acute colonic (pseudo)obstruction [48], cecal volvulus, vasovagal reactions, endocarditis, and ischemic colitis, the latter being caused by intravascular volume depletion [49]. Sepsis and other infections following colonoscopy are rare. Also subcutaneous emphysema [50, 51], pneumatosis coli, pneumoscrotum, pneumopericardium, and pneumothorax [24, 52] may occur. These are caused by insufflated gas passing into the subcutaneous tissues (subcutaneous emphysema), bowel wall (pneumotosis coli), or retroperitoneum due to polypectomy and/or colonic perforation.

References

1. Fisher D, Maple J, Ben-Menachem T, et al. Complications of colonoscopy. *Gastrointest. Endosc.* 2011;**74**(4):745–52.
2. Waye JD, Kahn O, Auerbach ME. Complications of colonoscopy and flexible sigmoidoscopy. *Gastrointest. Endosc. Clin. N. Am.* 1996;**6**:343–77.
3. Ko CW, Dominitz JA. Complications of colonoscopy: magnitude and management. *Gastrointest. Endosc. Clin. N. Am.* 2010;**20**:659–71.
4. Warren JL, Klabunde CN, Mariotto AB, et al. Adverse events after outpatient colonoscopy in het Medicare population. *Ann. Intern. Med.* 2009;**150**:849–57, W152.
5. Gibbs DH, Opelka FG, Beck DE, Hicks TC. Postpolypectomy colonic hemorrhage. *Dis. Colon Rectum* 1996;**39**:806.
6. Singh M, Mehta N, Murthy UK, et al. Postpolypectomy bleeding in patients undergoing colonoscopy on uninterrupted clopidogrel therapy. *Gastrointest. Endosc.* 2010;**71**:998–1005.
7. Witt DM, Delate T, McCool KH, et al. Incidence and predictors of bleeding or thrombosis after polypectomy in patients receiving and not receiving anticoagulation therapy. *J. Thromb. Haemost.* 2009;**7**:1982–9.
8. Sorbi D, Norton I, Conio M, et al. Postpolypectomy lower GI bleeding: descriptive analysis. *Gastrointest. Endosc.* 2000;**51**:690–6.
9. Buddingh KT, Herngreen T, Haringsma J, et al. Location in the right hemi-colon is an independent risk factor for delayed post-polypectomy hemorrhage: a multi-center case-control study. *Am. J. Gastroenterol.* 2011;**106**:1119–24.
10. Metz AJ, Bourke MJ, Moss A, et al. Factors that prdict bleeding following endoscopic mucosal resection of large colonic lesions. *Endoscopy* 2011;**43**:506–11.
11. Anderson Ma, Ben-Menachem T, Gan SI, et al. Management of antithrombitic agents for endoscopic procedures. *Gastrointest. Endosc.* 2009;**70**:1060–70.
12. Waye JD, Lewis BS, Yessayan S. Colonoscopy: a prospective report of complications. *J. Clin. Gastroenterol.* 1992;**15**:347.
13. Dobrowolski S, Dobosz M, Babicki A, Dymecki D, Hac S. Prophylactic submucosal saline–adrenaline injection in colonoscopic polypectomy: Prospective randomized study. *Surg. Endosc.* 2004;**18**:990–3.
14. Iishi H, Tatsuta M, Narahara H, Iseki K, Sakai N. Endoscopic resection of large pedunculated colorectal polyps using a detachable snare. *Gastrointest. Endosc.* 1996;**44**:594–7.
15. Di Giorgio P, De Luca L, Calcagno G, Rivellini G, Mandato M, De Luca B. Detachable snare versus epinephrine injection in the prevention of postpolypectomy bleeding: A randomized and controlled study. *Endoscopy* 2004;**36**:860–3.
16. 16.Liaquat H, Rohn E, Rex DK. Prophylactic clip closure reduced the risk of delayed postpolypectomy hemorrhage: experience in 277 clipped large sessile or flat colorectal lesions and 247 control lesions. *Gastrointest. Endosc.* 2013;**77**:401–7.
17. Shioji K, Suzuki Y, Kobayashi M, et al. Prophylactic clip application dos not decrease delayed bleeding after colonoscopic polypectomy. *Gastrointest. Endosc.* 2003;**57**:691–4.
18. Kavic SM, Basson MD. Complications of endoscopy. *Am. J. Surg.* 2001;**181**:319–32.
19. Nelson DB, McQuaid KR, Bond JH, Lieberman DA, Weiss DG, Johnston TK. Procedural success and complications of large-scale screening colonoscopy. *Gastrointest. Endosc.* 2002;**55**:307–14.
20. Levin TR, Zhao W, Conell C, et al. Complications of colonoscopy in an integrated health care delivery system. *Ann. Intern. Med.* 2006;**145**:880–6.
21. Rathgaber SW, Wick TM. Colonoscopy completion and complication rates in a community gastroenterology practice. *Gastrointest. Endosc.* 2002;**55**:307–14.
22. Viiala CH, Zimmerman M, Cullen DJ, et al. Complication rates of colonoscopy in an Australian teaching hospital environment. *Intern. Med. J.* 2003;**33**:355–9.
23. Lohsiriwat V, Sujarittanakarn S, Akaraviputh T, Lertakyamanee N, Lohsiriwat D, Kachinthorn U. What are the risk factors of colonoscopic perforation? *BMC Gastroenterol.* 2009;**9**:71.
24. Ho HC, Burchell S, Morris P, Yu M. Colon perforation, bilateral pneumothoraces, pneumopericardium, pneumomediastinum, and subcutaneous emphysema complicating endoscopic polypectomy: anatomic and management considerations. *Am. Surg.* 1996;**62**:770–774.

25. Kavin H, Sinicrope F, Esker AH. Management of perforation of the colon at colonoscopy. *Am. J. Gastroenterol.* 1992;**87**: 161–7.

26. Ker TS, Wasserberg N, Baert Jr RW. Colonoscopic perforation and bleeding of the colon can be treated safely without surgery. *Am. Surg.* 2004;**70**(10):992–4.

27. Hall C, Dorricott NJ, Donovan IA, Neuptolomos JP. Colon perforation during colonoscopy: surgery versus conservative management. *Br. J. Surg.* 1991;**78**:542–4.

28. Stapakis JC, Thickman D. Diagnosis of pneumoperitoneum: abdominal CT vs. upright chest film. J. Comput. Assist. *Tomogr.* 1992;**16**:713–16.

29. Araghizadeh FY, Timmcke AE, Opelka FG, Hichs TC, Beck DE. Colonoscopic perforations. *Dis. Colon Rectum* 2001; **44**(5):713–16.

30. Anderson ML, Pasha TM, Leighton JA. Endoscopic perforation of the colon: lessons from a 10-year study. *Am. J. Gastroenterol.* 2000;**95**:3418–22.

31. Iqbal CW, Cullinane DC, Schiller HJ, et al. Surgical management and outcomes of 165 colonic perforations from a single institution. *Arch. Surg.* 2008;**143**:701–7.

32. Panteris V, Haringsma J, Kuipers EJ. Colonoscopy perforation rate, mechanisms and outcome: from diagnostic to therapeutic colonoscopy. *Endoscopy* 2009;**41**:941–51.

33. Saito Y, Fukuzawa M, Matsuda T, et al. Clinical outcome of endoscopic submucosal dissection versus endoscopic mucosal resection of large colorectal tumors as determined by curative resection. *Surg. Endosc.* 2010;**24**:343–52.

34. Heldwein W, Dollhopf M, Rösch T, et al. The Munich Polypectomy Study (MUPS): prospective analysis of complications and risk factors in 4000 colonic snare polypectomies. *Endoscopy* 2005;**37**:1116–22.

35. Taku K, Sano Y, Fu K, Saito Y. Iatrogenic perforation at therapeutic colonoscopy: should the endoscopist attempt closure using endoclips or transfer immediately to surgery? *Endoscopy* 2006;**38**:428.

36. Cotton PB, Eisen GM, Aabakken L, et al. A lexicon for endoscopic adverse events: report of an ASGE workshop. *Gastrointest. Endosc.* 2010;**71**:446–54.

37. Baudet JS, Diaz-Bethencourt D, Aviles J, et al. Minor adverse events of colonoscopy on ambulatory patients: the impact of moderate sedation. *Eur. J. Gastroenterol. Hepatol.* 2009;**21**:656–61.

38. Vargo JJ, Holub JL, Faigel DO, et al. Risk factors for cardiopulmonary events during propofol-mediated upper endoscopy and colonoscopy. *Aliment. Pharmacol. Ther.* 2006;**24**:955–63.

39. Ko CW, Riffle S, Mochaels L, et al. Serious complications within 30 days of screening and surveillance colonoscopy are uncommon. *Clin. Gastroenterol. Hepatol.* 2010;**8**: 166–73.

40. Avgerinos A, Kalantzis N, Rekoumis G, et al. Bowel preparation and the risk of explosion during colonoscopic polypectomy. *Gut* 1984;**25**:361–4.

41. La Brooy SJ, Avgerinos A, Fendick CL, et al. Potentially explosive colonic concentrations of hydrogen after bowel preparation with mannitol. *Lancet* 1981;**1**:634–6.

42. Monahan DW, Peluso FE, Goldner F. Combustible colonic gas levels during flexible sigmoidoscopy and colonoscopy. *Gastrointest. Endosc.* 1992;**38**:40–3.

43. Kamath AS, Iqbal CW, Sarr MG, et al. Colonoscopic splenic injuries: incidence and management. *J. Gastrointest. Surg.* 2009;**13**:2136–40.

44. Michetti CP, Smeltzer E, Fakhry SM. Splenic injury due to colonoscopy: analysis of the world literature, a new case report, and recommendations for management. *Am. Surg.* 2010;**76**:1198–204.

45. Ahmed A, Eller PM, Schiffman FJ. Splenic rupture: an unusual complication of colonoscopy. *Am. J. Gastroenterol.* 1997;**92**:1201–4.

46. Hirata K, Noguchi J, Yoshikawa I, et al. Acute appendicitis immediately after colonoscopy. *Am. J. Gastroenterol.* 1996;**91**: 2239–40.

47. Caprilli R, Viscido A, Frieri G, et al. Acute colitis following colonoscopy. *Endoscopy* 1998;**30**:428–31.

48. Saunders MD. Acute colonic pseudo-obstruction. *Gastrointest. Endosc. Clin. N. Am.* 2007;**17**(2):341–60.

49. Cheng Y, Wu C, Lee C, Lee T, Hsiao K. Rare complication following screening colonoscopy: ischemic colitis. *Dig. Endosc.* 2012;**24**:379.

50. Bakker K, van Kersen F, Bellaar Spruyt J. Pneumopericardium and pneumomediastinum after polypectomy. *Endoscopy* 1991;**23**:46–7.

51. Humphreys F, Hewetson KA, Dellipiani AW. Massive subcutaneous emphysema following colonoscopy. *Endoscopy* 1984;**16**:160–1.

52. Lovisetto F, Zonta S, Rota E, et al. Left pneumothorax secondary to colonoscopic perforation of the sigmoid colon: a case report. *Surg. Laparosc. Endosc. Percutan. Tech.* 2007; **17**(1):62–4.

CHAPTER 15

Complications of capsule endoscopy

Roy Soetikno[1,2] and Andres Sanchez-Yague[3,4]

[1] Stanford University, Stanford, CA, USA
[2] Veterans Affairs Palo Alto Health Care System, Palo Alto, CA, USA
[3] Vithas Xanit International Hospital, Benalmadena, Spain
[4] Hospital Costa del Sol, Marbella, Spain

Introduction

Endoscopic evaluation of the small bowel has been a challenge because of its significant length and difficulty to reach it with conventional endoscopes. Capsule endoscopy (CE) is a non-invasive technology that allows diagnostic imaging of the entire length of the small bowel [1]. The capsule moves passively through the small bowel, obtaining images that approximate its physiologic state, as it does not inflate the bowel visualizing the mucosa in its collapsed state. It has become the gold standard in evaluating suspected disease of the small intestines [2].

Capsule endoscopy differs from regular endoscopic examinations in many ways mainly due to the inability to control the capsule once swallowed.

Contraindications represent prior conditions that require some kind of action to perform the examination (relative contraindications) or completely preclude it (absolute contraindications). Limitations are conditions that occur during the procedure and somehow affect its outcome; some of those limitations could be considered complications. Limitations can be divided into: technical limitations, if they affect the normal function of any of the components of the diagnostic system; and clinical limitations, if they are related to physiological or pathological conditions of the patient [3]. Some authors have referred to CE limitations as pitfalls [4].

Contraindications

Absolute contraindications

Pregnancy

Pregnancy remains an absolute contraindication to CE mainly due to the presence of limited data in this setting. An anecdotical case report highlights that it can be performed in selected patients [5]. No damage to newborns has been reported to date.

Known or suspected gastrointestinal obstruction

The presence of known or suspected gastrointestinal obstruction represents a contraindication due to the risk of capsule retention. Although CE has shown some role in the study of those patients [6] and a retained capsule has been used to identify the strictured segment prior to surgery in some cases [7], it should not be performed unless the patient is fully informed and willing to undergo surgery.

Programmed magnetic resonance imaging before capsule excretion

Magentic resonance imaging (MRI) should not be performed prior to capsule excretion due to the risk of capsule migration and subsequent internal organ injury though it has not been reported to date [8]. To date there are no MRI-compatible capsules. Capsule excretion should be confirmed with plain abdominal X-ray prior to MRI.

Gastrointestinal Emergencies, Third Edition. Edited by Tony C. K. Tham, John S. A. Collins, and Roy Soetikno.
© 2016 John Wiley & Sons, Ltd. Published 2016 by John Wiley & Sons, Ltd.

Relative contraindications
Patients with cardiac pacemakers or other implanted electromedical devices

Most capsule endoscopes use a frequency of 440 MHz to transmit images. Theoretically, this system may interfere with the normal operation of cardiac pacemakers. The manufacturers have included a written warning that the capsule should not be used in patients with pacemakers. Electromagnetic interference may alter the operation of pacemakers, potentially causing problems in several ways: [1] interference with the ventricular channel includes oversensing, which may result in ventricular pacing inhibition, resulting in bradycardia with dizziness and syncope; undersensing, which may lead to competition with the native QRS complexes possibly resulting in induction of tachyarrhythmias; and induction of asynchronous ventricular (noise mode) function; [2] interference with the atrial channel resulting in oversensing of electromagnetic signals, with a subsequent increase in ventricular pacing rate.

However, there have been studies showing that the capsule is safe to use in patients with implanted cardiac pacemakers and defibrillators [9]. Although electromagnetic interference has been observed this was not clinically significant and no potentially dangerous pacemaker inhibition was observed. On the other hand, recording gaps in the capsule video have been observed [10].

There is one capsule endoscopy model that uses human body communication to transmit the images. A small series showed it was safe in patients with caridac pacemakers and implantable cardiac defibrillators [11].

Patients with swallowing disorders

Patients with swallowing disorders may be unable to ingest the capsule or in case they do they may be at risk for aspiration of the capsule endoscopy into the airway. The initial capsule endoscope measured 11 by 26 mm, and that was considered as a large candy. Available capsule endoscopes present similar dimensions (diameters: 11–13 mm; lengths: 24–31 mm) [12]. Therefore before CE simple questions about eating habits may suffice to determine if the capsule could be ingested. In patients unable to swallow the capsule it may be possible to insert it using a net, polypectomy snare, or even a translucent cap [13]; however, the use of a dedicated delivery device is now preferred [14] even in pediatric patients [15] and in some cases guided by a real-time viewer [16].

Limitations

Technical limitations
Inability to activate the capsule

This limitation although rare is easily overcome using another capsule.

Battery problems

These were more common in the early days of CE. The main problem is a decrease in recording time that can lead to an incomplete examination.

Recording problems

These have been observed in less than 1% of capsule studies in two series [3,4] and anecdotally in patients using telemetry sensors [10]. These problems are usually manifest in small recorded segments and do not prevent completion of the procedure.

Errors during download

These were observed in less than 1% of capsule studies [3,4]. The problem can be usually solved by the company at its headquarters but can result in a significant delay.

Clinical limitations

The main clinical limitation is an incomplete study, in which the capsule fails to reach the cecum during the battery life. This has been attibuted to aspiration into the airway, delayed gastrointestinal passage without a known cause, and capsule retention.

Aspiration into the airway

CE aspiration into the airway is rare. occurring in 1 out of 800–1000 procedures [17]. Although generally benign, it is a potentially fatal complication [18]. A thorough clinical history and ingestion habits could be useful to prevent this complication. In patients unable to swallow the capsule it may be possible to insert it using the techniques as described in the section on patients with swallowing disorders.

Delayed gastrointestinal passage

In a large series of 728 patients failure to reach the cecum was observed in 48 cases (6.59%) with no obvious cause found. Attributed causes of this problem have been a capsule staying in the stomach for the entire recording time in 17 (2.34%) and delayed passage into the duodenum (over 90 minutes from ingestion of the capsule) in 30 (4.12%) though the capsules were excreted uneventfully in all of them later [4].

Inpatients present a higher risk of incomplete small bowel examinations [19] compared to outpatients. Intensive care unit (ICU) patients also present a higher proportion of incomplete exams compared to general medical floor patients. Most of those are related to delayed gastrointestinal passage.

A longer-lasting battery life has shown a increased rate of capsule completion rate [20]. A protocol based on the use of the real-time viewer improved the capsule completion rate from 72.5% to 90%. It included administration of prokinetics if the capsule was still located in the stomach at 60 min or a prokinetic and polyethylene glycol if it had reached the small bowel [21].

Capsule retention

A major risk associated with capsule endoscopy is capsule retention [2]. The ICCE 2005 Consensus for Capsule Retention [2] defined capsule retention as having a capsule endoscope remain in the digestive tract for a minimum of 2 weeks. Capsule retention was further defined as the capsule remaining in the bowel lumen unless directed medical, endoscopic or surgical intervention was undertaken. Clinically significant retention is different from regional transit abnormalities wherein the capsule remains for at least 60 minutes in a single segment of bowel that may or may not have evidence of visible mucosal abnormality. Clinically significant retention is seen in less than 2% of patients [3,4,22], although the rate of capsule retention varies from 0% in healthy patients to 21% in patients with suspected small bowel obstruction [23]. Rare complications include impaction and fracture of the capsule endoscope and intestinal perforation secondary to a retained capsule device.

Causes of capsule retention include Crohn's disease, non-steroidal anti-inflammatory drug (NSAID)-related strictures, small bowel tumors (Fig. 15.1) radiation enteritis, and surgical anastomotic strictures. Retention has not been reported in patients with a "normal" anatomy [1] although it has in those with anatomical variants such as Zenker's diverticulum [24], duodenal diverticulums [25], and colonic diverticulums [26].

Impaction and subsequent fracture of the CE device is a rare complication that has only been reported once [27]. The capsule was retained for 6 months without

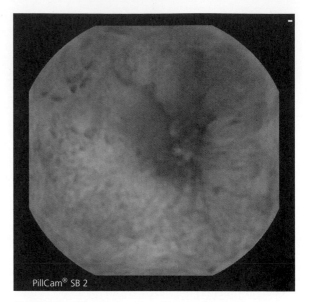

PillCam® SB 2

Fig. 15.1 Small bowel tumor causing capsule retention. (*see insert for color representation of the figure.*)

symptoms but the patient developed abdominal pain. A computerized tomography enterography identified four capsule fragments in the distal small bowel. Exploratory laparotomy was performed with resection of 40 cm of small bowel. The patient did well with no recurrence of abdominal pain.

Only one case of intestinal perforation due to a retained capsule endoscope device has been published [28]. Two months after capsule retention the patient presented with diffuse peritonitis secondary to a distal ileum perforation. The capsule was found in the area of the perforated ileum. The ileal segment was resected. Post-operative course was unremarkable and the patient was discharged.

Management of patients with capsule retention follows some simple steps. Most patients are asymptomatic [29,30], while development of pain usually heralds passage through a tight stricture. If retention is suspected the capsule images should be carefully reviewed as retention can be suspected from the interpretation of capsule images. A clear image of the obstructing lesion may be seen or repetitive views of the same mucosal areas may be visualized. Failure to see the colon during the examination is also an indication, although this is not diagnostic since 10–20% of capsule examinations fail to enter the colon during an 8-hour procedure time. If capsule retention is suspected or if the colon is not entered during the acquisition time, an abdominal or KUB X-ray should be obtained after 2 weeks [2].

Endoscopic or surgical intervention has been shown to be effective for capsule removal [2]. Apart from removal of the retained capsule, surgical intervention has the added advantage of treatment and/or resection of the offending pathology that caused the capsule retention (e.g. strictures).

Although effective in anecdotical reports, larger studies have shown that initiation of medical therapies s(steroids, infliximab, discontinuing NSAIDs, etc.) are not successful in managing capsule retention.

There is no guaranteed screening method to completely prevent capsule retention. Obtaining a good medical history with identification of risk factors remains to be the single best method [2]. Risk factors include known Crohn's disease, history of chronic NSAID use, history of previous small bowel obstruction as well as small bowel resection, previous abdominal surgery, and history of abdominal radiation. Patients with abdominal pain, distention, and nausea should be suspected of having a potential for capsule retention.

Imaging techniques can show long or medium-sized strictures but lack the ability to detect short strictures. Most case reports of capsule retention had prior imaging techniques that were normal [31]. Therefore normal imaging techniques do not rule out the existence of smal bowel strictures. On the other hand, studies on patients with significant strictures on imaging techniques have shown that some of those could undergo capsule endoscopy safely [32].

Another attempt to avoid capsule retention has been the development of the "patency capsule" (Given Imaging, Yoqneam, Israel) [1,2]. This is a self-dissolving capsule that has the same dimensions of the capsule endoscopy device (11 × 26 mm) and consists of a radio-frequency identification (RFID) tag (3 × 13 mm) surrounded by a lactose–barium body and an insoluble outer membrane. The capsule features a timer plug in one of the ends. When retained in a fluid filled environment, the capsule begins dissolving by the aforementioned timer after approximately 40 hours and completes the process in 80 hours, thus allowing the insoluble outer membrane to collapse and pass. The RFID tag is detected by a hand-held RFID scanner. Detection of a signal by the hand-held scanner indicates that the capsule is still retained in the gastrointestinal tract. If the capsule was recovered intact then a regular CE could be performed

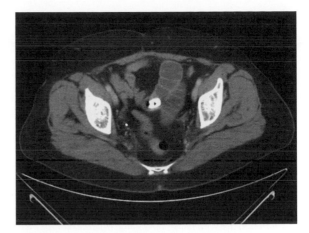

Fig. 15.2 Agile patency capsule causing small bowel obstruction before disintegration. The capsule dissolved on the specified time and symptoms were relieved.

but if the patient developed abdominal pain or the capsule was excreted deformed then a regular capsule examination was contraindicated. This patency capsule did not dissolve in several patients with long strictures and it was thought to be secondary to impaction of the timer plug in the stricture thus preventing disintegration of the capsule [33]. This observation led to the development of the Agile patency capsule (Given Imaging, Yoqneam, Israel) that features timer plugs at both ends potentially preventing that complication (Fig. 15.2). The Agile patency capsule has demonstrated a 100% accuracy in determining which patients could undergo a regular capsule [32]. The small bowel is considered patent for CE if the RFID tag is not detected at 30hours after ingestion or if the Agile is excreted intact.

References

1. Mishkin, D, Chuttani, R, Croffie, J, et al. ASGE Technology Status Evaluation Report: wireless capsule endoscopy. *Gastrointest. Endosc.* 2006;**63**(4):5394–5.
2. Cave, D, Legnani, P, de Franchis, R, Lewis, BS. ICCE Consensus for Capsule Retention. *Endoscopy* 2005;**37**(10):10656–7.
3. Sanchez-Yague A, Romero-Vazquez J, Caunedo-Alvarez A, et al. Limitations in capsule endoscopy examinations. *Gastrointest. Endosc.* 2007;**63**(5):AB114.
4. Rondonotti E, Herrerias JM, Pennazio M, Caunedo A, Mascarenhas-Saraiva M, de Franchis R. Complications, limitations, and failures of capsule endoscopy: a review of 733 cases. *Gastrointest. Endosc.* 2005;**62**(5):712–16.

5. Hogan RB, Ahmad N, Hogan RB 3rd, et al. Video capsule endoscopy detection of jejunal carcinoid in life-threatening hemorrhage, first trimester pregnancy. *Gastrointest Endosc* 2007;**66**(1):205–7.

6. Yang XY, Chen CX, Zhang BL, et al. Diagnostic effect of capsule endoscopy in 31 cases of subacute small bowel obstruction. *World J. Gastroenterol.* 2009;**15**(19):2401–5.

7. Cheon JH, Kim YS, Lee IS, et al. Can we predict spontaneous capsule passage after retention? A nationwide study to evaluate the incidence and clinical outcomes of capsule retention. *Endoscopy* 2007;**39**(12):1046–52.

8. Berry PA, Srirajaskanthan R, Anderson SH. An urgent call to the magnetic resonance scanner: potential dangers of capsule endoscopy. *Clin. Gastroenterol. Hepatol.* 2010;**8**(5):A26.

9. Dubner, S, Dubner, Y, Gallino, S, et al. Electromagnetic interference with implantable cardiac pacemakers by video capsule. *Gastrointest. Endosc.* 2005;**61**(2):250–4.

10. Bandorski D, Lotterer E, Hartmann D, et al. Capsule endoscopy in patients with cardiac pacemakers and implantable cardioverter-defibrillators - a retrospective multicenter investigation. *J. Gastrointest. Liver Dis.* 2011;**20**(1):33–7.

11. Chung JW, Hwang HJ, Chung MJ, Park JY, Pak HN, Song SY. Safety of capsule endoscopy using human body communication in patients with cardiac devices. *Dig. Dis. Sci.* 2012;**57**(6):1719–23.

12. Koulaouzidis A, Rondonotti E, Karargyris A. Small-bowel capsule endoscopy: a ten-point contemporary review. *World J. Gastroenterol.* 2013;**19**(24):3726–46.

13. Almeida N, Figueiredo P, Lopes S, et al. Capsule endoscopy assisted by traditional upper endoscopy. *Rev. Esp. Enferm. Dig.* 2008;**100**(12):758–63.

14. Holden JP, Dureja P, Pfau PR, et al. Endoscopic placement of the small-bowel video capsule by using a capsule endoscope delivery device. *Gastrointest. Endosc.* 2007;**65**(6):842–7.

15. Uko V, Atay O, Mahajan L, Kay M, Hupertz V, Wyllie R. Endoscopic deployment of the wireless capsule using a capsule delivery device in pediatric patients: a case series. *Endoscopy* 2009;**41**(4):380–2.

16. Bass LM, Misiewicz L. Use of a real-time viewer for endoscopic deployment of capsule endoscope in the pediatric population. *J. Pediatr. Gastroenterol. Nutr.* 2012;**55**(5):552–5.

17. Lucendo AJ, González-Castillo S, Fernández-Fuente M, De Rezende LC. Tracheal aspiration of a capsule endoscope: a new case report and literature compilation of an increasingly reported complication. *Dig. Dis. Sci.* 2011;**56**(9):2758–62.

18. Parker C, Davison C, Panter S. Tracheal aspiration of a capsule endoscope: not always a benign event. *Dig. Dis. Sci.* 2012;**57**(6):1727–8.

19. Yazici C, Losurdo J, Brown MD, et al. Inpatient capsule endoscopy leads to frequent incomplete small bowel examinations. *World J. Gastroenterol.* 2012;**18**(36):5051–7.

20. Park JY, Kim HM, Choi YA, et al. Longer capsule endoscopy operation time increases the rate of complete examination of the small bowel. *Hepatogastroenterology* 2010;**57**(101):746–50.

21. Hosono K, Endo H, Sakai E, et al. Optimal approach for small bowel capsule endoscopy using polyethylene glycol and metoclopramide with the assistance of a real-time viewer. *Digestion* 2011;**84**(2):119–25.

22. Liao Z, Gao R, Xu C, Li ZS. Indications and detection, completion, and retention rates of small-bowel capsule endoscopy: a systematic review. *Gastrointest. Endosc.* 2010;**71**(2):280–6.

23. Cheifetz AS, Lewis BS. Capsule endoscopy retention: is it a complication? *J. Clin. Gastroenterol.* 2006;**40**(8):688–91.

24. Ziachehabi A, Maieron A, Hoheisel U, Bachl A, Hagenauer R, Schöfl R. Capsule retention in a Zenker's diverticulum. *Endoscopy* 2011;**43** Suppl 2 UCTN:E387.

25. Ordubadi P, Blaha B, Schmid A, Krampla W, Hinterberger W, Gschwantler M. Capsule endoscopy with retention of the capsule in a duodenal diverticulum. *Endoscopy* 2008;**40** Suppl 2:E247–8.

26. Anderson BW, Liang JJ, Dejesus RS. Capsule endoscopy device retention and magnetic resonance imaging. *Proc. (Bayl. Univ. Med. Cent.)* 2013;**26**(3):270–1.

27. Fry, LC, De Petris, G, Swain,JM, Fleischer, DE. Impaction and fracture of a video capsule in the small bowel requiring laparotomy for removal of the capsule fragments. *Endoscopy* 2005; **37**(7):674–6.

28. Gonzalez Carro, P, Picazo Yuste, J, Fernandez Diez, S, Perez Roldan, F, Roncero Garcia-Escribano, O. Intestinal perforation due to a retained wireless capsule endoscope. *Endoscopy* 2005; **37**:684.

29. Baichi, M, Arifuddin, R, Mantry, PS. What we have learned from 5 cases of permanent capsule retention. *Gastrointest. Endosc.* 2006; **64**(2):283–7.

30. Sears, DM, Avots-Avotins, A, Culp, K, Gavin, MW. Frequency and clinical outcome of capsule retention during capsule endoscopy for GI bleeding of obscure origin. *Gastrointest. Endosc.* 2004; **60**(5):822–7.

31. Li F, Gurudu SR, De Petris G, Sharma VK, et al. Retention of the capsule endoscope: a single-center experience of 1000 capsule endoscopy procedures. *Gastrointest. Endosc.* 2008;**68**(1):174–80.

32. Herrerias JM, Leighton JA, Costamagna G, et al. Agile patency system eliminates risk of capsule retention in patients with known intestinal strictures who undergo capsule endoscopy. *Gastrointest. Endosc.* 2008;**67**(6):902–9.

33. Caunedo-Alvarez A, Romero-Vazquez J, Herrerias-Gutierrez JM. Patency and Agile capsules. *World J. Gastroenterol.* 2008;**14**(34):5269–73.

CHAPTER 16

Complications of endoscopic ultrasound

Maria Cecilia M. Sison-Oh,[1] Andres Sanchez-Yague,[2,3] and Roy Soetikno[4,5]

[1] Medical Center Manila, Manila, Philippines
[2] Vithas Xanit International Hospital, Benalmadena, Spain
[3] Hospital Costa del Sol, Marbella, Spain
[4] Stanford University, Stanford, CA, USA
[5] Veterans Affairs Palo Alto Health Care System, Palo Alto, CA, USA

Introduction

From its conceptualization more than 30 years ago, endoscopic ultrasonography (EUS) has evolved from a novel diagnostic imaging tool to a standard diagnostic and therapeutic modality. It has made a significant impact on the diagnosis and management of gastrointestinal and non-gastrointestinal diseases. These advances are due to the development of the linear array echoendoscope, which allows the placement of devices into the ultrasound plane of view, permitting various interventions to be accomplished. Among these interventions is the endoscopic ultrasound guided fine needle aspiration of lesions that are too small to be visualized by computerized tomography (CT) scan or magnetic resonance imaging (MRI) or lesions that are well encased by surrounding vascular structures.

EUS and EUS-guided fine needle aspiration (FNA) biopsy have emerged as accurate and safe methods for diagnosing and staging gastrointestinal and selected non-gastrointestinal malignancies [1]. EUS-FNA has a complication rate of approximately 1% [2]. Reported complications are related to biopsy of cystic and solid lesions [3]. In a large multicenter trial involving 554 consecutive mass or lymph node biopsies, only five (0.9%) complications were reported, all of which were non-fatal [4]. These complications were endoscope-induced perforation, superimposed infection of aspirated cystic lesions, and hemorrhage. EUS-FNA morbidity reported in a review of prospective series ranged between 0–2.5%; there was one death among 2468 patients (0.04%), with complications mostly from infection, bleeding and acute pancreatitis [2]. Major complications were observed in 2.5% of 355 patients who underwent EUS-FNA for solid pancreatic masses in another series [5], including infection and acute pancreatitis. There were no deaths reported.

In recent years, non-surgical EUS-guided drainage of pancreatic pseudocysts and pancreatic fluid collections has emerged and more clinicians prefer this mode of treatment over the more invasive surgical methods, since surgery is associated with a significant percentage of complications, and even mortality [6]. Reviews and retrospective studies report non-life-threatening immediate and medium-term complications of abdominal pain (78%, 47/55), jaundice (9%, 5/55), stent clogging (5%, 3/55), infection (5%, 3/55), and pseudocyst recurrence (10%, 6/55) [1,6].

The advent of endosonography has also resulted in the development of advances in palliative pain management. Through endoscopic ultrasound, the celiac plexus is visualized, then neurolysis is performed using the transgastric route, achieving results, comparable, if not better than percutaneous neurolysis. Currently, it is an accepted alternative method for celiac plexus neurolysis. There are reports, however, of serious neurological complications in 2% of patients such as paralysis, paresis, paresthesia of the lower extremities, hypotonia, as well as some minor complications such as pain immediately postprocedure and transient orthostasis, as well as self-limited diarrhea [8]. Isolated cases of retroperitoneal abscess formation after EUS guided celiac plexus block have likewise been reported [1].

Gastrointestinal Emergencies, Third Edition. Edited by Tony C. K. Tham, John S. A. Collins, and Roy Soetikno.
© 2016 John Wiley & Sons, Ltd. Published 2016 by John Wiley & Sons, Ltd.

The purpose of this chapter is to provide a review of complications seen in diagnostic and therapeutic endoscopic ultrasonography.

Complications

Hemorrhage

Hemorrhagic complications including extraluminal bleeding and intracystic hemorrhage are uncommon in EUS-FNA procedures as well as EUS-guided drainage procedures of pancreatic pseudocysts and fluid collections [2]. The mechanism for post EUS-guided FNA bleeding probably relates to injuring the blood supply to the aspirated lesion [9]. Extraluminal bleeding has been reported to occur from 1.3%-4% [1,2]. In a series of 50 patients who underwent EUS-guided FNA of pancreatic cystic lesions, three (6%) developed acute intracystic hemorrhage. Bleeding in all three cases stopped spontaneously after several minutes [10]. In a retroprospective study of 148 patients, one patient with underlying acquired factor VIII inhibitors developed bleeding [11]. A case report of arterial bleeding during EUS-guided pseudocyst drainage was also reported [12]. In another study of 208 patients who underwent EUS-guided FNA, two (~1%) patients developed hemorrhage [13]. Only one (0.18%) patient developed hemorrhage in a trial of 554 patients who underwent EUS-guided FNA [4].

Endosonographic appearance

Extraluminal hemorrhage is recognized by the development of an expanding echopoor zone surrounding the site of needle puncture of the targeted lesion [14]. The appearance is compatible with that of an hematoma. This is supported by the aspiration of blood tinged-fluid [14] in the aspirating syringe. In a study conducted by Varadarajulu et al. [10] intracystic hemorrhage was readily recognized during EUS-FNA as an expanding hyperechoic area around the site of needle puncture within the targeted cyst (Fig 16.1). This is again supported by aspiration of blood-tinged fluid.

Management

- Immediate recognition of this complication is important because it permits immediate termination of the procedure.
- The lesion should be observed endosonographically for cessation of bleeding.

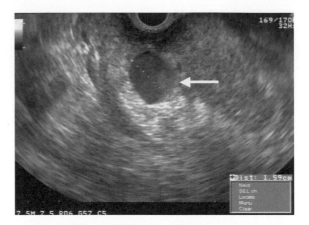

Fig. 16.1 Intracystic hemorrhage after fine needle aspiration using a 22 gauge needle of a pancreatic cyst.

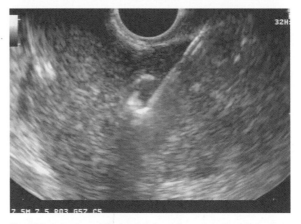

Fig. 16.2 Injection of fibrin glue into the cyst cavity after an arterial bleeding occurred and did not stop spontaneously 20 minutes after EUS FNA of a pancreatic cyst. The bleeding stopped instantaneously after injection of fibrin glue.

- If bleeding does not cease after a short period of time, pressure may be applied for 15–25 minutes at the needle puncture site by inflation of the balloon and by tip deflection of the echoendoscope [14].
- EUS-guided injection of epinephrine at the bleeding site may be performed [11].
- Another option is to inject fibrin glue into the cyst cavity in the region of the bleeding vessel, which can be identified by a pulsating vascular flow (Fig 16.2).

Prevention

Doppler imaging is vital in identifying vascular structures that need to be avoided during EUS interventional procedures. For example, the presence of large vessels in the center of a solid mass may be clarified using Doppler imaging [15]. As such, the risk of bleeding may be reduced by initially targeting only the periphery of the lesion and to move centrally only if inadequate samples are obtained [14]. The endoscopist must also ensure that smaller and easily compressible blood vessels are not within the needle path, as these are easily obscured and may not appear during Doppler imaging. In the event that a blood vessel was traversed, unintentionally or otherwise, care should taken to avoid torquing the echoendoscope as this may lacerate the blood vessel wall and increase the bleeding risk [15].

Patient factors also influence the risk of bleeding. A prospective controlled study by Kien-Fong et al. [16] evaluating bleeding rates after EUS-FNA in patients taking aspirin/non-steroidal anti-inflammatory drugs (NSAIDs) and low-molecular-weight heparin (LMWH) showed that bleeding was significantly more likely in patients on low molecular weight heparin than in patients not taking any antithrombotic agents. ASGE guidelines [17] recommend that for a planned high-risk procedure, such as EUS-FNA, the clinician may elect to discontinue aspirin and/or NSAIDs 5 to 7 days before the procedure. In other guidelines, EUS-FNA of solid masses and lymph nodes may be performed on patients taking aspirin or NSAIDs. However, EUS-FNA of cystic lesions should be avoided in patients taking any antiplatelet agent [18]. Warfarin, LMWH, oral thienopyridines (e.g. clopidogrel) should be discontinued prior to any EUS sampling procedure [17,19]. Moreover, a platelet count of >50 000/mm and an International Normalized Ratio (INR) <1.5 prior to EUS-FNA are recommended [15].

Pancreatitis

EUS-FNA of a pancreatic lesion carries the risk of pancreatitis as the needle traverses through healthy pancreatic tissue and/or ducts to reach the target lesion, or from inflammation as a result of intracystic hemorrhage [9,15]. Pancreatitis was noted to occur more commonly after EUS-FNA of pancreatic cystic lesions located in the pancreatic head or uncinate process [9]. In a pooled analysis of 19 centers involving 4909 EUS-guided FNAs of solid pancreatic lesions, pancreatitis occurred in 14 cases (0.29%) [20]. In another trial of 355 patients who underwent EUS-FNA for a solid pancreatic mass, three patients developed pancreatitis [5]. In a systematic review and recent meta-analysis of EUS-FNA morbidity

and mortality, acute pancreatitis occurred in 36 of 8246 patients (0.44%). Twenty-seven of these patients had mild pancreatitis, 6 had moderate pancreatitis, and 3 had severe pancreatitis [21].

Clinical features
- Presents within the first 24 hours after the procedure.
- Epigastric abdominal pain.
- Abdominal tenderness and guarding are also common.
- Nausea and vomiting.
- Elevated pancreatic enzymes at least 3x the upper limit of normal.

Management
The management of patients with pancreatitis after EUS-FNA of the pancreas is similar to the management of patients with pancreatitis due to other causes.

Prevention
Although there is no proven evidence, waiting 6 weeks after clinical resolution of the prior episode of acute pancreatitis may decrease the risk of developing acute pancreatitis with EUS-FNA [15]. The indication for pancreatic EUS-FNA should also be taken into account as studies suggest that nonmalignant pancreatic pathology is associated with an increased risk of acute pancreatitis [15]. In addition, in a review by Jenssen et al., it is recommended that EUS-FNA of pancreatic masses should be restricted to patients in whom a definitive cytopathological diagnosis is likely to alter management significantly [18].

Perforation
Cases of perforation have been described after EUS-FNA [3,10]. This is thought to be related to the passage of the echoendoscope rather than the FNA itself [3], and this may be due to the oblique-viewing optics of the scope [3]. Other factors associated with perforation during EUS procedures include the natural anatomical areas of angulation (e.g. hypopharynx, hiatal hernia, tip of duodenal bulb, rectosigmoid junction), presence of unexpected anatomical alterations such as an esophageal or duodenal diverticula, and luminal obstruction (e.g. gastrointestinal malignancies) [18]. The esophagus and duodenum are the most common sites for perforation (Fig. 16.3).

A single-center study in the United States enrolled patients undergoing upper gastrointestinal EUS over a

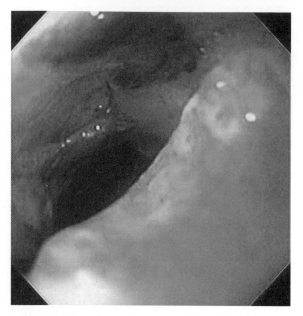

Fig. 16.3 Esophageal tear after passage of the echoendoscope. (*see insert for color representation of the figure.*)

Table 16.1 Guidelines for medical and surgical management of esophageal perforation.

Medical (non-operative) management	Surgical management
• Patients who are clinically stable (minimal pain, normotension, minimal fever, mild leukocytosis) • Instrumental perforations of patient on NPO* status and perforation detected within 2 hours • Perforations with a long delay in diagnosis such that the patient has already demonstrated a tolerance for the perforation • Perforations that are well contained and drain into the esophageal lumen (i.e. no crepitus, pneumothorax, pneumoperitoneum, or leak into the abdominal cavity)	• Patients who are clinically unstable (sepsis, respiratory failure, hypotension) • Non-contained perforations with contamination of the mediastinum or pleural space • Perforation of the intra-abdominal esophagus • Associated pneumothorax • Perforations with retained foreign bodies • Perforations from esophageal diseases for which elective surgery would be considered in the absence of a perforation (achalasia, stricture, carcinoma)

* NPO, nothing by mouth.

7-year period. Cervical esophageal perforations occurred in 3 out of 4844 patients (0.03%) [18]. A survey of German centers performing EUS was conducted from 2004 to 2006, and data showed a total of 8 cases of esophageal perforation out 85 084 (0.009%) EUS procedures. The study also showed 19 cases of duodenal perforation (0.022%) [18,22]. Perforation at the site of transmural stenting during EUS guided drainage of pancreatic fluid collections has also been reported (2/148, 1.3%) [11].

Clinical features of esophageal perforation (see Chapter 21, Oesophageal Perforation)

- Characteristic features include the triad of pain, fever, and subcutaneous or mediastinal air.
- The pain is usually localized to the site of perforation.
- In the elderly or very young, symptoms may be less severe.
- Chest and upright abdominal X-ray films should be obtained.
  - Although plain radiographs indicate abnormal findings in up to 90% of esophageal perforations, findings may be normal soon after perforation.
  - Films may reveal subcutaneous emphysema, pneumomediastinum, mediastinal air-fluid levels, mediastinal widening, pneumothorax, hydrothorax, pleural effusion, or pulmonary infiltrates.

- Contrast radiographic studies should be performed in cases of clinically suspected esophageal perforation.
  - Water-soluble contrast medium should be used in small boluses at first to prevent aspiration because of this agent's pulmonary toxicity. Although barium contrast material clearly is superior in demonstrating small perforations, it causes an inflammatory response in the mediastinal, pleural, and peritoneal cavities.
  - Films may show findings of extravasation of contrast in the area of perforation.

Management (see Table 16.1)

Non-surgical endoscopic management options for perforation have been reported and recent evidence shows that a substantial number of esophageal perforation patients can be managed using these means (Table 16.1). Patients with small, well-defined tears and minimal extraesophageal involvement may be better managed by non-operative methods [22]. The criteria for non-surgical management, as enumerated by Altorjay et. al. [23], include early diagnosis or late diagnosis

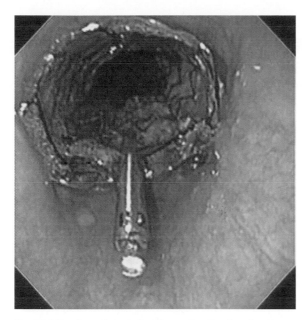

Fig. 16.4 Esophageal stent placed over the site of perforation. (*see insert for color representation of the figure.*)

with contained leak, perforation not in the abdomen, contained perforation in the mediastinum, content of the perforation draining back to the esophagus, perforation does not involve neoplasm or obstruction of the esophagus, absence of sepsis, and presence of experienced thoracic surgeon and contrast imaging in the hospital.

Non-surgical management options include the placement of removable covered expandable metallic stents over the area of perforation. With the use of these stents, both primary and secondary esophageal leaks are being treated with reduced hospital stay, fewer adjunctive procedures, and early resumption of oral intake [24]. In a study by Johnsson et al. [25], 22 consecutive patients with esophageal perforation were managed by the placement of a covered expandable metallic stent. Of the 22 cases, five (23%) patients died within 30 days of perforation. The remaining 17 were successfully managed with the expandable metal stent. In a different study conducted by White et al. [26], nine esophageal cancer patients with iatrogenic perforation were treated with a coated self-expanding metal stents (Fig. 16.4). All the patients had an unremarkable hospital course and were discharged on soft diet. On follow-up, all the patients had no signs of infection or recurrent dysphagia.

Fibrin sealant has also been used in the treatment of esophageal perforations. In addition, successful endoscopic closure of perforations with metallic clips has been reported for perforations associated with instrumentation [24].

Surgical management remains to be the main modality of treatment for esophageal perforations (Table 16.1). There is no clear-cut recommendation for indication of surgery but it includes hemodynamic instability, intraabdominal perforation, extravasation of contrast material into the different body cavities, and presence of underlying malignancy, obstruction, or stricture in the region of the perforation [24,27]. There are different procedures for the repair of esophageal perforations. However, the choice of procedure depends on the surgeon's experience, etiology of perforation, time from injury to diagnosis, and site of perforation [24].

• Conservative/non-operative management [23]
  ○ Nothing per mouth
  ○ Total parenteral nutrition should be initiated if a prolonged course is anticipated
  ○ Large-bore intravenous access
  ○ Intravenous fluids with normal saline to replace fluid volume loss.
  ○ Placement of nasogastric tube to clear gastric contents and limit further contamination
  ○ Early administration of broad-spectrum IV antibiotics and it should be given for a minimum of 7–10 days
  ○ Adequate analgesia
• Surgery.

Prevention

It is important to have an understanding of any anatomic or structural features that may increase the risk of perforation. Knowledge of prior difficult examinations is helpful in planning future examinations [15]. In stenosing tumors and for specific anatomical locations, care should be take in maneuvering the echoendoscope. Furthermore, dilation to achieve echoendoscope passage through malignant strictures should only be performed in select cases, with dilation restricted to15mm only to limit the risk of perforation [15,24].

Superimposed infection

Clinical infectious complications after EUS-FNA of solid lesions are uncommon, with rates of 0–0.6% in large prospective studies [4,10,19,22,28,29]. As such, prophylactic antibiotic therapy is not routinely recommended for EUS-FNA of solid masses and lymph nodes [1]. It is generally accepted, however, that EUS-FNA of cystic or fluid collections is associated with a higher risk of infection, and therefore warrants antibiotic prophylaxis followed by a short postprocedure antibiotic course [1,2,11,19,30]. Mediastinal cysts are at risk for infection during EUS-FNA, despite administration of prophylactic antibiotic therapy, and infections from the procedure may result in life-threatening mediastinitis [1,15,19,30]. For this reason and because of limited clinical impact, EUS-FNA of simple mediastinal cysts is usually contraindicated [2]. There have also been isolated reports of retroperitoneal abscesses after EUS guided celiac plexus block [1].

Management
- Broad-spectrum antibiotics for 7–14 days.
- In cases, where an abscess develops, abscess drainage procedures are performed in addition to the administration of broad-spectrum antibiotics [1,19].

Prevention
Current guidelines do not recommend antibiotic prophylaxis in average risk patients undergoing EUS-FNA of solid masses or lymph nodes [15]. However, antibiotic prophylaxis should be administered in patients undergoing EUS-FNA of cystic lesions and fluid collections [1,2,19].

Aspiration
Aspiration of food or fluid into the lungs is an uncommon complication. In a Danish prospective study, tracheal suction was needed in 5.1% of patients (15/293), but only one patient aspirated during the procedure (0.3%) [28].

Management
- Terminate the procedure.
- Perform aggressive chest physiotherapy.
- Oxygen support through a nasal cannula or a face mask.
  - If the patient, remains hypoxic, consider ventilatory support.
- Request for a chest X-ray.
- Broad-spectrum antibiotics.
- Other labs
  - Hemogram
  - Metabolic panel
  - Sputum culture and sensitivity.

Prevention
- No food or drink at least 6 hours prior to procedure.
- Suction oral secretions.
- If possible, keep patient on his/her left side throughout the entire procedure.
- When filling the lumen of the gastrointestinal tract with water, elevate the head of the bed to about 30 degrees.
- Water filling in the upper gastrointestinal tract should be restricted to the minimum amount necessary and the endoscopy unit and team should be prepared to do nasopharyngeal suction [19].

Oversedation
Providing adequate sedation and analgesia is a vital part in the practice of gastrointestinal endoscopy. Most endoscopic procedures are performed under "conscious sedation". At this level of sedation, the patient is able to make a purposeful response to tactile and verbal stimulation. At the same time, pulmonary and cardiovascular function are maintained [7]. This type of sedation is accomplished with the use of a benzodiazepine alone or in combination with an opiate. The most commonly used benzodiazepines are midazolam and diazepam. Midazolam is favored by most endoscopists for its fast onset of action, high amnestic properties, and shorter duration of action [7]. Opiates such as fentanyl and meperidine provide both sedation and analgesia. Fentanyl has a faster onset of action and clearance as well as a reduced incidence of nausea compared to meperidine. Combination of these agents are frequently utilized, especially during longer procedures. However, such combinations increase the risk of oversedation, oxygen desaturation and cardiorespiratory complications.

Only a few studies report on the frequency of sedation-associated complications in EUS and EUS-FNA. In the German Prospective EUS Registry, oxygen desaturation ($SpO_2 < 80\%$) was reported in 0.39% of patients, but majority of patients did not require intubation or mechanical ventilation [19]. In a retrospective study on the safety of nurse-administered propofol sedation for upper gastrointestinal EUS, 6 out of 806 patients (0.7%) experienced oxygen desaturation ($SpO_2 < 90\%$), and 4 patients (0.5%) required assisted positive pressure ventilation [31].

Management
- Reversal agents
  - Flumazenil (Romazicon), an imidazobenzodiazepine derivative, is a competitive benzodiazepine

antagonist. It has been shown to effectively antagonize benzodiazepine-induced sedation and ventilatory depression, as well as psychomotor impairment and retrograde amnesia. Doses of 0.1–0.2 mg produce partial antagonism, whereas higher doses of 0.4–1.0 mg usually produce complete antagonism in patients who have received the usual amount of sedation. Reversal effect is evident within 1–2 minutes after administration, and the peak effect is seen in 6–10 minutes after injection.

○ Naloxone (Narcan) is a competitive opioid antagonist. It reverses opioid-induced respiratory depression, sedation and hypotension. When administered intravenously, the onset of action is apparent within 2 minutes. The usual initial dose is 0.4–2 mg IV. If there is no apparent response or if response is inadequate, doses may be repeated at 2–3 minute intervals. The maximum dosage is 10 mg.

Prevention

Guidelines for conscious sedation and monitoring during endoscopy [7] were formulated by the American Society for Gastrointestinal Endoscopy to minimize complications associated with oversedation. A summary of these guidelines include:

- A focused history and physical examination is required prior to the administration of moderate sedation.
- Routine monitoring of patient's pulse rate, blood pressure, and oxygen saturation are useful in identifying early problems [7,14].
- The use of benzodiazepines and/or opiates will result in a satisfactory outcome in nearly all patients.
- Specific antagonists of opiates (naloxone) and benzodiazepines (flumazenil) are available and should be present in every endoscopy unit to treat over-sedated patients.

Summary

Endoscopic ultrasound and EUS-guided interventional procedures are generally safe and effective modalities. However, adverse events do develop, and as these procedures assume more defining roles in the diagnosis and management of gastrointestinal and non-gastrointestinal diseases, the potential for these adverse events will likely increase. Adherence to guidelines on indications and contraindications, adequate education as well as in-depth training are vital conditions necessary for enhancing the safety and efficacy of EUS procedures. Knowledge of potential complications, their expected frequency and associated risk factors may help minimize their occurrence. Steps should be actively taken to minimize the frequency and severity of these complications, but if they do occur, early recognition and timely intervention may minimize morbidity and mortality and result in improved outcomes.

References

1. ASGE Guideline: Adverse events associated with EUS and EUS FNA. *Gastrointest. Endosc.* 2013;**77**(6):839–43.
2. Polkowski M, Larghi A, Weynand B, Giovannini M, Pujol B, Dumonceau J-M. Learning, techniques, and complications of endoscopic ultrasound (EUS)-guided sampling in gastroenterology: European Society of Gastrointestinal Endoscopy (ESGE) Technical Guideline. *Endoscopy* 2012;**44**:190–205.
3. Gress, F, Bhattacharya, I. *Endoscopic Ultrasonography*. Blackwell Science: Oxford, 2001.
4. Wiersema, MJ, Villmann, P, Giovannini, M, et al. Endosonography-guided fine-needle aspiration biopsy: Diagnostic accuracy and complication assessment. *Gastroenterology* 1997;**112**:1087.
5. Eloubeidi, MA, Tamhane, A, Varadarajulu, S, Wilcox, CM. Frequency of major complications after EUS-guided FNA of solid pancreatic masses: A prospective evaluation. *Gastrointest. Endosc.* 2006;**63**:622.
6. Ng PY, Rasmussen DN, Vilmann P, et al. Endoscopic ultrasound-guided drainage of pancreatic pseudocysts: Medium-term assessment of outcomes and complications. *Endosc. Ultrasound* 2013;**2**(4):199–203.
7. Guidelines for conscious sedation and monitoring during gastrointestinal endoscopy. *Gastrointest. Endosc.* 2003;**53**(3):317–22.
8. Wiechowska-Kozlowska A, Boer K, Wójcicki M, et al. The efficacy and safety of endoscopic ultrasound-guided celiac plexus neurolysis for treatment of pain in patients with pancreatic cancer. Gastroenterol. Res. Pract. 2012;1–5.
9. O'Toole, D, Palazzo, L, Arotcarena, R, Dancour, A, Aubert, A, Hammel P Amaris, J. Ruszniewski, P, Assessment of complications of EUS-guided fine-needle aspiration. *Gastrointest. Endosc.* 2001;**53**(4):470.
10. Varadarajulu, S, Eloubeidi, MA. Frequency and significance of acute intracystic hemorrhage during EUS-FNA of cystic lesions of the pancreas. *Gastrointest. Endosc.* 2004;**60**(4):631–5.
11. Varadarajulu S, Christein JD, Wilcox CM. Frequency of complications during EUS-guided drainage of pancreatic fluid collections in 148 consecutive patients. *J. Gastroenterol. Hepatol.* 2011;**26**(10):1504 8.

12. Săftoiu A, Ciobanu L, Seicean A, Tantău M. Arterial bleeding during EUS-guided pseudocyst drainage stopped by placement of a covered self-expandable metal stent. *BMC Gastroenterology* 2013;**13**:93.

13. Gress, FG, Hawes, RH, Savides, TJ, Ikenberry, SO, Lehman, GO. Endoscopic ultrasound-guided fine-needle aspiration using linear array and radial scanning endosonography. *Gastrointest. Endosc.* 1997;**45**:243–50.

14. Affi, A, Vasquez-Sequeiros, E, Norton,I, Clain, J, Wiersema, M. Acute extraluminal hemorrhage associated with EUS-guided fine needle aspiration: Frequency and clinical significance. *Gastrointest. Endosc.* 2001;**53**(2):221–5.

15. Fujii L, Levy M. Basic techniques in endoscopic ultrasound-guided fine needle aspiration for solid lesions: Adverse events and avoiding them. *Endosc. Ultrasound* 2014;**3**(1):35–45.

16. Kien-Fong V, Chang F, Doig L, et al. A prospective control study of the safety and cellular yield of EUS-guided FNA or Trucut biopsy in patients taking aspirin, nonsteroidal anti-inflammatory drugs, or prophylactic low molecular weight heparin. *Gastrointest. Endosc.* 2006;**63**:808–13.

17. ASGE Guideline: Management of antithrombotic agents for endoscopic procedures. *Gastrointest. Endosc.* 2009;**70**(6): 1060–70.

18. Jenssen C, Alvarez-Sánchez MV, Napoléon B, et al. Diagnostic endoscopic ultrasonography: Assessment of safety and prevention of complications. *World J. Gastroenterol.* 2012;**18**(34):4659–76.

19. Boustiére C, Veitch A, Vanbiervliet G, et al. Endoscopy and antiplatelet agents. European Society of Gastrointestinal Endoscopy ESGE Guideline. *Endoscopy* 2011;**43**:445–61.

20. Eloubeidi, MA, Gress, FG, Savides, TJ, Wiersema, MJ. Acute pancreatitis after EUS-guided FNA of solid pancreatic masses: A pooled analysis from EUS centers in the United States. *Gastrointest. Endosc.* 2004; **60**:385.

21. Wang KX, Ben QW, Jin ZD, et al. Assessment of morbidity and mortality associated with EUS-guided FNA: a systematic review. *Gastrointest. Endosc.* 2011;**73**(2): 283–90.

22. Jenssen C, Faiss S, Nürnberg D. [Complications of endoscopic ultrasound and endoscopic ultrasound-guided interventions – results of a survey among German centers]. Z. *Gastroenterol.* 2008;**46**:1177–84.

23. Altorjay A, Kiss J, Voros A, et al. Nonoperative management of eosphageal perforations: Is it justified? *Ann. Surg.* 1997;**225**(4):415–21.

24. Kaman L, Iqbal J, Kundil B, et al. Management of esophageal perforation in adults. *Gastroenterol. Res.* 2010;**3**(6):235–44.

25. Johnsson, E, Lundell, L, Liedman, B. Sealing of esophageal perforation or rupture with expandable metal stents: A prospective controlled study on treatment efficacy and limitations. *Dis. Esophagus* 2005; **18**(4):262–6.

26. White, RE, Munqatana, C, Topazian, M. Expandable metal stent for iatrogenic perforation of esophageal malignancies. *Gastrointest. Surg.* 2003;**7**(6):715–9.

27. Gupta NM, Kaman L. Personal management of 57 consecutive patients with esophageal perforation. *Am J Surg* 2004; **187**(1):58–63.

28. Mortensen MD, Fristrup C, Holm FS, et al. Prospective evaluation of patient tolerability, satisfaction with patient information, and complications in endoscopic ultrasonography. *Endoscopy* 2005;**37**(2):146–53.

29. Al-Haddad M, Wallace MB, Woodward TA, et al. The safety of fine-needle aspiration guided by endoscopic ultrasound: a prospective study. *Endoscopy* 2008;**40**:204–8.

30. Diehl D, Cheruvattath R, Facktor M, Go BD. Infection after endoscopic ultrasound-guided aspiration of mediastinal cysts. *Interactive Cardiovasc. Thorac. Surg.* 2010;**10**: 338–40.

31. Fatima H, DeWitt J, LeBlanc J, et al. Nurse-administered propofol sedation for upper endoscopic ultrasonography. *Am. J. Gastroenterol.* 2008;**103**:1649–56.

CHAPTER 17

Complications of Endoscopic Mucosal Resection (EMR) and Endoscopic Submucosal Dissection (ESD)

Ichiro Oda, Haruhisa Suzuki, and Seiichiro Abe

National Cancer Center Hospital, Tokyo, Japan

Introduction

Endoscopic resection has been accepted as a less-invasive method for local resection of superficial gastrointestinal tumors having a negligible risk of lymph-node metastasis [1–3]. The methods vary from polypectomy, endoscopic mucosal resection (EMR) to endoscopic submucosal dissection (ESD). EMR procedures include inject and cut, strip biopsy, EMR with a cap-fitted endoscope, endoscopic aspiration mucosectomy, and EMR with a ligating device; ESD is a relatively new endoscopic resection method that facilitates one-piece resection. The appropriate endoscopic resection technique should be safe, effective and suitable to a variety of clinical situations. Endoscopic resection is associated with various complication risks such as bleeding and perforation. In this chapter, we describe the endoscopic resection related complications and the methods for managing them.

Stomach

Perforation

The rates of perforation during gastric EMR and ESD have been reported as 0.5–5.3% and 1.2–9.6%, respectively [4–16]. The risk factors of gastric perforations during ESD have been reported as: lesions in the upper third of the stomach, larger size lesions and lesions with ulcer findings [9,15,16]. In terms of delayed perforations occurring after completion of gastric ESD, such perforations occur in approximately 0.5% [17].

Closure of a perforation using endoscopic clips after snare excision of a gastric leiomyoma was first reported by Binmoeller et al. in 1993 [18]. In 2006, endoscopic closure with endoscopic clips for EMR/ESD-related gastric perforations was reported to be effective in a large series of consecutive cases [6]. Two methods of endoscopic closure have been reported including the "single-closure method" and the "omental-patch method" using endo-clips with a right-angle hook (HX-610–090, HX-610-090L; Olympus Medical Systems Corp., Tokyo, Japan) [6]. The single-closure method is performed to treat small defects and starts from the edge of the perforation rather than the center. The omental-patch method is performed on relatively larger defects by suctioning either the greater omentum or the lesser omentum into the stomach lumen and then clipping the omentum as a patch to the edges of the perforation. (Fig. 17.1).

Bleeding

Bleeding complications can be subdivided into immediate (intraoperative) bleeding, occurring during the procedure, and delayed bleeding, taking place after the procedure with respect to the time of onset. Immediate bleeding is infrequent with EMR techniques, but is common with ESD. Management of immediate bleeding plays a critical role in the successful completion of ESD. It is difficult to measure precisely the volume of bleeding during endoscopic resection, so significant immediate bleeding was defined in a previous study as the diminution of ≥2 g/dL in hemoglobin (Hb) comparing preprocedure and next-day levels. Evidence of significant immediate bleeding was found in 63 of 945 patients

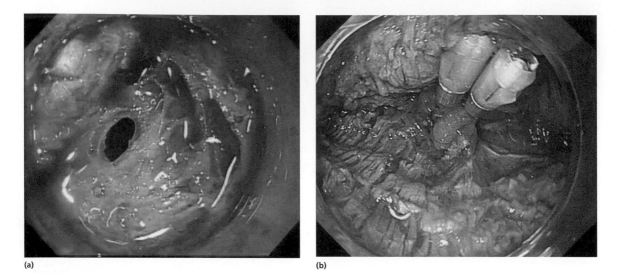

Fig. 17.1 (a) Perforation occurred during gastric ESD. (b) Perforation closed successfully with "omental-patch method" using endoclips. (*see insert for color representation of the figure.*)

(7%) in that particular study [9]. The rates of significant immediate bleeding in the upper and middle thirds of the stomach are higher than in the lower third of the stomach because of the larger diameter of the submucosal arteries in the upper and middle thirds of the stomach [19].

The reported rate of delayed bleeding after EMR is 3.9–5.3% [4,7,8,20]. Delayed bleeding after ESD has been reported to range from 0 to 15.6% [5,7–14,21]. This wide variation is partly due to differences in the definition of delayed bleeding as used in the reported studies. For example, the definition of delayed bleeding can vary from bleeding with a clinical symptom such as hematemesis and melena, bleeding necessitating endoscopic treatment to bleeding requiring a blood transfusion. Delayed bleeding has been reported to relate to lesion location, size, patient age and procedure time [9,22,23]. In our previously published case series, 76% of patients experienced delayed bleeding within 24 hours after ESD and the remaining 24% between 2 and 15 days following the procedure [9].

Electrocautery is used for hemostasis of immediate bleeding during ESD because endoscopic clips interfere with the subsequent resection procedure [19,24]. Electrocautery is usually performed using different devices, depending on the degree of bleeding. Minor oozing can be controlled by electrocautery using a cutting device such as the IT knife2, Hook knife, Dual knife (KD-611L, KD-620LR, KD-650L; Olympus Medical Systems Corp.,

Tokyo, Japan), FlushKnife BT, or SAFEKnifeV (DK2618JB, DK2518DV; Fujifilm Corp., Tokyo, Japan). Electrocautery using hemostatic forceps such as the Coagrasper (FD-410LR; Olympus Medical Systems Corp., Tokyo, Japan) or hot biopsy forceps (Radial Jaw; Boston Scientific Japan Corp., Tokyo, Japan) is suitable for arterial bleeding. (Fig. 17.2) The critical step in achieving effective hemostasis is identification of the exact bleeding point using water flushing. Endoscopes equipped with water-jet systems (GIF-Q260J; Olympus Medical Systems Corp., Tokyo, Japan) (EG-450RD5; Fujifilm Corp., Tokyo, Japan) have been available for use to precisely identify the bleeding point. It is also necessary to pre-coagulate to prevent bleeding when vessels are found during the procedure.

All endoscopic treatment modalities can also be used individually or in combination for hemostasis of delayed bleeding after endoscopic resection. Different modalities are applied according to the period of delayed bleeding. In the early days of delayed bleeding, the artificial ulcer floor is still soft with less granulation tissue so endoscopic clips or electrocautery using hemostatic forceps can be applied to control this complication. In the later days of delayed bleeding, the artificial ulcer floor hardens with granulation tissue so the injection method is preferable.

In an effort to prevent delayed bleeding, it has been reported that prophylactic post-ESD coagulation of visible vessels in the resection area was useful regardless

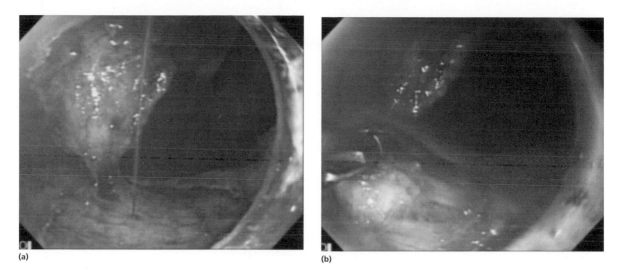

(a)   (b)

Fig. 17.2 (a) Arterial bleeding during gastric ESD. (b) Arterial bleeding managed by electrocautery using hemostatic forceps. (*see insert for color representation of the figure.*)

of active bleeding [21]. The effectiveness of second-look endoscopy after hemostasis of peptic ulcer bleeding has previously been shown, although the effectiveness of second-look endoscopy after gastric cancer ESD based on a retrospective analysis is still controversial and a prospective study is needed in the future [25–27].

Other complications

The risk of stenosis has been reported to range from 0.7 to 1.9% in all gastric ESD cases [28,29]. In particular, endoscopists should be careful of stenosis occurring after ESD for lesions located near the cardia and pylorus. Stenosis was found in 17% of the cardiac ESD cases and 7% of the cases involving lesions located near the pylorus. Circumferential extent of a mucosal defect >3/4 and longitudinal extent >5 cm were each significantly related to the occurrence of post-ESD stenosis in both cardiac and pyloric resections [28,29].

Gastric ESD is usually performed under deep sedation without tracheal intubation, so there is a slight risk of aspiration pneumonia. The risk of such pneumonia has been reported to range from 0.8 to 1.6% for gastric ESD [14,30].

There have also been several case reports about air embolism which is uncommon, but is a potentially fatal complication associated with gastric ESD [31,32]. In order to minimize such fatal occurrences, some institutions have started to use CO_2 insufflation as an added safety measure [33].

Colon

Perforation

During therapeutic colonoscopy, perforation is the most serious complication and requires rapid and appropriate management. The rate of perforations has varied from 0.07 to 1.3% [34–42]. Oka et al. reported the perforation according to the methods of therapeutic colonoscopies in the questionnaire survey from 107 Japanese institutions [41]. The overall occurrence of perforation was 0.07% (64/85,586). Perforation by ESD (3.3%; 23/688) showed a significantly higher rate than that by hot biopsy (0.01%; 2/14,382), polypectomy (0.02%; 6/34,433) and EMR (0.09%; 33/36,083). A more recent Japanese multicenter study for early colorectal neoplasia ≥20 mm in size reported that perforations were observed in 0.8% (8/1,029) in snare technique (polypectomy/EMR) and 2.0% (16/816) in ESD [42].

Surgery is generally the first choice of treatment because it is difficult to manage chemical or bacterial peritonitis due to intraperitoneal leakage of intestinal fluid; this contains chemical substances such as digestive enzymes and fecal fluid containing large amounts of bacteria via the perforated site [43,44]. Patients who developed sepsis and died of peritonitis due to delayed initiation of surgery have also been reported [45]. However, recent reports have shown the usefulness of endoscopic clipping to prevent leakage of intestinal contents in patients with perforation associated with endoscopic treatment [40–42,46,47].

Bleeding

Delayed bleeding is the most common complication associated with therapeutic colonoscopies. In the questionnaire survey from 107 Japanese institutions, the overall occurrence of delayed bleeding was 1.2% (1014/85 586). Delayed bleeding occurred in 0.3% (38/14 382) for hot biopsy, 1.3% (444/34 433) for polypectomy, 1.4% (520/36 083) for EMR and 1.7%, (12/688) for ESD [41].

A variety of techniques are useful for controlling bleeding related to therapeutic colonoscopies. These include application of the endoclip or endoloop, use of the Argon Plasma Coagulator injection of diluted epinephrine, cauterization using monopolar or bipolar instruments, and repeat application of the snare or hot-forceps biopsy to grasp the remnant stalk of pedunculated polyp [48,49].

Esophagus

Perforation

The reported rates of perforation induced by EMR and ESD in the esophagus are 0–2.5% and 0–10%, respectively [50–60]. Shimizu et al. reported 3 cases of successful closures of esophageal perforations after EMR with endoscopically applied clips [51]. Perforations during esophageal ESD were also managed by conservative medical treatment [53]. Esophageal perforation may, however, cause severe or fatal conditions, such as severe mediastinal emphysema and severe mediastinitis. In order to minimize such fatal occurrences, it is better to use CO_2 insufflation from the beginning of the procedure because of its prophylactic effect just in case of perforation [33].

Bleeding

Sgourakis et al. reported 0.6% of the rate of bleeding requiring intervention in the systematic review of EMR and ESD in the management of superficial esophageal neoplasia including dysplasia, adenocarcinoma, and squamous cell carcinoma [61]. A variety of techniques are useful for controlling bleeding related to esophageal EMR/ESD. These include application of the endoclip, use of APC and cauterization using monopolar or bipolar instruments.

Stenosis

Esophageal stenosis after endoscopic resection is an important late complication, as it results in severe dysphagia. In the esophageal EMR/ESD cases, the luminal circumference and longitudinal length of the mucosal defect related to risk factors of developing stenosis [54,62–64].

Patients with esophageal stenosis experienced dysphagia and require endoscopic balloon dilatation. Although the dysphagia usually resolve in response to repeated balloon dilatation, a number of repeated balloon dilatations are necessary [62,65,66]. Recently, there have been several reports on preventive effect for esophageal stenosis after widespread ESD using endoscopic injection of triamcinolone, which is a long-acting steroid derivative, or oral prednisolone [67–69].

References

1. Rembacken BJ, Gotoda T, Fujii T, et al. Endoscopic mucosal resection. *Endoscopy* 2001;**33**:709–18.
2. Soetikno R, Gotoda T, Nakanishi Y, et al. Endoscopic mucosal resection. *Gastrointest. Endosc.* 2003;**57**:567–79.
3. Soetikno R, Kaltenbach T, Yeh R, et al. Endoscopic mucosal resection for early cancers of the upper gastrointestinal tract. *J. Clin. Oncol.* 2005;**23**:4490–8.
4. Oka S, Tanaka S, Kaneko I, et al. Advantage of endoscopic submucosal dissection compared with EMR for early gastric cancer. *Gastrointest. Endosc.* 2006;**64**:877–83.
5. Oda I, Saito D, Tada M, et al. A multicenter retrospective study of endoscopic resection for early gastric cancer. *Gastric Cancer* 2006;**9**:262–70.
6. Minami S, Gotoda T, Ono H, et al. Complete endoscopic closure of gastric perforation induced by endoscopic resection of early gastric cancer using endoclips can prevent surgery. *Gastrointest. Endosc.* 2006;**63**:596–601.
7. Hoteya S, Iizuka T, Kikuchi D, et al. Benefits of endoscopic submucosal dissection according to size and location of gastric neoplasm, compared with conventional mucosal resection. *J. Gastroenterol. Hepatol.* 2009;**24**:1102–6.
8. Ahn JY, Jung HY, Choi KD, et al. Endoscopic and oncologic outcomes after endoscopic resection for early gastric cancer: 1370 cases of absolute and extended indications. *Gastrointest. Endosc.* 2011;**74**:485–93.
9. Oda I, Gotoda T, Hamanaka H, et al. Endoscopic submucosal dissection for early gastric cancer: Technical feasibility, operation time and complications from a large consecutive series. *Dig. Endosc.* 2005;**17**:54–8.
10. Jung HY, Choi KD, Song HJ, et al. Risk management in endoscopic submucosal dissection using needle knife in Korea. *Dig. Endosc.* 2007;**19**(Suppl. 1):S5–8.
11. Ono H, Hasuike N, Inui T, et al. Usefulness of a novel electrosurgical knife, the insulation-tipped diathermic knife-2, for endoscopic submucosal dissection of early gastric cancer. *Gastric Cancer* 2008;**11**:47–52.

12. Chung IK, Lee JH, Lee SH, et al. Therapeutic outcomes in 1000 cases of endoscopic submucosal dissection for early gastric neoplasms: Korean ESD Study Group multicenter study. *Gastrointest. Endosc.* 2009;**69**:1228–35.

13. Mannen K, Tsunada S, Hara M, et al. Risk factors for complications of endoscopic submucosal dissection in gastric tumors: analysis of 478 lesions. *J. Gastroenterol.* 2010;**45**:30–6.

14. Akasaka T, Nishida T, Tsutsui S, et al. Short-term outcomes of endoscopic submucosal dissection (ESD) for early gastric neoplasm: multicenter survey by osaka university ESD study group. *Dig. Endosc.* 2011;**23**:73–7.

15. Ohta T, Ishihara R, Uedo N, et al. Factors predicting perforation during endoscopic submucosal dissection for gastric cancer. *Gastrointest. Endosc.* 2012;**75**:1159–65.

16. Yoo JH, Shin SJ, Lee KM, et al. Risk factors for perforations associated with endoscopic submucosal dissection in gastric lesions: emphasis on perforation type. *Surg. Endosc.* 2012;**26**:2456–64.

17. Hanaoka N, Uedo N, Ishihara R, et al. Clinical features and outcomes of delayed perforation after endoscopic submucosal dissection for early gastric cancer. *Endoscopy* 2010;**42**:1112–5.

18. Binmoellar KF, Grimm H, Soehendra N. Endoscopic closure of a perforation using metallic clips after snare excision of gastric leiomyoma. *Gastrointest. Endosc.* 1993;**39**:172–4.

19. Toyonaga T, Nishino E, Hirooka T, et al. Intraoperative bleeding in endoscopic submucosal dissection in the stomach and strategy for prevention and treatment. *Dig. Endosc.* 2006;**18**:S123–7.

20. Okano A, Hajiro K, Takakuwa H, et al. Predictors of bleeding after endoscopic mucosal resection of gastric tumors. *Gastrointest. Endosc.* 2003;**57**:687–90.

21. Takizawa K, Oda I, Gotoda T, et al. Routine coagulation of visible vessels may prevent delayed bleeding after endoscopic submucosal dissection–an analysis of risk factors. *Endoscopy* 2008;**40**:179–83.

22. Okada K, Yamamoto Y, Kasuga A, et al. Risk factors for delayed bleeding after endoscopic submucosal dissection for gastric neoplasm. *Surg. Endosc.* 2011;**25**:98–107.

23. Toyokawa T, Inaba T, Omote S, et al. Risk factors for perforation and delayed bleeding associated with endoscopic submucosal dissection for early gastric neoplasms; analysis of 1123 lesions. *J. Gastroenterol. Hepatol* 2012;**27**:907–12.

24. Muraki Y, Enomoto S, Iguchi M, et al. Management of bleeding and artificial gastric ulcers associated with endoscopic submucosal dissection. *World J. Gastrointest. Endosc.* 2012;**16**:1–8.

25. Villanueva C, Balanzó J, Torras X, et al. Value of second-look endoscopy after injection therapy for bleeding peptic ulcer: a prospective and randomized trial. *Gastrointest. Endosc.* 1994;**40**:34–9.

26. Chiu PW, Lam CY, Lee SW, et al. Effect of scheduled second therapeutic endoscopy on peptic ulcer rebleeding: a prospective randomised trial. *Gut* 2003;**52**:1403–7.

27. Goto O, Fujishiro M, Kodashima S, et al. A second-look endoscopy after endoscopic submucosal dissection for gastric epithelial neoplasm may be unnecessary: a retrospective analysis of postendoscopic submucosal dissection bleeding. *Gastrointest. Endosc.* 2010;**71**:241–8.

28. Tsunada S, Ogata S, Mannen K, et al. Case series of endoscopic balloon dilation to treat a stricture caused by circumferential resection of the gastric antrum by endoscopic submucosal dissection. *Gastrointest. Endosc.* 2008;**67**:979–83.

29. Coda S, Oda I, Gotoda T, et al. Risk factors for cardiac and pyloric stenosis after endoscopic submucosal dissection, and efficacy of endoscopic balloon dilation treatment. *Endoscopy* 2009;**41**:421–6.

30. Isomoto H, Ohnita K, Yamaguchi N, et al. Clinical outcomes of endoscopic submucosal dissection in elderly patients with early gastric cancer. *Eur. J. Gastroenterol. Hepatol.* 2010;**22**:311–7.

31. Kawahara Y, Okada H, Yamamoto K. Two cases of air embolism during ESD. *Gastroenterol. Endosc.* 2009;**51**(Suppl. 2):2086 (Abstract in Japanese).

32. Takeuchi H, Abe N, Sugiyama M. A case of air embolism during gastric ESD. *Gastroenterol Endosc* 2012;**54**(Suppl. 1):893 (Abstract in Japanese).

33. Nonaka S, Saito Y, Takisawa H, et al. Safety of carbon dioxide insufflation for upper gastrointestinal tract endoscopic treatment of patients under deep sedation. *Surg. Endosc.* 2010;**24**:1638–45.

34. Kavin H, Sinicrope F, Esker AH. Management of perforation of the colon at colonoscopy. *Am. J. Gastroenterol.* 1992;**87**:161–7.

35. Farley DR, Bannon MP, Zietlow SP, et al. Management of colonoscopic perforations. *Mayo Clin. Proc.* 1997;**72**:729–33.

36. Waye JD, Kahn O, Auerbach ME. Complications of colonoscopy and flexible sigmoidoscopy. *Gastrointest. Endosc. Clin. N. Am.* 1996;**6**:343–77.

37. Putcha RV, Burdick JS. Management of iatrogenic perforation. *Gastroenterol. Clin. N. Am.* 2003;**32**:1289–309.

38. Orsoni P, Berdah S, Verrier C, et al. Colonic perforation due to colonoscopy: a retrospective study of 48 cases. *Endoscopy* 1997;**29**:160–4.

39. Anderson ML, Pasha TM, et al. Endoscopic perforation of the colon: lessons from a 10-year study. *Am. J. Gastroenterol.* 2000;**95**:3418–22.

40. Taku K, Sano Y, Fu KI, et al. Iatrogenic perforation associated with therapeutic colonoscopy: a multicenter study in Japan. *J. Gastroenterol. Hepatol.* 2007;**22**:1409–14.

41. Oka S, Tanaka S, Kanao H, et al. Current status in the occurrence of postoperative bleeding, perforation and residual/local recurrence during colonoscopic treatment in Japan. *Dig. Endosc.* 2010;**22**:376–80.

42. Nakajima T, Saito Y, Tanaka S, et al. Current status of endoscopic resection strategy for large, early colorectal neoplasia in Japan. *Surg. Endosc.* 2013;**27**:3262–70.

43. Lo AY, Beaton HL. Selective management of colonoscopic perforations. *J. Am. Coll. Surg.* 1994;**179**:333–7.

44. Hall C, Dorricott NJ, Donovan IA, et al. Colon perforation during colonoscopy: surgical versus conservative management. *Br. J. Surg.* 1991;**78**:542–4.

45. Soliman A, Grundman M. Conservative management of colonoscopic perforation can be misleading. *Endoscopy* 1998;**30**:790–2.

46. Mana F, De Vogelaere K, Urban D. Iatrogenic perforation of the colon during diagnostic colonoscopy: endoscopic treatment with clips. *Gastrointest. Endosc.* 2001;**54**:258–9.

47. Fu KI, Sano Y, Sigeharu K, et al. Colonic Perforation after endoscopic biopsy of a submucosal tumor: successful conservative treatment. *Dig. Endosc.* 2002;**14**:181–3.

48. Soetikno R, Friedland S, Matsuda T, et al. Colonoscopic polypectomy and mucosal resection. In Clinical Gastrointestinal Endoscopy, Ginsberg GG, Kochman ML, Norton I, et al. (eds). Elsevier Saunders, Philadelphia, 2005:549–68.

49. Parra-Blanco A, Kaminaga N, Kojima T, et al. Hemoclipping for postpolypectomy and postbiopsy colonic bleeding. *Gastrointest. Endosc.* 2000;**51**:37–41.

50. Inoue H, Tani M, Nagai K, et al. Treatment of esophageal and gastric tumors. *Endoscopy* 1999;**31**:47–55.

51. Shimizu Y, Kato M, Yamamoto J, et al. Endoscopic clip application for closure of esophageal perforations caused by EMR. *Gastrointest. Endosc.* 2004;**60**:636–9.

52. Tomizawa Y, Iyer PG, Wong Kee Song LM, et al. Safety of Endoscopic mucosal resection for Barrett's esophagus. *Am. J. Gastroenterol.* 2013;**8**(9):1440–7; quiz 1448.

53. Takahashi H, Arimura Y, Masao H, et al. Endoscopic submucosal dissection is superior to conventional endoscopic resection as a curative treatment for early squamous cell carcinoma of the esophagus. *Gastrointest. Endosc.* 2010;**72**:255–64.

54. Ono S, Fujishiro M, Niimi K, et al. Long-term outcomes of endoscopic submucosal dissection for superficial esophageal squamous cell neoplasms. *Gastrointest Endosc* 2009;**70**:860–6.

55. Oyama T, Tomori A, Hotta K, et al. Endoscopic submucosal dissection of early esophageal cancer. *Clin. Gastroenterol. Hepatol.* 2005;**3**:S67–70.

56. Hirasawa K, Kokawa A, Oka H, et al. Superficial adenocarcinoma of the esophagogastric junction: Long-term results of endoscopic submucosal dissection. *Gastrointest. Endosc.* 2010;**72**:960–6.

57. Ishii N, Horiki N, Itoh T, et al. Endoscopic submucosal dissection with a combination of small-caliber-tip transparent hood and flex knife is a safe and effective treatment for superficial esophageal neoplasias. *Surg. Endosc.* 2010;**24**:335–42.

58. Ishihara R, Iishi H, Uedo N, et al. Comparison of EMR and endoscopic submucosal dissection for en bloc resection of early esophageal cancers in Japan. *Gastrointest. Endosc.* 2008;**68**:1066–72.

59. Repici A, Hassan C, Carlino A, et al. Endoscopic submucosal dissection in patients with early esophageal squamous cell carcinoma: Results from a prospective Western series. *Gastrointest. Endosc.* 2010;**71**:715–21.

60. Isomoto H, Yamaguchi N, Minami H, et al. Management of complications associated with endoscopic submucosal dissection/ endoscopic mucosal resection for esophageal cancer. *Dig. Endosc.* 2013;**25**(Suppl. 1):29–38.

61. Sgourakis G, Gockel I, Lang H. Endoscopic and surgical resection of T1a/T1b esophageal neoplasms: a systematic review. *World J. Gastroenterol.* 2013;**19**:1424–37.

62. Katada C, Muto M, Manabe T, et al. Esophageal stenosis after endoscopic mucosal resection of superficial esophageal lesions. *Gastrointest. Endosc.* 2003;**57**:165–9.

63. Lewis JJ, Rubenstein JH, Singal AG, et al. Factors associated with esophageal stricture formation after endoscopic mucosal resection for neoplastic Barrett's esophagus. *Gastrointest. Endosc.* 2011;**74**:753–60.

64. Mizuta H, Nishimori I, Kuratani Y, et al. Predictive factors for esophageal stenosis after endoscopic submucosal dissection for superficial esophageal cancer. *Dis. Esophagus* 2009;**22**:626–31.

65. Ezoe Y, Muto M, Horimatsu T, et al. Efficacy of preventive endoscopic balloon dilation for esophageal stricture after endoscopic resection. *J. Clin. Gastroenterol.* 2011;**45**:222–7.

66. Takahashi H, Arimura Y, Okahara S, et al. Risk of perforation during dilation for esophageal strictures after endoscopic resection in patients with early squamous cell carcinoma. *Endoscopy* 2011;**43**:184–9.

67. Hashimoto S, Kobayashi M, Takeuchi M, et al. The efficacy of endoscopic triamcinolone injection for the prevention of esophageal stricture after endoscopic submucosal dissection. *Gastrointest. Endosc.* 2011;**74**:1389–93.

68. Hanaoka N, Ishihara R, Takeuchi Y, et al. Intralesional steroid injection to prevent stricture after endoscopic submucosal dissection for esophageal cancer: a controlled prospective study. *Endoscopy* 2012;**44**:1007–11.

69. Yamaguchi N, Isomoto H, Nakayama T, et al. Usefulness of oral prednisolone in the treatment of esophageal stricture after endoscopic submucosal dissection for superficial esophageal squamous cell carcinoma. *Gastrointest. Endosc.* 2011;**73**:1115–21.

CHAPTER 18

Complications of bariatric surgery

Allison R. Schulman, Michele B. Ryan, and Christopher C. Thompson

Brigham and Women's Hospital, Harvard Medical School, Boston, MA, USA

Introduction

The increasing worldwide prevalence of severe obesity and associated comorbidities has resulted in a substantial increase in the number of bariatric procedures performed every year [1,2]. In fact, bariatric surgery has become one of the fastest growing operative procedures performed worldwide, and has gained acceptance as the leading sustained weight-loss option for morbid obesity [3]. Furthermore, studies have demonstrated an increase in survival and a decrease in weight-related comorbid illness such as diabetes and cardiovascular disease for those undergoing bariatric surgery, as compared with nonsurgical cohorts [4]. While the performance of bariatric surgery has continued to improve over the past decade, complications from the procedures are not uncommon, and have been estimated to occur in as many as 40% of patients [5,6].

The type of complications and overall risk of adverse outcomes vary according to baseline patient characteristics, the duration of time since the operation, and the type of bariatric surgery performed. Several studies have shown increased mortality rates in patients who are male, over the age of 50 years, or have heart failure, peripheral vascular disease, or chronic renal failure. Excessive obesity may also increase postoperative mortality, although results are conflicting [7,8]. Early complications refer to morbidity that occurs within 30 days of the procedure, and rates vary between 3.4 and 12 percent of patients [6,9–12]. These complications include venous or pulmonary thromboembolism, postoperative pneumonia, or respiratory, which are more common in a postoperative state, and those that are specific to bariatric procedures [13,14]. Complications that occur after 30 days are referred to as late complications, and vary considerably based on the procedure performed [15]. This chapter will review the major complications, early and late, associated with the most commonly performed bariatric surgeries.

Roux-en-Y gastric bypass

The Roux-en-Y gastric bypass has been the most common bariatric surgery procedure performed, accounting for almost half of all bariatric procedures performed worldwide [16]. The surgery involves the creation of a small gastric pouch and an anastomosis to a Roux limb of the jejunum that bypasses 75–150 cm of small bowel (Fig. 18.1a). This new anatomy leads to restriction of food intake and limited absorption, leading to the benefit of weight loss. However, there are several complications associated with this procedure, some of which are related to the altered anatomy, and others of which are specific to the surgical technique or approach (i.e. laparoscopic versus open).

Gastric remnant distension

One uncommon but potentially life-threatening postoperative complication is acute gastric remnant distension, occurring in 0 to 0.8% of cases [17–22]. The portion of the stomach that is excluded during the creation of the pouch is known as the gastric remnant, and has the potential to distend in the setting of a paralytic ileus or

---

Gastrointestinal Emergencies, Third Edition. Edited by Tony C. K. Tham, John S. A. Collins, and Roy Soetikno.
© 2016 John Wiley & Sons, Ltd. Published 2016 by John Wiley & Sons, Ltd.

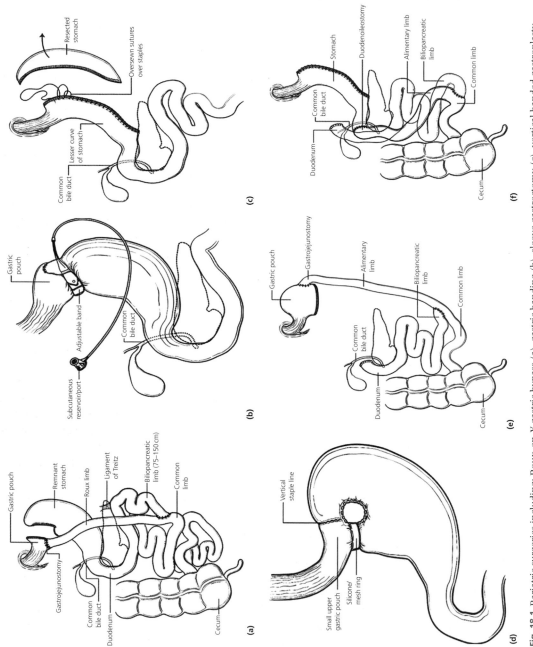

Fig. 18.1 Bariatric surgeries including: Roux-en-Y gastric bypass (a), gastric banding (b), sleeve gastrectomy (c), vertical banded gastroplasty (d), biliopancreatic-diversion (e), and biliopancreatic diversion with duodenal switch (f).

(a)
Gastric pouch
Remnant stomach
Roux limb
Ligament of Treitz
Biliopancreatic limb (75–150 cm)
Common limb
Gastrojejunostomy
Common bile duct
Duodenum
Cecum

(b)
Gastric pouch
Adjustable band
Common bile duct
Subcutaneous reservoir/port

(c)
Resected stomach
Oversewn sutures over staples
Lesser curve of stomach
Common bile duct

(d)
Vertical staple line
Small upper gastric pouch
Silicone/ mesh ring

(e)
Gastric pouch
Gastrojejunostomy
Alimentary limb
Biliopancreatic limb
Common limb
Common bile duct
Duodenum
Cecum

(f)
Stomach
Duodenoileostomy
Alimentary limb
Biliopancreatic limb
Common limb
Common bile duct
Duodenum
Cecum

distal mechanical obstruction, typically as a consequence of gastric remnant ulcer formation or at the site of the jejunojejunostomy. Iatrogenic injury to the vagal nerve may also contribute to the pathogenesis.

The typical clinical presentation involves left upper quadrant abdominal pain and tympany, hiccups, shoulder discomfort, abdominal distention, and persistent tachycardia. A large gastric air bubble can be seen on chest radiographs. Although rare, delayed diagnosis may lead to rupture, organ failure, sepsis, and death, given the volume and composition of the contents that are spilled into the peritoneum [22,23]. Emergent operative decompression and possible exploration is often required. Some authors have advocated that prophylactic drainage of the gastric remnant via gastrostomy may be effective at preventing this complication, and should be considered in the elderly and those who have diabetic gastroparesis [23].

Anastomotic leaks

One of the most serious complications of bariatric surgery are postoperative leaks at the anastomosis site, which often occur within one week of surgery, but can appear as late as one month after the operation. The incidence ranges from 0.1 to 5.6%, and is much higher after revision surgery [10,24]. The clinical presentation can range from low-grade fevers or tachycardia, which can be treated conservatively to hemodynamic instability or sepsis, which requires emergent operative exploration and treatment. Endoscopic placement of self-expandable stents is emerging as a minimally invasive, safe, and effective alternative in the management of leaks after bariatric surgery, thereby minimizing the need for surgical revision [25].

Gastrojejunostomy anastomotic stricture/ stomal stenosis

Stricture of the gastrojejunal anastomosis (also known as stomal stenosis) has been reported in 2.9–23% of patients who have undergone Roux-en-Y gastric bypass surgery [26,27]. Tension or ischemia at the site of anastomosis, coupled with an individual patient's capacity to heal, likely contributes to the development of this complication. The laparoscopic Roux-en-Y gastric bypass procedure has been particularly linked to occurrence of stomal stenosis, possibly attributed to the use of small-diameter circular staplers during the construction of the gastrojejunostomy, although this continues to be a debated [24,26–29].

Patients with gastrojejunostomy anastomotic strictures typically present weeks to months postoperatively, although the time to stricture development may depend on the surgical approach. One study showed patients who have undergone open procedures present significantly later than those who have had laparoscopic surgeries (114.2 and 48.5 days, respectively) [28]. Clinical symptoms include progressive dysphagia, nausea, vomiting, and inability to tolerate oral intake. Abdominal pain is typically not present [30]. The classic presenting symptoms usually lead to direct endoscopic visualization as the first diagnostic tool and rarely mandate extensive additional workup [30].

Endoscopic balloon dilation of the stricture is used almost exclusively to treat this complication, with surgical revision required in less than 0.05% of cases [26–28,30,31]. Dilation to at least 15 mm is safe and decreases the need for repeat procedures [32]. The majority of patients require only one endoscopic dilation, and the complication rate is less than 3% [31,33–35].

Marginal ulcerations

Marginal ulceration at the site of the gastrojejunal anastomosis is a recognized complication and has been reported in up to 16% of patients after gastric bypass surgery [36,37] (Fig. 18.2a). Although these ulcerations can occur at any time postoperatively, the highest risk period is within the first 30 days following the procedure. The clinical presentation can range from being asymptomatic to having severe pain and obstructive symptoms or gastrointestinal bleeding, and rarely, can present as perforation. The mechanisms underlying the development of marginal ulceration have not been fully elucidated, and the etiology of this complication is likely multifactorial [38–41] (Table 18.1). Patients must stop smoking or ulcers will not heal.

There is substantial evidence that acidity plays a major role in the disease pathophysiology, given that the jejunum receives the acidic chyme from the stomach pouch in the absence of the duodenum's intrinsic acid-buffering properties. Studies have demonstrated that patients with increased acid in the stomach pouch and increased exposure to an acidic pH were at increased risk for marginal ulceration [36]. Furthermore, a recent systemic review and meta-analysis found significant incremental benefit of use of prophylactic proton-pump inhibitors (PPIs) in reducing marginal ulceration after gastric bypass surgery [42].

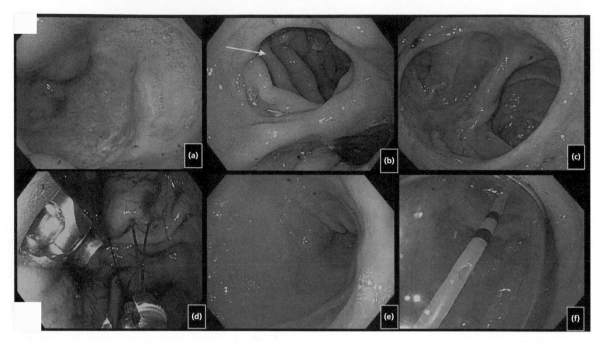

Fig. 18.2 Endoscopic examples of complications and/or treatments including marginal ulceration (a), gastrogastric fistula (b), dilated gastrojejunal anastamosis (c), and an endoscopic suturing procedure to decrease stoma size (d) following Roux-en-Y gastric bypass, and gastric outlet obstruction at the incisura angularis (e) with subsequent endoscopic balloon dilation (f) following sleeve gastrectomy. (*see insert for color representation of the figure.*)

Table 18.1 Etiology of marginal ulceration.

Predisposing factors
- Surgical technique
  - Type of gastric bypass (divided vs. non-divided
  - Route (antecolic vs. retrocolic)
  - Type of anastomosis (hand sewn, linear stapled, circular stapled)
  - Orientation of the pouch
  - Experience of the surgeon
  - Suture material used (absorbable vs. non-absorbable)
- Smoking
- NSAID use
- Alcohol
- Lack of PPI use

Factors implicated in the physiopathology
- *Helicobacter pylori*
- Inflammation
- Foreign body reaction
- Acid secretion
- Bile reflux
- Fistula
- Ischemia

The majority of patients with marginal ulcerations respond to medical therapy, in addition to smoking cessation and indefinite discontinuation of non-steroidal anti-inflammatory drugs (NSAIDs) [43]. Surgical revision of the gastrojejunostomy with truncal vagotomy has traditionally been performed in the small percentage of patients who do not improve, however, reoperation carries significant morbidity and a 7.7% recurrence rate [40]. Endoscopic suturing techniques have recently been developed and appear promising in the treatment of recalcitrant marginal ulceration. While the mechanism by which this work is unclear, the first successful case series showed that the procedure was technically feasible, safe, and efficacious [44].

Cholelithiasis

The development of cholelithiasis is not uncommon following Roux-en-Y gastric bypass, and is estimated to occur in 28 to 71% of patients within 6 months following surgery, with up to 40% of these patients becoming symptomatic [45]. Rapid weight loss has been shown to contribute to the formation of gallstones by increasing the cholesterol saturation in the bile and the gallbladder mucin concentration [46,47]. Postoperative anatomical changes and compromised gallbladder emptying are also thought to play a role [45,48–51].

Choledocholithiasis after Roux-en-Y gastric bypass can be particularly challenging to treat via endoscopic retrograde cholangiopancreatography (ERCP) due to the relative inaccessibility of the duodenum [52,53]. Traditional alternative approaches include surgical or transhepatic percutaneous access or placement of a prophylactic gastrostomy tube into the bypassed stomach [54,55]. More recently, endoscopic ultrasound (EUS)-assisted percutaneous gastric access for single-session ERCP has been described, which can be performed in the endoscopy suite and appears safe, effective, and allows for subsequent ERCPs if needed [56].

In light of the increased incidence of cholelithiasis in the morbidly obese population, it is not uncommon to perform a cholecystectomy at the time of bypass if the patient has symptomatic gallstones preoperatively. In asymptomatic patients, the surgical opinion is more divided, with only some studies demonstrating a benefit [57–59]. The use of a synthetic bile salt, ursodeoxycholic acid, has also been found to significantly decrease gallstone formation following gastric bypass surgery [60].

Hernias

Ventral incisional hernias occur much less frequently in laparoscopic Roux-en-Y gastric bypass than in the traditional open technique, and typically present with an enlarging bulge, pain or obstructive symptoms [21,61]. Repair is often deferred if symptoms are minimal until after significant weight loss has been achieved.

Internal hernias can also occur, mostly involving small bowel and occurring at spaces between a mesenteric defect at the jejunojejunostomy, the transverse mesocolon and Roux-limb mesentery (Peterson's hernias), or the transverse mesocolon if the Roux-limb is passed retrocolic. These can difficult to detect radiographically given their intermittent nature, but the computerized tomography (CT) finding of swirled vessels or fat at the root of the mesentery has the highest sensitivity and specificity of diagnosis [62,63].

Nutritional abnormalities

Metabolic and nutritional derangements are not uncommon following Roux-en-Y gastric bypass, since reversing underlying obesity leads to reduced oral intake

Table 18.2 Recommended supplement doses after bariatric surgery.

Nutritional supplement	Dosage
Multivitamin (with folic acid)	1–2 daily (400 µg daily)
Calcium citrate + vitamin D	1200–2000 mg daily +400–800 U daily
Elemental iron with vitamin D	40–650 mg daily
Vitamin B12	Oral: ≥350 µg daily *or* Intramuscular injection: 1000 µg monthly *or* 3000 µg every 6 months *or* Intranasal injection: 500 µg weekly

and/or excessive losses secondary to reconfiguration of gastrointestinal motility, pH, and enzymatic profiles [64]. Anemia from iron, folate, and vitamin B12 deficiencies is the most common complication and is estimated to occur in 20–49% of patients. Major deficits can also occur with magnesium, calcium, zinc, 25-hydroxyvitamin D, thiamine, and β carotene, and appropriate nutrient supplementation is essential [65] (Table 18.2). Furthermore, hyperoxaluria and subsequent nephrolithiasis or renal failure have also been reported following Roux-en-Y gastric bypass [66].

Short bowel syndrome

Short bowel syndrome is defined as a malabsorptive state that follows massive resection of the small intestine, and is a particular problem with the rarer malabsorptive procedures discussed in subsequent sections [67]. A small percentage of patients are prone to developing this syndrome after complicated bypass procedures in which hernias or adhesions necessitate additional bowel resections. While the condition is not uniformly fatal, it might lead to life-threatening complications, with the basic goals of medical treatment being to maintain fluid, electrolyte, and nutrient balances.

Dumping syndrome

Early and late dumping syndrome can occur in up to half of patients who undergo gastric bypass surgery when large quantities of simple carbohydrates are ingested. Early dumping typically occurs within 15 minutes of ingestion and has been attributed to rapid fluid shifts from the plasma into the bowel from hyperosmolality of

Table 18.3 Symptoms of early and late dumping.

Early dumping
- Gastrointestinal symptoms
  - Abdominal pain
  - Diarrhea
  - Borborygmi
  - Bloating
  - Nausea
- Vasomotor symptoms
  - Flushing
  - Palpitations
  - Perspiration
  - Tachycardia
  - Hypotension
  - Syncope

Late dumping
- Hypoglycemia
  - Perspiration
  - Palpitations
  - Hunger
  - Weakness
  - Confusion
  - Tremor
  - Syncope

the food. Late dumping, on the other hand, results from hyperglycemia and the subsequent insulin response leading to hypoglycemia, and occurs several hours after eating [68]. Each of these conditions may present as a spectrum of symptoms that are shown in Table 18.3. A more extreme condition that can develop is that of pancreatic nesidioblastosis, a form of acquired hyperinsulinism in a post-bypass patient that leads to postprandial neuroglycopenic hyperinsulinemic hypoglycemia and requires surgical management [69].

Failure to lose weight

Late weight regain occurs in up to 20% of patients who have undergone Roux-en-Y gastric bypass [70]. Typically this is due to progressive dietary non-compliance, but anatomical changes can also occur which promote weight gain. A gastrogastric fistula (GGF) is an abnormal connection between the gastric pouch and the excluded stomach (Fig. 18.2b). The most common presenting symptom is weight gain or inability to lose weight, although pain, nausea, and emesis are often reported. Endoscopy and upper gastrointestinal series should be performed to make the diagnosis. If

present, maximum medical therapy should be instituted, with over one third of patients experiencing symptom resolution. If the GGF remains symptomatic, then procedural intervention is required. Traditionally, this has been accomplished via a surgical approach. Recent, less-invasive endoscopic approaches using suturing systems or clips have shown to be successful in some patients, however, results are less than optimal [71,72].

Dilation of the gastric pouch or the gastrojejunal anastomosis also leads to weight regain (Fig. 18.2c). Recent studies suggest that endoscopic suturing to tighten the stoma appear technically feasible and safe, and offer a new and less invasive treatment option for post-bypass weight regain [73–76] (Fig. 18.2d).

Gastric banding

Adjustable gastric banding is a restrictive procedure that restricts the upper part of the gastric cavity by inserting an adjustable, prosthetic band over the cardia of the stomach to form a gastric pouch with roughly 15 milliliter capacity (Fig. 18.1b). The gastric band consists of a silicone ring connected to an infusion port, the latter of which remains in the subcutaneous tissue and can be easily accessed for saline injections to increase the degree of restriction [77]. These types of procedures bring the added advantage of allowing regulation of the outlet size, thus rendering it flexible to meet the changing needs of the patient. However, the disadvantages of the restriction methods are the presence of a foreign body, and a greater dependence on patient compliance. Adjustable gastric banding it is most commonly performed laparoscopically, and has the lowest perioperative complication rate and mortality among all bariatric procedures [78]. However, its use has decreased over the last decade due to the high revision rate and weight regain [16,79].

Band-related complications

Band erosion, or intragastric migration, is a severe complication of adjustable banding procedures and has been shown in the majority of studies to occur in less than 6.8% of patients [80]. Band erosion may occur early within weeks, or can be seen months and even years after operation, with the mean time to occurrence of 22.5 months [80,81]. Early erosions are usually secondary to undetected gastric perforations during surgery or early infection, while late erosions are generally the consequence of gastric wall ischemia from an excessively tight band or other mechanism. Clinical manifestations of this complication can range from weight gain, to nausea and vomiting, to life-threatening sepsis. Furthermore, if the site of erosion occurs into the posterior part of the stomach near the cardioesophageal junction, than the gastric artery can be involved and massive hematemesis can occur [82]. Cellulitis at the port site also indicates likely band erosion and warrants further investigation. Diagnosis can be made endoscopically, and depending on what portion of the band is visible, removal may be accomplished at the time of the procedure [83,84]. Otherwise, laparoscopy is required for treatment.

Band slippage is among the most prevalent late complication, leading to prolapse of a portion of the stomach through the band. When the band migrates cephalad, an acute angle between the stomach pouch and the esophagus is created, which can lead to gastric obstruction. Alternatively, when the stomach migrates cephalad, the band is displaced caudally and a new gastric pouch can be created. Patients often present with vomiting and epigastric pain, and require urgent or emergent surgical management [85,86].

Laparoscopic adjustable gastric band (LAGB) procedures have also been associated with acute stomal obstruction, defined as an obstruction to the flow of food from the gastric pouch to the rest of the stomach. These events can occur in up to 14% of patients [87,88]. Depending on the surgical approach, stomal obstruction can be the result of smaller bands applied over a thick gastroesophageal junction (GEJ), incorporation of too much tissue inside the band, or malpositioning of the band itself [88]. Symptoms include dysphagia, chest or abdominal pain, and inability to tolerate oral intake or secretions. An upper gastrointestinal series is often diagnostic. For patients with partial obstruction, initial treatment is often conservative, but in the setting of complete obstruction, exploratory laparoscopy is warranted [88].

Port-related complications

The mechanical port component of the adjustable band device exposes the patients to infectious complications given the presence of a foreign body, in addition to the inevitable consequences of device weathering, which can lead to its failure [89,90]. Infections in the subcutaneous port reservoir occur in less than 10% of patients

[91,92]. Typically, the infected port is removed with reimplantation of a new port once the infection clears. Band erosion should also be considered as a potential etiology and evaluated as indicated.

Port malfunction can also occur. Leakage, faulty or perforated tubing, or port dislocation, occur with a frequency of 0.4–7% of patients who undergo the adjustable banding procedure [93,94]. Often, these problems are diagnosed when there is arrest of weight loss, or weight regain, and curtailment of the restrictive action. Suturing the port into a polypropylene mesh and attaching it to the rectus fascia has been demonstrated to reduce port dislocation [95].

Esophageal-related complications

Esophagitis and reflux have been reported as complications following banding procedures with varying prevalence throughout the literature, and typically require acid-suppression therapy and deflation of the band [96–98]. An achalasia-like syndrome can also occur in less than ten percent of patients and results from esophageal dilation proximal to the band [99]. Excessive inflation of the band or excessive food intake can precipitate this condition and cause symptoms of reflux, epigastric discomfort, and inability to tolerate oral intake. Typically, treatment involves deflation of the band and diet modification, but worsening esophageal dilation and inadequate weight loss mandate replacement of the band in a new location or conversion to an alternative bariatric procedure.

Sleeve gastrectomy

Laparoscopic sleeve gastrectomy is a restrictive procedure in which a large portion of the greater curvature of the stomach is removed, leaving just a small tube along the lesser curvature and in so doing resecting fundal ghrelin-producing cells to decrease appetite [100] (Fig. 18.1c). It was initially designed for high-risk patients to achieve a significant reduction in weight loss and co-morbidities and increase the safety of a second operation [101–103]. However, given its favorable outcomes, coupled with preservation of the pylorus, maintenance of physiological food passage, and avoidance of foreign material, laparoscopic sleeve gastrectomy is increasingly being performed as a standalone procedure with very promising results [103].

Stenosis

Gastric outlet obstruction can occur as a result of stenosis, which classically occurs at the incisura angularis or the gastroesophageal junction following a sleeve gastrectomy (Fig. 18.2e). The incidence has been reported to be 0.7–4% [101,104]. Over-sewing the staple line or using a bougie that is too small both predispose to narrowing at these locations. Symptoms of obstruction can occur depending on the severity of the narrowing. This diagnosis is typically made by an upper gastrointestinal series, and endoscopic dilation is the primary mode of management, however, surgical intervention is often required (Fig. 18.2f).

Gastric leaks

Gastric leaks have been reported in up to 5.3% of patients, and usually occur along the superior aspect of the staple line just below the GEJ. Leaks can be the result of inadequate healing of the gastric tissue from poor blood supply and oxygenation, or from heat generated from cautery during dissection of the greater curvature [105]. This complication is one of the most serious, and often requires reoperation [105]. Recently, endoscopic approaches using stents and clips have proven successful, and offers a less invasive first line therapy for many patients [106].

Vertical banded gastroplasty

Vertical banded gastroplasty (VBG) is a purely restrictive procedure that involves the creation of a small proximal gastric pouch less than 50 mL lined by a vertical staple line and a tight prosthetic mesh that is sutured to itself but not the stomach (Fig. 18.1d). This surgery has the benefit of providing an outlet diameter that remains constant [107].

While this type of procedure has largely been replaced by other procedures, familiarity with the complications is still important. Staple line dehiscence can result in a fistula to the fundus, often leading to weight gain and found in as many as half of all patients on routine postoperative endoscopy [108]. Obstruction from stomal stenosis can occur and be managed by endoscopic balloon dilation, although results are often short-lived and revision may be necessary when symptoms persist [109]. Erosion of the mesh band is a late complication of this procedure, and can be removed via an endoscopic approach, but may ultimately require surgical revision [110,111].

Biliopancreatic-diversion with or without duodenal switch

Biliopancreatic diversion (BPD) is a relatively uncommon procedure because of its technical complexity and high complication rates (Fig. 18.1e). It is a malabsorptive procedure, in which absorption is limited to a short segment of small intestine, in addition to the gastric reservoir being decreased in size [112]. The BPD with duodenal switch (BPD-DS) is a variation of the BPD in which a sleeve of stomach remains in which the pylorus remains connected duodenum (Fig. 18.1f). While these procedures achieve excellent weight loss, they have high surgical morbidity and mortality rates, including long-term nutritional deficiencies.

Conclusion

Obesity is one of the most rapidly emerging health problems world-wide. Due to the fact that medical, nutritional, and behavioral weight loss management methods have had a low success rate, bariatric surgery has become the primary treatment for morbid obesity. Despite improvement in the performance of these procedures, complications are not uncommon, and estimated to occur in as many as 40% of patients. The type of complications and overall risk of adverse outcomes vary according to baseline patient characteristics, the duration of time since the operation, and the type of bariatric surgery performed. In the coming decades, more knowledge will be gained regarding the long-term sustainability of these techniques and subsequent improvement in obesity-related comorbid disease. With the development of novel and less invasive procedures, including emerging endoscopic bariatric treatments, the morbidity of these procedures may decrease substantially.

References

1. Uy MC, Talingdan-Te MC, Espinosa WZ, Daez ML, Ong JP. Ursodeoxycholic acid in the prevention of gallstone formation after bariatric surgery: a meta-analysis. *Obes. Surg.* 2008;**18**(12):1532–8.
2. Nougou A, Suter M. Almost routine prophylactic cholecystectomy during laparoscopic gastric bypass is safe. *Obes. Surg.* 2008;**18**(5):535–9.
3. Buchwald H, Oien DM. Metabolic/bariatric surgery worldwide 2008. *Obes. Surg.* 2009;**19**(12):1605–11.

4. Perry CD, Hutter MM, Smith DB, Newhouse JP, McNeil BJ. Survival and changes in comorbidities after bariatric surgery. *Ann. Surg.* 2008;**247**(1):21–7.

5. Encinosa WE, Bernard DM, Du D, Steiner CA. Recent improvements in bariatric surgery outcomes. *Med. Care* 2009;**47**(5):531–5.

6. Flum DR, Belle SH, King WC, et al. Perioperative safety in the longitudinal assessment of bariatric surgery. *N. Engl. J. Med.* 2009;**361**(5):445–54.

7. Arterburn D, Livingston EH, Schifftner T, Kahwati LC, Henderson WG, Maciejewski ML. Predictors of long-term mortality after bariatric surgery performed in Veterans Affairs medial centers. *Arch. Surg.* 2009;**144**(10):914–20.

8. Stephens DJ, Saunders JK, Belsley S, et al. Short-term outcomes for super-super obese (BMI > or =60 kg/m²) patients undergoing weight loss surgery at a high-volume bariatric surgery center: laparoscopic adjustable gastric banding, laparoscopic gastric bypass, and open tubular gastric bypass. *Surg. Obes. Relat. Dis.* 2008;**4**(3):408–15.

9. Stenberg E, Szabo E, Agren G, et al. Early complications after laparoscopic gastric bypass surgery: results From the Scandinavian Obesity Surgery Registry. *Ann. Surg.* 2014;**260**(6):1040–7.

10. Nelson DW, Blair KS, Martin MJ. Analysis of obesity-related outcomes and bariatric failure rates with the duodenal switch vs gastric bypass for morbid obesity. *Arch. Surg.* 2012;**147**(9):847–54.

11. Topart P, Becouarn G, Ritz P. Comparative early outcomes of three laparoscopic bariatric procedures: sleeve gastrectomy, Roux-en-Y gastric bypass, and biliopancreatic diversion with duodenal switch. *Surg. Obes. Relat. Dis.* 2012;**8**(3):250–4.

12. Kehagias I, Karamanakos SN, Argentou M, Kalfarentzos F. Randomized clinical trial of laparoscopic Roux-en-Y gastric bypass versus laparoscopic sleeve gastrectomy for the management of patients with BMI < 50 kg/m². *Obes. Surg.* 2011;**21**(11):1650–6.

13. Jones KB Jr, Afram JD, Benotti PN, et al. Open versus laparoscopic Roux-en-Y gastric bypass: a comparative study of over 25,000 open cases and the major laparoscopic bariatric reported series. *Obes. Surg.* 2006;**16**(6):721–7.

14. Podnos YD, Jimenez JC, Wilson SE, Stevens CM, Nguyen NT. Complications after laparoscopic gastric bypass: a review of 3464 cases. *Arch. Surg.* 2003;**138**(9):957–61.

15. Carlin AM, Zeni TM, English WJ, et al. The comparative effectiveness of sleeve gastrectomy, gastric bypass, and adjustable gastric banding procedures for the treatment of morbid obesity. *Ann. Surg.* 2013;**257**(5):791–7.

16. Buchwald H, Oien DM. Metabolic/bariatric surgery worldwide 2011. *Obes. Surg.* 2013;**23**(4):427–36.

17. Oliak D, Ballantyne GH, Weber P, Wasielewski A, Davies RJ, Schmidt HJ. Laparoscopic Roux-en-Y gastric bypass: defining the learning curve. *Surg. Endosc.* 2003;**17**(3):405–8.

18. Schauer P, Ikramuddin S, Hamad G, Gourash W. The learning curve for laparoscopic Roux-en-Y gastric bypass is 100 cases. *Surg. Endosc.* 2003;**17**(2):212–5.

19. Suter M, Giusti V, Héraief E, Zysset F, Calmes JM. Laparoscopic Roux-en-Y gastric bypass: initial 2-year experience. *Surg. Endosc.* 2003;**17**(4):603–9.

20. DeMaria EJ, Schweitzer MA, Kellum JM, Meador J, Wolfe L, Sugerman HJ. Results of 281 consecutive total laparoscopic Roux-en-Y gastric bypasses to treat morbid obesity. *Ann. Surg.* 2002;**235**(5):640–5; discussion 645–7.

21. Higa KD, Boone KB, Ho T, Davies OG. Laparoscopic Roux-en-Y gastric bypass for morbid obesity: technique and preliminary results of our first 400 patients. *Arch. Surg.* 2000;**135**(9):1029–33; discussion 1033–4.

22. Papasavas PK, Caushaj PF, McCormick JT, et al. Laparoscopic management of complications following laparoscopic Roux-en-Y gastric bypass for morbid obesity. *Surg Endosc,* 2003. **17**(4):610–4.

23. Han SH, White S, Patel K, Dutson E, Gracia C, Mehran A. Acute gastric remnant dilation after laparoscopic Roux-en-Y gastric bypass operation in long-standing type I diabetic patient: Case report and literature review. *Surg Obes Relat Dis,* 2006. **2**(6):664–6.

24. Gonzalez R, Nelson LG, Gallagher SF, Murr MM. Anastomotic leaks after laparoscopic gastric bypass. *Obes Surg,* 2004. **14**(10):1299–307.

25. Puli, S.R., I.S. Spofford, and C.C. Thompson, Use of self-expandable stents in the treatment of bariatric surgery leaks: a systematic review and meta-analysis. *Gastrointest Endosc,* 2012. **75**(2):287–93.

26. Alasfar F, Sabnis AA, Liu RC, Chand B. Stricture rate after laparoscopic Roux-en-Y Gastric bypass with a 21-mm circular stapler: the Cleveland Clinic experience. *Med. Princ. Pract.* 2009;**18**(5):364–7.

27. Mathew A, Veliuona MA, DePalma FJ, Cooney RN. Gastrojejunal stricture after gastric bypass and efficacy of endoscopic intervention. *Dig. Dis. Sci.* 2009;**54**(9):1971–8.

28. Kravetz AJ, Reddy S, Murtaza G, Yenumula P. A comparative study of handsewn versus stapled gastrojejunal anastomosis in laparoscopic Roux-en-Y gastric bypass. *Surg. Endosc.* 2011;**25**(4):1287–92.

29. Carrodeguas L, et al. Gastrojejunal anastomotic strictures following laparoscopic Roux-en-Y gastric bypass surgery: analysis of 1291 patients. *Surg. Obes. Relat. Dis.* 2006;**2**(2):92–7.

30. Goitein D, Papasavas PK, Gagné D, Ahmad S, Caushaj PF. Gastrojejunal strictures following laparoscopic Roux-en-Y gastric bypass for morbid obesity. *Surg. Endosc.* 2005; **19**(5):628–32.

31. Nguyen NT, Stevens CM, Wolfe BM. Incidence and outcome of anastomotic stricture after laparoscopic gastric bypass. *J. Gastrointest. Surg.* 2003;**7**(8):997–1003; discussion 1003.

32. Peifer KJ, Shiels AJ, Azar R, Rivera RE, Eagon JC, Jonnalagadda S. Successful endoscopic management of gastrojejunal anastomotic strictures after Roux-en-Y gastric bypass. *Gastrointest. Endosc.* 2007;**66**(2):248–52.

33. Ahmad J, Martin J, Ikramuddin S, Schauer P, Slivka A. Endoscopic balloon dilation of gastroenteric anastomotic stricture after laparoscopic gastric bypass. *Endoscopy* 2003;**35**(9):725–8.

34. Barba CA, Butensky MS, Lorenzo M, Newman R. Endoscopic dilation of gastroesophageal anastomosis stricture after gastric bypass. *Surg.Endosc.* 2003;**17**(3):416–20.

35. Go MR, Muscarella P 2nd, Needleman BJ, Cook CH, Melvin WS. Endoscopic management of stomal stenosis after Roux-en-Y gastric bypass. Surg. *Endosc.* 2004;**18**(1):56–9.

36. MacLean LD, Rhode BM, Nohr C, Katz S, McLean AP. Stomal ulcer after gastric bypass. *J. Am. Coll. Surg.* 1997;**185**(1):1–7.

37. Sapala JA, Wood MH, Sapala MA, Flake TM Jr. Marginal ulcer after gastric bypass: a prospective 3-year study of 173 patients. *Obes. Surg.* 1998;**8**(5):505–16.

38. Dallal, R.M. and L.A. Bailey, Ulcer disease after gastric bypass surgery. *Surg Obes Relat Dis*, 2006. **2**(4):455–9.

39. Rasmussen JJ, Fuller W, Ali MR. Marginal ulceration after laparoscopic gastric bypass: an analysis of predisposing factors in 260 patients. *Surg. Endosc.* 2007;**21**(7):1090–4.

40. Patel, R.A., R.E. Brolin, and A. Gandhi, Revisional operations for marginal ulcer after Roux-en-Y gastric bypass. *Surg. Obes Relat Dis*, 2009. **5**(3):317–22.

41. Azagury DE, Abu Dayyeh BK, Greenwalt IT, Thompson CC. Marginal ulceration after Roux-en-Y gastric bypass surgery: characteristics, risk factors, treatment, and outcomes. *Endoscopy*, 2011. **43**(11):950–4.

42. Ying VW, Kim SH, Khan KJ, et al. Prophylactic PPI help reduce marginal ulcers after gastric bypass surgery: a systematic review and meta-analysis of cohort studies. Surg. Endosc. 2014.

43. Sanyal AJ1, Sugerman HJ, Kellum JM, Engle KM, Wolfe L Stomal complications of gastric bypass: incidence and outcome of therapy. *Am. J. Gastroenterologyterol.* 1992;**87**(9): 1165–9.

44. Jirapinyo P, Watson RR, Thompson CC. Use of a novel endoscopic suturing device to treat recalcitrant marginal ulceration (with video). *Gastrointest. Endosc.* 2012;**76**(2):435–9.

45. Shiffman ML, Sugerman HJ, Kellum JM, Brewer WH, Moore EW. Gallstone formation after rapid weight loss: a prospective study in patients undergoing gastric bypass surgery for treatment of morbid obesity. *Am. J. Gastroenterol.* 1991;**86**(8):1000–5.

46. Shiffman ML, Sugerman HJ, Kellum JM, Moore EW. Changes in gallbladder bile composition following gallstone formation and weight reduction. *Gastroenterology* 1992; **103**(1):214–21.

47. Worobetz LJ, Inglis FG, Shaffer EA. The effect of ursodeoxycholic acid therapy on gallstone formation in the morbidly obese during rapid weight loss. *Am. J. Gastroenterol.* 1993;**88**(10):1705–10.

48. Iglezias Brandao de Oliveira C, Adami Chaim E, da Silva BB. Impact of rapid weight reduction on risk of cholelithiasis after bariatric surgery. *Obes. Surg.* 2003;**13**(4):625–8.

49. Everhart JE. Contributions of obesity and weight loss to gallstone disease. *Ann. Intern. Med.* 1993;**119**(10):1029–35.

50. Ahmed AR, O'Malley W, Johnson J, Boss T. Cholecystectomy during laparoscopic gastric bypass has no effect on duration of hospital stay. *Obes. Surg.* 2007;**17**(8):1075–9.

51. Bastouly M, Arasaki CH, Ferreira JB, Zanoto A, Borges FG, Del Grande JC. Early changes in postprandial gallbladder emptying in morbidly obese patients undergoing Roux-en-Y gastric bypass: correlation with the occurrence of biliary sludge and gallstones. *Obes. Surg.* 2009;**19**(1):22–8.

52. Baron TH, Vickers SM. Surgical gastrostomy placement as access for diagnostic and therapeutic ERCP. *Gastrointest. Endosc.* 1998;**48**(6):640–1.

53. Wright BE, Cass OW, Freeman ML. ERCP in patients with long-limb Roux-en-Y gastrojejunostomy and intact papilla. *Gastrointest. Endosc.* 2002;**56**(2):225–32.

54. Fobi MA, Chicola K, Lee H. Access to the bypassed stomach after gastric bypass. *Obes. Surg.* 1998;**8**(3):289–95.

55. Gutierrez JM, Lederer H, Krook JC, Kinney TP, Freeman ML, Jensen EH. Surgical gastrostomy for pancreatobiliary and duodenal access following Roux en Y gastric bypass. *J. Gastrointest. Surg.* 2009;**13**(12):2170–5.

56. Thompson CC, Ryou MK, Kumar N, Slattery J, Aihara H, Ryan MB. Single-session EUS-guided transgastric ERCP in the gastric bypass patient. *Gastrointest.Endosc.* 2014;**80**(3):517.

57. Tarantino I, Warschkow R, Steffen T, Bisang P, Schultes B, Thurnheer M. Is routine cholecystectomy justified in severely obese patients undergoing a laparoscopic Roux-en-Y gastric bypass procedure? A comparative cohort study. *Obes. Surg.* 2011;**21**(12):1870–8.

58. Villegas L, Schneider B, Provost D, et al. Is routine cholecystectomy required during laparoscopic gastric bypass? *Obes. Surg.* 2004;**14**(2):206–11.

59. Hamad GG, Ikramuddin S, Gourash WF, Schauer PR. Elective cholecystectomy during laparoscopic Roux-en-Y gastric bypass: is it worth the wait? *Obes. Surg.* 2003;**13**(1): 76–81.

60. Sugerman HJ, Brewer WH, Shiffman ML, et al. A multicenter, placebo-controlled, randomized, double-blind, prospective trial of prophylactic ursodiol for the prevention of gallstone formation following gastric-bypass-induced rapid weight loss. *Am. J. Surg.* 1995;**169**(1):91–6; discussion 96–7.

61. Nguyen NT, Goldman C, Rosenquist CJ. Laparoscopic versus open gastric bypass: a randomized study of outcomes, quality of life, and costs. *Ann. Surg.* 2001;**234**(3):279–89; discussion 289–91.

62. Iannuccilli JD, Grand D, Murphy BL, Evangelista P, Roye GD, Mayo-Smith W. Sensitivity and specificity of eight CT signs in the preoperative diagnosis of internal mesenteric hernia following Roux-en-Y gastric bypass surgery. *Clin. Radiol.* 2009;**64**(4):373–80.

63. Lockhart ME, Tessler FN, Canon CL, et al. Internal hernia after gastric bypass: sensitivity and specificity of seven CT signs with surgical correlation and controls. *AJR Am. J. Roentgenol.* 2007;**188**(3):745–50.

64. Dalcanale L, Oliveira CP, Faintuch J, et al. Long-term nutritional outcome after gastric bypass. *Obes. Surg.* 2010;**20**(2):181–7.

65. Odom J, Zalesin KC, Washington TL, et al. Behavioral predictors of weight regain after bariatric surgery. *Obes. Surg.* 2010;**20**(3):349–56.

66. Kumar R, Lieske JC, Collazo-Clavell ML, et al. Fat malabsorption and increased intestinal oxalate absorption are common after Roux-en-Y gastric bypass surgery. *Surgery* 2011;**149**(5):654–61.

67. O'Keefe SJ, Buchman AL, Fishbein TM, Jeejeebhoy KN, Jeppesen PB, Shaffer J. Short bowel syndrome and intestinal failure: consensus definitions and overview. *Clin. Gastroenterol. Hepatol.* 2006;**4**(1):6–10.

68. Ukleja A, Dumping syndrome: pathophysiology and treatment. *Nutr. Clin. Pract.* 2005;**20**(5):517–25.

69. Clancy TE, Moore FD, Jr, Zinner MJ. Post gastric bypass hyperinsulinism with nesidioblastosis: subtotal or total pancreatectomy may be needed to prevent recurrent hypoglycemia. *J. Gastrointest. Surg.* 2006;**10**(8):1116–9.

70. Kalarchian MA, Marcus MD, Wilson GT, Labouvie EW, Brolin RE, LaMarca LB. Binge eating among gastric bypass patients at long-term follow-up. *Obes. Surg.* 2002; **12**(2):270–5.

71. Fernandez-Esparrach G, Lautz DB, Thompson CC. Endoscopic repair of gastrogastric fistula after Roux-en-Y gastric bypass: a less-invasive approach. *Surg. Obes. Relat. Dis.* 2010;**6**(3):282–8.

72. Haito-Chavez Y, Law JK, Kratt T, et al. International multicenter experience with an over-the-scope clipping device for endoscopic management of GI defects (with video). *Gastrointest. Endosc.* 2014;**80**(4):610–22.

73. . Thompson CC, Slattery J, Bundga ME, Lautz DB. Peroral endoscopic reduction of dilated gastrojejunal anastomosis after Roux-en-Y gastric bypass: a possible new option for patients with weight regain. *Surg. Endosc.* 2006;**20**(11): 1744–8.

74. Thompson CC, Chand B, Chen YK, et al. Endoscopic suturing for transoral outlet reduction increases weight loss after Roux-en-Y gastric bypass surgery. *Gastroenterology* 2013;**145**(1):129–137 e3.

75. Kumar N, Thompson CC. Comparison of a superficial suturing device with a full-thickness suturing device for transoral outlet reduction (with videos). *Gastrointest. Endosc.* 2014;**79**(6):984–9.

76. Jirapinyo P, Slattery J, Ryan MB, Abu Dayyeh BK, Lautz DB, Thompson CC.Evaluation of an endoscopic suturing device for transoral outlet reduction in patients with weight regain following Roux-en-Y gastric bypass. *Endoscopy* 2013;**45**(7):532–6.

77. O'Brien PE, Brown WA, Smith A, McMurrick PJ, Stephens M. Prospective study of a laparoscopically placed, adjustable gastric band in the treatment of morbid obesity. *Br. J. Surg.* 1999;**86**(1):113–8.

78. O'Brien PE. Laparoscopic adjustable gastric banding: a real option for a real problem. *ANZ J. Surg.* 2003;**73**(8):562.

79. Cummins AG, LaBrooy JT, Stanley DP, Rowland R, Shearman DJ. Quantitative histological study of enteropathy associated with HIV infection. *Gut* 1990;**31**(3): 317–21.

80. Suter M, Giusti V, Héraief E, Calmes JM Band erosion after laparoscopic gastric banding: occurrence and results after conversion to Roux-en-Y gastric bypass. *Obes. Surg.* 2004;**14**(3):381–6.

81. Abu-Abeid S, Keidar A, Gavert N, Blanc A, Szold A. The clinical spectrum of band erosion following laparoscopic adjustable silicone gastric banding for morbid obesity. *Surg. Endosc.* 2003;**17**(6):861–3.

82. Png KS, Rao J, Lim KH, Chia KH. Lap-band causing left gastric artery erosion presenting with torrential hemorrhage. *Obes. Surg.* 2008;**18**(8):1050–2.

83. Neto MP, Ramos AC, Campos JM, et al. Endoscopic removal of eroded adjustable gastric band: lessons learned after 5 years and 78 cases. *Surg. Obes. Relat. Dis.* 2010;**6**(4):423–7.

84. Blero D, Eisendrath P, Vandermeeren A, et al. Endoscopic removal of dysfunctioning bands or rings after restrictive bariatric procedures. *Gastrointest. Endosc.* 2010;**71**(3): 468–74.

85. Sherwinter DA, Powers CJ, Geiss AC, Howard M, Warman J. Posterior prolapse: an important entity even in the modern age of the pars flaccida approach to lap-band placement. *Obes. Surg.* 2006;**16**(10):1312–7.

86. Abuzeid AW, Banerjea A, Timmis B, Hashemi M. Gastric slippage as an emergency: diagnosis and management. *Obes. Surg.* 2007;**17**(4):559–61.

87. Gravante G, Araco A, Araco F, Delogu D, De Lorenzo A, Cervelli V. Laparoscopic adjustable gastric bandings: a prospective randomized study of 400 operations performed with 2 different devices. *Arch. Surg.* 2007;**142**(10): 958–61.

88. Spivak H, Favretti F. Avoiding postoperative complications with the LAP-BAND system. *Am. J. Surg.* 2002; **184**(6B):31S–37S.

89. Abu-Abeid S, Szold A. Results and complications of laparoscopic adjustable gastric banding: an early and intermediate experience. *Obes. Surg.* 1999;**9**(2):188–90.

90. Belachew M, et al. Laparoscopic placement of adjustable silicone gastric band in the treatment of morbid obesity: how to do it. *Obes. Surg.* 1995;**5**(1):66–70.

91. Keidar A, Carmon E, Szold A, Abu-Abeid S. Port complications following laparoscopic adjustable gastric banding for morbid obesity. *Obes. Surg.* 2005;**15**(3):361–5.

92. Angrisani L, Furbetta F, Doldi SB, et al. Lap Band adjustable gastric banding system: the Italian experience with 1863 patients operated on 6 years. *Surg. Endosc.* 2003;**17**(3):409–12.

93. Ren CJ, Horgan S, Ponce J. US experience with the LAP-BAND system. *Am. J. Surg.* 2002;**184**(6B):46S-50S.

94. Dargent J. Laparoscopic adjustable gastric banding: lessons from the first 500 patients in a single institution. *Obes. Surg.* 1999;**9**(5):446–52.

95. Fabry H, Van Hee R, Hendrickx L, Totté E. A technique for prevention of port complications after laparoscopic adjustable silicone gastric banding. *Obes. Surg.* 2002;**12**(2): 285–8.

96. Rubenstein RB. Laparoscopic adjustable gastric banding at a US center with up to 3-year follow-up. *Obes. Surg.* 2002;**12**(3):380–4.

97. Ovrebø KK, Hatlebakk JG, Viste A, Bassøe HH, Svanes K. Gastroesophageal reflux in morbidly obese patients treated with gastric banding or vertical banded gastroplasty. *Ann. Surg.* 1998;**228**(1):51–8.

98. Doherty C, Maher JW, Heitshusen DS. Prospective investigation of complications, reoperations, and sustained weight loss with an adjustable gastric banding device for treatment of morbid obesity. *J. Gastrointest. Surg.* 1998;**2**(1):102–8.

99. DeMaria EJ. Laparoscopic adjustable silicone gastric banding: complications. *J. Laparoendosc. Adv. Surg. Tech. A* 2003;**13**(4): 271–7.

100. Gumbs AA, Gagner M, Dakin G, Pomp A. Sleeve gastrectomy for morbid obesity. *Obes. Surg.* 2007;**17**(7): 962–9.

101. Cottam D, Qureshi FG, Mattar SG,et al Laparoscopic sleeve gastrectomy as an initial weight-loss procedure for high-risk patients with morbid obesity. *Surg. Endosc.* 2006;**20**(6):859–63.

102. Regan JP, Inabnet WB, Gagner M, Pomp A. Early experience with two-stage laparoscopic Roux-en-Y gastric bypass as an alternative in the super-super obese patient. *Obes. Surg.* 2003;**13**(6):861–4.

103. Gagner M, Deitel M, Kalberer TL, Erickson AL, Crosby RD. The Second International Consensus Summit for Sleeve Gastrectomy, March 19–21, 2009. *Surg. Obes. Relat. Dis.* 2009;**5**(4):476–85.

104. Lalor PF, Tucker ON, Szomstein S, Rosenthal RJ. Complications after laparoscopic sleeve gastrectomy. *Surg. Obes. Relat. Dis.* 2008;**4**(1):33–8.

105. Burgos AM, Braghetto I, Csendes A, et al. Gastric leak after laparoscopic-sleeve gastrectomy for obesity. *Obes. Surg.* 2009;**19**(12):1672–7.

106. Ritter LA, Wang AY, Sauer BG, Kleiner DE. Healing of complicated gastric leaks in bariatric patients using endoscopic clips. *JSLS* 2013;**17**(3):481–3.

107. Mason EE. Vertical banded gastroplasty for obesity. *Arch. Surg.* 1982;**117**(5):701–6.

108. MacLean LD, Rhode BM, Sampalis J, Forse RA. Results of the surgical treatment of obesity. *Am. J. Surg.* 1993; **165**(1):155–60; discussion 160–2.

109. Sataloff DM, Lieber CP, Seinige UL. Strictures following gastric stapling for morbid obesity. Results of endoscopic dilatation. Am. *Surg.* 1990;**56**(3):167–74.

110. Moreno P1, Alastrué A, Rull M. Band erosion in patients who have undergone vertical banded gastroplasty: incidence and technical solutions. *Arch. Surg.* 1998;**133**(2):189–93.

111. El-Hayek K, Timratana P, Brethauer SA, Chand B. Complete endoscopic/transgastric retrieval of eroded gastric band: description of a novel technique and review of the literature. *Surg. Endosc.* 2013;**27**(8):2974–9.

112. Guedea ME, Arribas del Amo D, Solanas JA. Results of biliopancreatic diversion after five years. *Obes. Surg.* 2004;**14**(6):766–72.

CHAPTER 19

Complications of drugs used in gastroenterology

Paul Kevin Hamilton[1] and Philip Toner[2]

[1] Belfast Health and Social Care Trust, Belfast, UK

[2] Belfast Health and Social Care Trust, Belfast City Hospital, Belfast, UK

The nature of drug complications

There are two main forms of drug complications, known more correctly as adverse drug reactions (ADRs). Type A reactions represent an augmentation of a drug's pharmacological actions and are therefore dose-dependent and predictable; type B reactions are bizarre events that cannot be predicted [1]. The patient with constipation who is treated over-zealously with laxatives and who subsequently develops diarrhea has suffered a type A reaction. In contrast, an occurrence of Stevens-Johnson syndrome in a patient treated with a proton pump inhibitor (PPI) is an example of a type B reaction.

It is alarming to consider that ADRs are responsible for around 7% of hospital admissions [2] and 6% of intensive care unit admissions [3]. Of patients requiring re-admission after a hospital stay, one in five cases is due to an ADR [4]. Interactions between medicines account for a significant proportion of ADRs, usually type A. This is of particular importance since polypharmacy, the use of many medications in the same patient, is a significant problem in modern medicine [5]. The more drugs a patient takes, the more likely those drugs are to interact with one another, and the more likely an ADR is to occur. The incidence of drug interactions and ADRs increases with advancing age [6], with polypharmacy playing a major role in this.

Drugs used in gastroenterology may not only cause gastrointestinal symptoms themselves, but can also lead to disease in other systems that can range from trivial to life-threatening. With the increasing use of powerful immunomodulating drugs, it is now more important than ever for gastroenterologists to have a good working knowledge of the complications that their drugs can cause. All prescribers should, however, be vigilant when prescribing any drug, since even the most benign-sounding entries in drug formularies have often been linked with unpleasant side effects.

An overview of ADRs for gastroenterology drugs

There are many sources of information detailing undesirable effects of therapeutic agents. Table 19.1 provides an overview of the most commonly occurring adverse drug reactions as detailed in the medicines' summaries of product characteristics. These are continually updated as new information becomes known. ADRs with frequencies currently listed as rare or very rare, and those with unknown frequencies are not detailed here. This should not detract from these of course, since it is often the effects that occur rarely that carry the most significance for patients that are affected by them.

Specific ADRs

There now follows a more in depth discussion of some recently publicised ADRs for very frequently prescribed agents, and an account of ADRs for agents with the most unfavourable safety profiles. The discussion is

Gastrointestinal Emergencies, Third Edition. Edited by Tony C. K. Tham, John S. A. Collins, and Roy Soetikno.
© 2016 John Wiley & Sons, Ltd. Published 2016 by John Wiley & Sons, Ltd.

Table 19.1 Adverse drug reactions attributed to drugs commonly used in gastroenterology.

	Expected frequency of adverse drug reaction		
	Very common (≥1/10)	**Common (≥1/100 to <1/10)**	**Uncommon (≥1/1000 to <1/100)**
Antacids			
All agents	Incidence of ADRs not known. Aluminium preparations tend to cause constipation. Magnesium preparations tend to cause diarrhea. Flatulence and vomiting may occur.		
Antimuscarinics			
Hyoscine butylbromide			Skin reactions Tachycardia Dry mouth Possible hypersensitivity reactions including anaphylaxis
Motility stimulants			
Metoclopramide	Incidence of ADRs not known. The following may occur: hyperprolactinemia (and its clinical effects), extrapyramidal symptoms, tardive dyskinesia, drowsiness, dizziness, tremor, visual disturbances, acute hypertension in patients with phaeochromocytoma, hypotension, dyspnea, diarrhea, skin reactions, edema		
Domperidone		Dry mouth	Headache, anxiety, sommolence, asthenia Diarrhea Rash, pruritus Loss of libido, galactorrhea, breast pain/ tenderness
Histamine-H₂ receptor antagonists			
Ranitidine			Abdominal pain, constipation, diarrhea, nausea
Cimetidine		Headache, dizziness, lethargy Diarrhea Skin rashes Myalgia	Depression, confusion, hallucinations Leukopenia Tachycardia Hepatitis Increased plasma creatinine Gynecomastia, impotence (at high dose)
Prostaglandin analogs			
Misoprostol	Diarrhea Rash	Headache, dizziness Abdominal pain, constipation, dyspepsia, flatulence, nausea, vomiting	Vaginal hemorrhage, menstrual disorders Pyrexia

Proton pump inhibitors

Esomeprazole	Headache	Edema
	Abdominal pain, constipation, diarrhea, flatulence, nausea, vomiting	Insomnia, dizziness, paraesthesia, somnolence, vertigo
		Dry mouth
		Increased liver enzymes
		Dermatitis, pruritus, rash, urticaria
		Fracture of the hip, wrist or spine
Lansoprazole	Headache, dizziness, fatigue	Edema
	Abdominal pain, constipation, diarrhea, flatulence, nausea, vomiting	Depression
	Dry mouth/ throat	Thrombocytopenia, eosinophilia, leukopenia
	Increased liver enzymes	Fracture of the hip, wrist or spine; arthralgia, myalgia
	Urticaria, itch, rash	
Omeprazole	Headache	Edema
	Abdominal pain, constipation, diarrhea, flatulence, nausea, vomiting	Insomnia, dizziness, paresthesia, somnolence, vertigo, malaise
		Increased liver enzymes
		Dermatitis, pruritus, rash, urticaria
		Fracture of the hip, wrist or spine
Pantoprazole		Sleep disorders, dizziness, asthenia, fatigue, malaise, headache
		Abdominal pain, constipation, diarrhea, nausea, vomiting, abdominal distension, bloating
		Dry mouth
		Increased liver enzymes
		Pruritus, rash, exanthema, eruption
		Fracture of the hip, wrist or spine
Rabeprazole	Headache, dizziness, insomnia, asthenia	Nervousness , somnolence
	Abdominal pain, constipation, diarrhea, flatulence, nausea, vomiting	Dyspepsia, eructation
	Infection. influenza like illness	Dry mouth
	Cough, pharyngitis, rhinitis	Increased liver enzymes
		Rash, erythema
		Bronchitis, sinusitis
		Non-specific pain, back pain, chest pain
		Chills, pyrexia

Anti-motility drugs

Loperamide	Headache,	Dizziness, somnolence
	Constipation, flatulence, nausea	Abdominal pain, vomiting, dyspepsia
		Dry mouth
		Rash

(Continued)

Table 19.1 (Continued)

	Expected frequency of adverse drug reaction		
	Very common (≥1/10)	Common (≥1/100 to <1/10)	Uncommon (≥1/1000 to <1/100)
Racecadotril		Headache	Rash, erythema
Antimicrobial drugs			
Vancomycin	ADRs uncommon when used orally. Patients with IBD, particularly those with renal impairment, are at risk of significant systemic absorption		
Metronidazole	Nil listed at these frequencies		
Ciprofloxacin	Nausea Diarrhea		Headache, dizziness, sleep disorders, taste disorders, anorexia, asthenia psychomotor hyperactivity/agitation, Abdominal pain, dyspepsia, flatulence, vomiting Increased liver enzymes Rash, pruritis, urticaria Mycotic superinfections Musculoskeletal pain, arthralgia Renal impairment Fever Increase in alkaline phosphatase, eosinophilia
Aminosalicylates			
Balsalazide/mesalazine		Headache Abdominal pain, diarrhea, vomiting, nausea Arthralgia/myalgia	
Olsalazine		Headache Diarrhea, nausea Rash Arthralgia	Dizziness, paresthesia, depression Vomiting, dyspepsia Increased liver enzymes Pruritus, alopecia, photosensitivity reactions, urticaria Thrombocytopenia Tachycardia Dyspnea Myalgia Pyrexia

Sulfasalazine	Gastric distress, nausea	Dizziness, headache, Insomnia, taste disorders, tinnitus Abdominal pain, diarrhea, vomiting, stomatitis Leukopenia, proteinuria Conjuctival and scleral injection Cough Pruritus Arthralgia Fever	Facial edema Depression, convulsions, vertigo Increased liver enzymes Dyspnea Alopecia, urticaria Thrombocytopenia Vasculitis
Corticosteroids	Incidence of ADRs not listed. Increased susceptibility and severity of infections with suppression of clinical symptoms and signs, opportunistic infections, recurrence of dormant tuberculosis. Abdominal distension, acute pancreatitis, dyspepsia, nausea, increased appetite, esophageal candidiasis, esophageal ulceration, peptic ulceration with perforation and hemorrhage, perforation of the small bowel, particularly in patients with inflammatory bowel disease. Cushingoid facies, hirsutism, impaired carbohydrate tolerance, menstrual irregularity and amenorrhea, negative protein and calcium balance, suppression of the hypothalamo–pituitary–adrenal axis, weight gain. Hypertension, nocturia, hypokalaemic alkalosis, potassium loss, sodium and water retention, risk of congestive heart failure in susceptible patients. Avascular osteonecrosis, osteoporosis, proximal myopathy, tencon rupture, vertebral and long bone fractures, muscle weakness, wasting and loss of muscle mass. Acne, bruising, impaired healing, skin atrophy, striae, telangiectasia. Wide range of psychiatric reactions including affective disorders and psychotic reactions, marked euphoria leading to dependence; aggravation of epilepsy, behavioral disturbances, irritability, nervousness, anxiety, sleep disturbances, and cognitive dysfunction. Psychological dependence. Corneal or scleral thinning, scleral perforation, exacerbation of ophthalmic viral or fungal disease, glaucoma, increased intraocular pressure, papilledema, posterior subcapsular cataracts. Hypersensitivity including anaphylaxis, leukocytosis, malaise, thromboembolism. Too rapid a reduction of corticostero dosage following prolonged treatment can lead to acute adrenal insufficiency, hypotension, and death. A "withdrawal syndrome" may also occur including arthralgia, conjunctivitis, fever, loss of weight, myalgia, painful itchy skin nodules and rhinitis.		
Other immunomodulators			
Azathioprine	Susceptibility to infection Nausea, anorexia, vomiting	Leukopenia, anemia, thrombocytopenia Pancreatitis, hepatic dysfunction Alopecia	Hypersensitivity reactions Steatorrhea, diarrhea
Methotrexate	Stomatitis, dyspepsia, nausea, anorexia. Elevated transaminases.	Headache, tiredness, drowsiness Oral ulcers, diarrhea Exanthema, erythema, pruritus Pneumonia, interstitial alveolitis/pneumonitis often associated with eosinophilia Leukopenia, anemia, thrombocytopenia	Dizziness, confusion, depression Pharyngitis, enteritis, vomiting Photosensitisation, alopecia, herpes zoster, vasculitis, herpetiform eruptions of the skin, urticaria Precipitation of diabetes mellitus Cirrhosis, fibrosis and fatty cegeneration of the liver, decrease in serum albumin Pancytopenia Inflammation and ulceration of the urinary bladder, renal impairment, disturbed micturition Inflammation and ulceration of the vagina Arthralgia, myalgia, osteoporosis

(Continued)

Table 19.1 (Continued)

	Expected frequency of adverse drug reaction		
	Very common (≥1/10)	Common (≥1/100 to <1/10)	Uncommon (≥1/1000 to <1/100)
Mercaptopurine	Bone marrow suppression, leukopenia, thrombocytopenia Nausea, vomiting, pancreatitis Biliary stasis, hepatotoxicity		Anorexia Anemia
Mycophenolate mofetil	Sepsis, gastrointestinal candidiasis, urinary tract infection, herpes simplex, herpes zoster Leukopenia, thrombocytopenia, anemia Abdominal pain, vomiting, diarrhea, nausea	Other infections Convulsions, hypertonia, tremor, somnolence, myasthenic syndrome, dizziness, headache, paresthesia, dysgeusia, anorexia Gastrointestinal hemorrhage, peritonitis, ileus, colitis, gastric ulcer, duodenal ulcer, gastritis, esophagitis, stomatitis, constipation, dyspepsia, flatulence, eructation, gingival hyperplasia, pancreatitis Hepatitis, jaundice, hyperbilirubinemia Skin neoplasia Pancytopenia, leukocytosis Acidosis, hyperkalaemia, hypokalaemia, hyperglycaemia, hypomagnesaemia, hypocalcaemia, hypercholesterolemia, hyperlipidaemia, hypophosphatemia, hyperuricemia, gout; increased creatinine , urea, blood lactate dehydrogenase, alkaline phosphatase Tachycardia, hypotension, hypertension, vasodilatation Pleural effusion, dyspnea, cough Skin hypertrophy, rash, acne, alopecia Arthralgia Renal impairment Edema, pyrexia, chills, pain, malaise, asthenia Weight loss	Agranulocytosis
Ciclosporin	Respiratory tract, urinary tract and cytomegalovirus infection Hyperlipidemia Tremor, headache including migraine. Hypertension Liver impairment Renal impairment	Paresthesia Nausea, vomiting, abdominal pain, diarrhea, gingival hyperplasia Sepsis, herpes infections, candidal infection. Skin papillomas, basal cell carcinoma, squamous cell carcinoma, Bowen's disease, Lymphoproliferative disorders. Anorexia, hyperuricemia, hyperkalemia, hypomagnesemia Hypertrichosis Muscle cramps, myalgia Fatigue	Anemia, thrombocytopenia. Encephalopathy. Allergic rashes. Edema, weight increase

Infliximab	Viral infections	Bacterial infections	Other infections
	Headache	Neutropenia, leucopenia, anaemia, lymphadenopathy.	Thrombocytopenia, lymphopenia, lymphocytosis
	Upper respiratory tract infection, sinusitis.	Allergic respiratory symptoms.	Anaphylactic reactions, lupus-like syndrome, serum sickness or serum sickness-like reaction
	Abdominal pain, nausea.	Depression, insomnia, vertigo, dizziness, hypoaesthesia, paraesthesia	Amnesia, agitation, confusion, somnolence, nervousness, seizure, neuropathy
	Infusion-related reactions	Conjunctivitis	Cardiac failure (new onset or worsening), arrhythmia, syncope, bradycardia.
		Tachycardia, palpitations, hypotension, hypertension	Peripheral ischemia, thrombophlebitis, hematoma.
		Ecchymosis, hot flush, flushing	Pulmonary edema, bronchospasm, pleurisy, pleural effusion.
		Dyspnea, epistaxis	Intestinal perforation, intestinal stenosis, diverticulitis, pancreatitis, cheilitis.
		Gastrointestinal hemorrhage, diarrhea, dyspepsia, gastroesophageal reflux, constipation	Hepatitis, hepatocellular damage, cholecystitis.
		Abnormal liver function	Bullous eruptions, onychomycosis, seborrhea, rosacea, skin papilloma, hyperkeratosis, abnormal skin pigmentation, keratitis, periorbital edema, hordeolum
		New onset or worsening of psoriasis, urticaria, rash, pruritus, hyperhidrosis, dry skin, fungal dermatitis, eczema, alopecia	Vaginitis
		Arthralgia, myalgia, back pain, chest pain, fatigue, fever, injection site reactions, chills, edema	Impaired healing.

(Continued)

Table 19.1 (Continued)

		Expected frequency of adverse drug reaction	
	Very common (≥1/10)	Common (≥1/100 to <1/10)	Uncommon (≥1/1000 to <1/100)
Adalimumab	Respiratory tract infections	Systemic infections	Other infections
	Leucopenia (including neutropenia and agranulocytos s), anaemia	Skin neoplasia	Diverticulitis
	Hyperlipidemia	Leukocytosis, thrombocytopenia	Lymphoma, solid organ neoplasia, melanoma
	Headache	Hypersensitivity, allergies	Idiopathic thrombocytopenic purpura
	Abdominal pain, nausea, vomiting	Hypokalaemia, hyperuricemia, abnormal sodium concentrations, hypocalcaemia, hyperglycemia, hypophosphatemia, dehydration	Sarcoidosis
	Raised liver enzymes	Paraesthesia, migraine, nerve root compression, vertigo	Stroke, tremor, neuropathy, diplopia, deafness, tinnitus
	Rash	Visual impairment, conjunctivitis, blepharitis, eye swelling	Myocardial infarction, arrhythmia, congestive heart failure, aortic aneurysm, vascular arterial occlusion, thrombophlebitis
	Musculoskeletal pain	Tachycardia, hypertension	Pulmonary embolism, interstitial lung disease, chronic obstructive pulmonary disease, pneumonitis, pleural effusion
	Injection site reactions	Flushing	Pancreatitis, dysphagia, edema
		Hematoma	Cholecystitis, cholelithiasis, hepatic steatosis, increased bilirubin
		Asthma, dyspnea, cough	Night sweats, scarring
		GI hemorrhage, dyspepsia, gastroesophageal reflux disease, sicca syndrome	Rhabdomyolysis, systemic lupus erythematosus
		Worsening or new onset of psoriasis, urticaria, bruising, dermatitis, onychoclasis, hyperhidrosis, alopecia, pruritus	Nocturia, erectile dysfunction
		Muscle spasms	Inflammation
		Renal impairment, hematuria	
		Chest pain, edema, pyrexia	
		Coagulation and bleeding disorders , positive autoantibody tests, blood lactate dehydrogenase increased	
		Impaired healing	
Laxatives			
Bisacodyl		Abdominal cramps/pain, diarrhea and nausea	Dizziness
			Hematochezia, vomiting, anorectal discomfort
Lactulose	Flatulence, abdominal pain	Nausea, vomiting	
Methylnaltrexone	Abdominal pain, nausea, diarrhea, flatulence	Dizziness	
		Injection site reactions	
		Hyperhidrosis	

Prucalopride	Headache	Anorexia, tremors
	Abdominal pain, diarrhea, nausea	Palpitations
		Fever, malaise
Linaclotide	Diarrhea	Faecal incontinence, defecation urgency
	Vomiting, dyspepsia, rectal hemorrhage, flatulence, abnormal bowel sounds	Hypokalemia
	Pollakiuria	Dehydration
	Dizziness	Decreased appetite
	Viral gastroenteritis, abdominal pain, flatulence, abdominal distension	Orthostatic hypotension
	Dizziness, fatigue	

Drugs affecting intestinal secretions

Pancreatin	Abdominal pain	Rash
	Nausea, vomiting, constipation, abdominal distension, diarrhea	
Colestyramine	Frequency of ADRs not listed. Constipation, diarrhea (in high dose). May interfere with the absorption of fat soluble vitamins. Possibly increased bleeding tendency due to Vitamin K deficiency. Hyperchloremic acidosis.	
Ursodeoxycholic acid	Pasty stools, diarrhea	

Source: Datapharm Communications Ltd.

limited to the treatment of adults. Toxicological aspects are beyond the scope of this book.

Proton pump inhibitors

Prescribed by most gastroenterologists on an almost daily basis, it is easy to become complacent when prescribing proton pump inhibitors (PPIs). This is compounded by their clinical efficacy, low cost (for most agents) and the fact that the most commonly occurring ADRs (headache and insignificant gastrointestinal upset) are relatively minor. As longer-term exposure to these agents increases, some interesting effects have, however, been reported.

The phenomenon of PPI-induced hypomagnesemia has received some attention recently. This electrolyte abnormality might occur due to drug-induced alterations in magnesium transport in intestinal cells [7]. Case reports suggest that this is a class-effect, that it occurs after a median of 5.5 years treatment, that it responds to PPI cessation and magnesium replacement, and that it returns upon reintroduction of the culprit drug [8]. Symptoms of hypomagnesemia include neuromuscular manifestations (e.g. twitching, cramps and spasms), neuropsychiatric features including seizures, and cardiovascular effects (e.g. arrhythmias and hypertension); low levels of potassium, calcium and phosphate may also result [9]. The UK's Medicines and Healthcare products Regulatory Agency (MHRA) recommend contemplating the "measurement of magnesium levels before starting PPI treatment and periodically during prolonged treatment, especially in those who will take a PPI concomitantly with digoxin or drugs that may cause hypomagnesaemia" [10]. They also suggest that people taking long-term treatment with a PPI should be advised to seek medical advice if they experience symptoms in keeping with this electrolyte disturbance.

Following several reports in the literature linking PPI use with bone fractures, two meta-analyses have shown that this heightened risk appears real. The odds ratio (95% confidence interval) for spinal fracture has been reported as 1.50 (1.32–1.72), hip fracture as between 1.23 (1.11–1.36) and 1.34 (1.09–1.66) and any fracture at between 1.20 (1.11–1.30) and 1.30 (1.15–1.48) [11,12]. One might suppose that the increased risk of fractures in patients taking PPIs relates to alterations in calcium absorption (due to alteration of the acidity of gastric secretions and subsequent effects on calcium

ionisation) and hence bone mineral density. However, conflicting reports detailing the effect of PPIs on bone mineral density have been published and the mechanism for the observed increased fracture effect remains unknown [13]. The MHRA recommends that "patients at risk of osteoporosis should be treated according to current clinical guidelines to ensure they have an adequate intake of vitamin D and calcium" [14].

Concerns have been raised that that use of PPIs might put patients at risk from *Clostridium difficile* infection (CDI). Although some studies report no association between PPI use and CDI [15,16], several meta-analyses and a systematic review of the literature suggest that the association is real [17–19]. In these studies the odds ratio for developing CDI whilst taking a PPI varied from 1.65 to 2.15. The literature suffers from publication bias and marked homogeneity between studies. Despite this, and although a cause–effect relationship cannot be assumed, there does appear to be a genuine link between the use of these agents and CDI. It could be suggested that altered effects of gastric secretions on *C. difficile* spores occur in the less acidic milieu that results from PPI use. Indeed, a quasi dose-response relationship between gastric pH and CDI incidence has been reported with an incidence of nosocomial CDI of 0.3% in those on no acid-suppressing medication, 0.6% in those on histamine-2 receptor antagonists, 0.9% on those on daily PPIs and 1.4% in those taking more frequent PPIs [20]. However, this hypothesis has not stood up to more rigorous experimental enquiry [21]. Further studies are required to further elucidate the potential link between PPIs and CDI and, at present, there is no firm guidance on whether to discontinue PPIs in patients who develop this infection.

Aminosalicylates

Aminosalicylates are anti-inflammatory drugs that are used in the treatment of inflammatory bowel disease (IBD). Sulfasalazine is the oldest and least expensive agent in its class; it comprises a sulfapyridine carrier molecule linked to salicylate, and is not as commonly prescribed today as the other agents because of the possibility of side-effects associated with the sulfapyridine group [22]. Other drugs in the class are generally very well tolerated. The most common ADRs include headache, nausea, epigastric pain, diarrhea, and oligospermia [23].

As with several other drugs used to treat IBD, patients taking aminosalicylates should be instructed to report any symptoms that might indicate an iatrogenic blood disorder (e.g. bruising, bleeding, symptoms of infection) [24]. It is also recommended that renal function should be checked before commencing these drugs and at regular intervals thereafter. Pancreatitis and interstitial nephritis appear significantly more common with mesalazine than the other agents [25]. Mesalazine may increase the risk of hematological toxicity when co-prescribed with azathioprine (AZA) and 6-mercaptopurine (6-MP), but this is not a common problem [22]. In approximately 3% of patients, acute intolerance to aminosalicylates may occur, with reactions resembling a flare of IBD; recurrence after re-challenging the patient may enable this ADR to be detected [23].

Corticosteroids

Used in the management of IBD since the late 1940s [26], corticosteroids are effective therapeutic agents that are unfortunately linked to many adverse effects. In Crohn's disease affecting the ileum and right colon, budesonide can be used – it is poorly absorbed from the gastrointestinal tract and has extensive first-pass metabolism, therefore reducing systemic side-effects [22]. The use of topical preparations should also limit the incidence of ADRs.

Adverse effects from corticosteroids are listed in Table 1 and are generally well known. Patients who will require a long duration of treatment should have periodic bone mineral density assessments, annual ophthalmologic examinations and monitoring for glucose intolerance and other metabolic abnormalities [27]. It has been suggested that patients taking as little as 10 mg prednisolone (or equivalent) for more than 3 weeks may have a suppressed hypothalamic–pituitary–adrenal axis for more than a year after stopping, and may need to receive supplemental steroids in further illness or surgery [22]. It is because of the extensive side effect profile of corticosteroids that efforts are often made to introduce other drugs as "steroid-sparing" treatments.

Thiopurines

AZA and 6-MP are thiopurine drugs that are cytotoxic and immunosuppressive. Both agents are pro-drugs that are metabolized to their active forms. Although fairly complex, an understanding of the metabolism of these agents is essential to fully appreciate their actions and some of their adverse effects. This is particularly important when it is considered that up to 40% of patients

with IBD fail to respond to these drugs [28] and almost 10% withdraw from treatment due to ADRs [29]. As detailed in Table 19.1, ADRs from these agents can be severe and even life-threatening. The commonest reactions are allergic in nature, although bone marrow toxicity and neoplasia are particularly concerning associations. Meta-analyses have yielded conflicting results with regard to the risk of malignancy with these agents [30,31], and it is felt that the absolute risk is small [23]. 6-MP is not licensed for the treatment of IBD in the United Kingdom, but is sometimes used in patients who cannot tolerate AZA due to nausea, diarrhea, or myalgia [22].

AZA is largely metabolised to 6-MP which is in turn acted on by 3 enzymes as detailed in Fig. 19.1. Xanthine oxidase (XO) activity results in the formation of inactive 6-thiouric acid; thiopurine S-methyl-transferase (TPMT) activity yields 6-methylmercaptopurine; and hypoxanthine guanine phosphoribosyltransferase catalyzes the formation of 6-thioinosine monophosphate (6-TIMP) [32]. 6-TIMP is further metabolized by TPMT to form 6-methylmercaptopurine ribonucleotides (6-MMP(R)) and by other enzymes to yield 6-thioguanine nucleotides (6-TGNs), which represent the active metabolites responsible for the drugs' immunosuppressant actions [33].

TPMT is the main regulatory enzyme utilized in the metabolism of AZA and 6-MP. Over 30 years ago it was shown that individuals differ in their intrinsic activity of this enzyme, with some having high activity, others having intermediate activity and a smaller proportion having undetectable activity [34]. It is now also known that some people have extremely high enzyme activity. This variation is seemingly mainly due to polymorphisms in the TPMT gene. Patients with low TPMT activity produce increased amounts of 6-TGN after administration of a dose of AZA or 6-MP and are therefore more likely to exhibit toxic effects (particularly in relation to cytopenia) [35]. Conversely, those with higher TPMT activity will form less 6-TGN, but will generate more 6-MMP(R). They would therefore be expected to exhibit inadequate responses to standard doses of agents and may develop hepatotoxicity due to 6-MMP(R).

The activity of AZA and 6-MP will be increased if co-prescribed with allopurinol, an inhibitor of XO. Accidental co-prescription of these drugs can lead to severe and potentially fatal bone marrow suppression [22]. Some patients with very high TMPT activity might

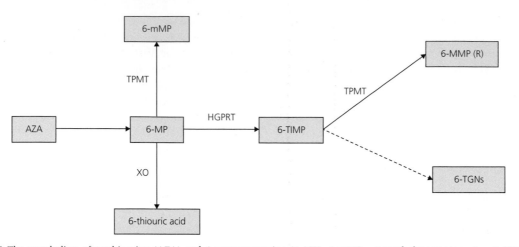

Fig. 19.1 The metabolism of azathioprine (AZA) and 6-mercaptopurine (6-MP). 6-mMP = 6-methylmercaptopurine, 6-MMP(R) = 6-methylmercaptopurine ribonucleotides, 6-TGNs = 6-thioguanine nucleotides, 6-TIMP = 6-thioinosine monophosphate, HGPRT = hypoxanthine guanine phosphoribosyltransferase, TPMT = thiopurine *S*-methyl-transferase, XO =xanthine oxidase.

benefit from the addition of allopurinol, however, but this approach requires a marked reduction in thiopurine dose and very frequent monitoring of blood cell counts [35]. Embarking on this therapeutic journey should only be under expert supervision.

Prescribers should strongly consider measuring TPMT activity before using these agents. Patients with absent activity should not receive the drugs; those with reduced activity may be treated under specialist supervision [24] and lower than normal doses would seem sensible. The precise role of measuring TPMT levels, however, remains controversial [23]. Weekly blood count monitoring for at least the first 4 weeks of therapy followed by checks at 8 weeks and then at least 3 monthly is recommended, and patients should be told to immediately report any symptoms that might reflect bone marrow suppression. In addition, patients should be advised to take precautions to avoid excessive sun exposure due to concerns over a link with skin cancer [23].

Methotrexate

Methotrexate is a folic acid antagonist that operates as an antimetabolite cytotoxic agent. Although marketing authorisation is lacking in the United Kingdom, methotrexate is sometimes used for the treatment of Crohn's disease.

In an early placebo-controlled trial of methotrexate for Crohn's disease 17% of patients on active treatment withdrew due to ADRs compared to 2% on placebo

[36]. The commonest reasons for withdrawal were asymptomatic elevation of serum aminotransferases and nausea although skin rash, pneumonia, and optic neuritis were also implicated. Less severe effects, not warranting withdrawal from treatment, occurred with a similar frequency to those in the placebo group. In a comparator trial between methotrexate and AZA for Crohn's disease, there was no difference in the rate of withdrawal from therapy between groups, although ADRs not requiring drug cessation were more common in the methotrexate group (44% vs. 7%) [37].

Prescribers should be wary of bone marrow suppression with methotrexate. This is a particular risk in patients of advanced age and those with renal impairment and concomitant use of other anti-folate drugs (e.g. trimethoprim) [24].

One major concern with methotrexate therapy is liver toxicity. A meta-analysis of 13 trials assessing this showed that the incidence of a rise in aminotransferase levels up to a two-fold increase over the upper limit of normal was 1.4 per 100 person-months, and the rate of more extreme elevations was 0.9 per 100 person-months, suggesting that the true incidence of this ADR is relatively low [38]. It has been suggested that methotrexate is avoided in patients with other significant risk factors for liver dysfunction, such as alcohol excess and obesity in an attempt to minimize liver toxicity [23].

Methotrexate can cause allergic, cytotoxic and immunological reactions that can result in pulmonary toxicity [39]. The exact incidence is unknown, but a prevalence of 2% has been suggested [40]. Clinical features are non-specific, and radiological evidence includes interstitial/alveolar infiltrates, increased interstitial markings, and pleural effusions [41]. Formal diagnostic criteria have been proposed [42,43]. Treatment generally involves withdrawal of methotrexate and consideration of corticosteroid treatment.

Patients should receive adequate education before commencing methotrexate. They should appreciate that the usual dosing regimen is once weekly, not daily. Patients should be asked to report symptoms that might suggest blood cell count abnormalities, liver toxicity and respiratory disease as soon as possible. A careful blood monitoring scheme must be in place for patients taking this drug. Full blood counts, renal, and liver function should be regularly checked, and detailed guidelines have been drawn up to assist practitioners with this [44]. It is recommended that patients prescribed methotrexate also take folate (either folic acid or folinic acid). A recent systematic review of the use of the drug for the treatment of rheumatoid arthritis showed that co-prescription of folate is associated with a 9% absolute risk reduction in the incidence of gastrointestinal ADRs, a 16% absolute risk reduction in transaminase elevation and 15.2% absolute risk reduction for drug withdrawal [45]. It seems reasonable to assume that a similar protective effect of folate exists when methotrexate is used for Crohn's disease.

Anti-tumor necrosis factor-α agents

Infliximab (IFX) and adalimumab (ADA) are anti-tumor necrosis factor-α (anti-TNF-α) monoclonal antibodies. Both drugs are used in the treatment of Crohn's disease, with IFX also being used in ulcerative colitis. The list of potential ADRs with these agents is long (Table 19.1), reflecting their powerful mechanisms of action and the fact that they are relatively new treatments that have been subjected to the scrutiny of modern drug licencing authorities. They should never be commenced without due consideration and discussion with the patient.

A major concern when using these drugs is the risk of infection, particularly since deaths from to infective complications have been reported [46]. Anti-TNF-α therapy has been known to trigger *Mycobacterium tuberculosis* infections, presumably in individuals harbouring dormant disease [47], and guidelines now exist to assist prescribers assess risk and manage *M. tuberculosis* prior to the initiation of immunosuppressant therapy [48]. The

use of these drugs has also been linked to reactivation of chronic hepatitis B, and prophylactic antiviral therapy has been suggested for those with positive serological markers [49]. For patients requiring surgery, bear in mind that a meta-analysis demonstrated a significant increase in postoperative complications [50].

A meta-analysis of the use of anti-TNF-α therapies for rheumatoid arthritis reported an odds ratio for malignancy of 3.3 (95% confidence interval 1.2–9.1), with the risk seemingly being dose-related [51]. The number needed to harm was 154 for one additional malignancy within a treatment period of 6–12 months. This marked increase in risk has however not been duplicated in all studies, and it has been suggested that the occurrence of cancer after these treatments is, in fact, quite rare [23].

Considerable patient education is necessary before commencing anti-TNF-α treatment. Any symptoms in keeping with infection, heart failure, or low blood cell counts should be reported immediately. Monitoring of blood cell counts, erythrocyte sedimentation rate, renal function, electrolytes, and liver function tests is also recommended.

Principles of prescribing

The literature detailing drug complications is dynamic, with the evidence base continually being updated as experience with the various agents increases. Prescribers are advised to keep up to date with new pharmacovigilance alerts for drugs that they commonly prescribe. Newer drugs in any field of medicine should always be adopted cautiously since it may not be possible to identify rare adverse effects in premarketing investigative trials. It is often post-marketing surveillance studies and pharmacovigilance alerts that give the first insight into less commonly occurring reactions. Prescribers are encouraged to engage in ADR reporting. All reactions to newer agents and serious reactions to established therapies should all be notified.

Some general principles of good prescribing apply in gastroenterology as in all medical disciplines, in an attempt to minimise drug complications for all patients. These include the following:
- Start new agents only when necessary.
- Use the lowest dose required, particularly at extremes of age.
- Minimise polypharmacy.

- Be mindful of drug interactions.
- Withdraw drugs that are ineffective and/or providing no benefit.
- Educate patients on common and serious adverse drug reactions, and what to do if they occur.

References

1. Pirmohamed M, Breckenridge AM, Kitteringham NR, et al. Adverse Drug Reactions. *BMJ* 1998;**316**:1295–8.
2. Pirmohamed M, James S, Meakin S, et al. Adverse drug reactions as cause of admission to hospital: prospective analysis of 18 820 patients. *BMJ* 2004;**329**:15–9.
3. Schwake L, Wollenschlager I, Stremmel W, et al. Adverse drug reactions and deliberate self-poisoning as cause of admission to the intensive care unit: a 1-year prospective observational cohort study. *Intensive Care Med.* 2009;**35**: 266–74.
4. Davies EC, Green CF, Mottram DR, et al. Emergency re-admissions to hospital due to adverse drug reactions within 1 year of the index admission. *Br. J. Clin. Pharmacol.* 2010;**70**:749–55.
5. Milton JC, Jackson SH. Inappropriate polypharmacy: reducing the burden of multiple medication. *Clin. Med.* 2007;**7**:514–7.
6. Rollason V, Vogt N. Reduction of Polypharmacy in the Elderly: A Systematic Review of the Role of the Pharmacist. *Drugs Aging* 2003;**20**:817–32.
7. Thongon N, Krishnamra N. Omeprazole decreases magnesium transport across Caco-2 monolayers. *World J. Gastroenterol.* 2011;**17**:1574–83.
8. Hess MW, Hoenderop JG, Bindels RJ, et al. Systematic review: hypomagnesaemia induced by proton pump inhibition. *Aliment. Pharmacol. Ther.* 2012;**36**:405–13.
9. Berkelhammer C, Bear RA. A Clinical approach to common electrolyte problems: 4. hypomagnesemia. *Can. Med. Assoc. J.* 1985;**132**:360–8.
10. MHRA. Drug Safety Update April 2012. 2012;**5**:A1.
11. Kwok CS, Yeong JK, Loke YK. Meta-analysis: risk of fractures with acid-suppressing medication. *Bone* 2011;**48**: 768–76.
12. Eom CS, Park SM, Myung SK, et al. Use of acid-suppressive drugs and risk of fracture: a meta-analysis of observational studies. *Ann. Fam. Med.* 2011;**9**:257–67.
13. Fournier MR, Targownik LE, Leslie WD. Proton Pump inhibitors, osteoporosis, and osteoporosis-related fractures. *Maturitas* 2009;**64**:9–13.
14. MHRA. Drug Safety Update April 2012. 2012;**5**:A2.
15. Leonard AD, Ho KM, Flexman J. Proton pump inhibitors and diarrhoea related to *Clostridium difficile* infection in hospitalised patients: a case-control study. *Int. Med. J.* 2012;**42**:591–4.
16. Naggie S, Miller BA, Zuzak KB, et al. A case-control study of community-associated *Clostridium difficile* infection: no role for proton pump inhibitors. *Am. J. Med.* 2011;**124**:276. e1,276.e7.
17. Tleyjeh IM, Bin Abdulhak AA, Riaz M, et al. Association between proton pump inhibitor therapy and *Clostridium difficile* infection: a contemporary systematic review and meta-analysis. *PLoS ONE* 2012;**7**:e50836.
18. Deshpande A, Pant C, Pasupuleti V, et al. Association between proton pump inhibitor therapy and *Clostridium difficile* infection in a meta-analysis. *Clin. Gastroenterol. Hepatol.* 2012;**10**:225–33.
19. Janarthanan S, Ditah I, Adler DG, et al. *Clostridium difficile*-associated diarrhea and proton pump inhibitor therapy: a meta-analysis. *Am. J. Gastroenterol.* 2012;**107**:1001–10.
20. Howell MD, Novack V, Grgurich P, et al. Iatrogenic gastric acid suppression and the risk of nosocomial *Clostridium difficile* infection. *Arch. Intern. Med.* 2010;**170**:784–90.
21. Nerandzic MM, Pultz MJ, Donskey CJ. Examination of potential mechanisms to explain the association between proton pump inhibitors and *Clostridium difficile* infection. *Antimicrob. Agents Chemother.* 2009;**53**:4133–7.
22. Taylor K, Wilkinson M. Recommended drug therapy for inflammatory bowel disease. *Prescriber* 2012;**23**:28–38.
23. Mowat C, Cole A, Windsor A, et al. Guidelines for the management of inflammatory bowel disease in adults. *Gut* 2011;**60**:571–607.
24. Joint Formulary Committee. *British national formulary (BNF) 65.* Pharmaceutical Press, London, 2013.
25. Ransford RA, Langman MJ. Sulphasalazine and mesalazine: serious adverse reactions re-evaluated on the basis of suspected adverse reaction reports to the Committee on Safety of Medicines. *Gut* 2002;**51**:536–9.
26. Buchman AL. Side effects of corticosteroid therapy. *J. Clin. Gastroenterol.* 2001;**33**:289–94.
27. Lichtenstein GR, Abreu MT, Cohen R, et al. American Gastroenterological Association Institute medical position statement on corticosteroids, immunomodulators, and infliximab in inflammatory bowel disease. *Gastroenterology* 2006;**130**:935–9.
28. Dubinsky MC, Yang H, Hassard PV, et al. 6-MP Metabolite profiles provide a biochemical explanation for 6-MP resistance in patients with inflammatory bowel disease. *Gastroenterology* 2002;**122**:904–15.
29. Timmer A, McDonald JW, Tsoulis DJ, et al. Azathioprine and 6-mercaptopurine for maintenance of remission in ulcerative colitis. *Cochrane Database of Systematic Reviews* 2012;**9**:000478.
30. Kandiel A, Fraser AG, Korelitz BI, et al. Increased risk of lymphoma among inflammatory bowel disease patients treated with azathioprine and 6-mercaptopurine. *Gut* 2005;**54**:1121–5.
31. Masunaga Y, Ohno K, Ogawa R, et al. Meta-analysis of risk of malignancy with immunosuppressive drugs in

inflammatory bowel disease. *Ann. Pharmacother.* 2007; **41**:21–8.

32. Chouchana L, Narjoz C, Beaune P, et al. Review article: the benefits of pharmacogenetics for improving thiopurine therapy in inflammatory bowel disease. *Aliment. Pharmacol. Ther.* 2012;**35**:15–36.

33. Sahasranaman S, Howard D, Roy S. Clinical pharmacology and pharmacogenetics of thiopurines. *Eur. J. Clin. Pharmacol.* 2008;**64**:753–67.

34. Weinshilboum RM, Sladek SL. Mercaptopurine pharmacogenetics: monogenic inheritance of erythrocyte thiopurine methyltransferase activity. *Am. J. Hum. Genet.* 1980;**32**:651–62.

35. Chouchana L, Roche D, Jian R, et al. Poor response to thiopurine in inflammatory bowel disease: how to overcome therapeutic resistance? *Clin. Chem.* 2013;**59**:1023–7.

36. Feagan BG, Rochon J, Fedorak RN, et al. Methotrexate for the treatment of Crohn's disease. The North American Crohn's Study Group Investigators. *N. Engl. J. Med.* 1995;**332**:292–7.

37. Ardizzone S, Bollani S, Manzionna G, et al. Comparison between methotrexate and azathioprine in the treatment of chronic active Crohn's disease: a randomised, investigator-blind study. *Dig. Liver Dis.* 2003;**35**:619–27.

38. Khan N, Abbas AM, Whang N, et al. Incidence of liver toxicity in inflammatory bowel disease patients treated with methotrexate: a meta-analysis of clinical trials. *Inflamm. Bowel Dis.* 2012;**18**:359–67.

39. Kim YJ, Song M, Ryu JC. Mechanisms underlying methotrexate-induced pulmonary toxicity. *Expert Opinion on Drug Safety* 2009;**8**:451–8.

40. St Clair EW, Rice JR, Snyderman R. Pneumonitis complicating low-dose methotrexate therapy in rheumatoid arthritis. *Arch. Intern. Med.* 1985;**145**:2035–8.

41. Cannon GW. Methotrexate pulmonary toxicity. *Rheum. Dis. Clin. North Am.* 1997;**23**:917–37.

42. Carson CW, Cannon GW, Egger MJ, et al. Pulmonary disease during the treatment of rheumatoid arthritis with low dose pulse methotrexate. *Semin. Arthr. Rheum* 1987;**16**:186–95.

43. Searles G, McKendry RJ. Methotrexate pneumonitis in rheumatoid arthritis: potential risk factors. Four case reports and a review of the literature. *J. Rheumatol.* 1987;**14**:1164–71.

44. Chakravarty K, McDonald H, Pullar T, et al. British Society for Rheumatology, British Health Professionals in Rheumatology Standards,Guidelines and Audit Working Group.British Association of Dermatologists (BAD). BSR/BHPR Guideline for Disease-Modifying Anti-Rheumatic Drug (DMARD) Therapy in Consultation with the British Association of Dermatologists. *Rheumatology* 2008;**47**:924–5.

45. Shea B, Swinden MV, Tanjong Ghogomu E, et al. Folic acid and folinic acid for reducing side effects in patients receiving methotrexate for rheumatoid arthritis. *Cochrane Database of Systematic Reviews* 2013;**5**:CD000951.

46. Lees CW, Heys D, Ho GT, et al. A retrospective analysis of the efficacy and safety of infliximab as rescue therapy in acute severe ulcerative colitis. *Aliment. Pharmacol. Ther.* 2007;**26**:411–9.

47. Keane J, Gershon S, Wise RP, et al. Tuberculosis associated with infliximab, a tumor necrosis factor alpha-neutralizing agent. *N. Engl. J. Med.* 2001;**345**:1098–104.

48. British Thoracic Society Standards of Care, Committee. BTS recommendations for assessing risk and for managing Mycobacterium tuberculosis infection and disease in patients due to start anti-TNF-alpha treatment. *Thorax* 2005;**60**:800–5.

49. Esteve M, Saro C, Gonzalez-Huix F, et al. Chronic hepatitis B reactivation following infliximab therapy in Crohn's disease patients: need for primary prophylaxis. *Gut* 2004;**53**:1363–5.

50. Yang Z, Wu Q, Wu K, et al. Meta-analysis: pre-operative infliximab treatment and short-term post-operative complications in patients with ulcerative colitis. *Aliment. Pharmacol. Ther.* 2010;**31**:486–92.

51. Bongartz T, Sutton AJ, Sweeting MJ, et al. Anti-TNF antibody therapy in rheumatoid arthritis and the risk of serious infections and malignancies: systematic review and meta-analysis of rare harmful effects in randomized controlled trials. *JAMA* 2006;**295**:2275–85.

52. Datapharm Communications Ltd. Electronic medicines compendium. [Online] http://www.medicines.org.uk/emc/ (accessed 13 July 2015).

SECTION 3
Specific conditions

CHAPTER 20

Foreign body impaction in the esophagus

George Triadafilopoulos

Stanford University School of Medicine, Stanford, CA, USA

Introduction

Foreign body impaction in the esophagus is associated with significant morbidity and, rarely, mortality due to perforation and sepsis. This emergency is encountered in both children and adults. The most common cause of esophageal foreign body obstruction in adults is meat bolus impaction above a pre-existing peptic or malignant esophageal stricture, distal esophageal (mucosal) ring, or eosinophilic esophagitis (Figs 20.1, 20.2, and 20.3) [1]. Eosinophilic esophagitis is increasingly found to responsible for meat bolus impactions in adults in the West, while peptic esophagitis and stricture formation accounts for almost a quarter of cases in Asia [2]. This reflects not only the different epidemiology of these diseases but also the frequent use of proton pump inhibitors that has dramatically decreased the prevalence of grades C and D esophagitis.

In contrast, more than 75% of esophageal foreign body obstructions in children are from coin ingestion [3]. Mentally-impaired, edentulous, or elderly subjects may also present with accidental foreign body, pill, or large food bolus impaction. Intentional ingestion of foreign bodies by psychiatric patients or prison inmates may also lead to esophageal foreign body impaction. Although the esophagus has four areas of "physiologic" narrowing (cricopharyngeus, aortic arch, left main stem bronchus, diaphragmatic hiatus) (Fig. 20.4), underlying, clinically-silent, structural or functional esophageal diseases (i.e. esophageal achalasia or scleroderma esophagus) (Figs 20.5 and 20.6) are frequently responsible for esophageal foreign body impaction. Table 20.1 shows the most common underlying conditions predisposing to esophageal body impactions.

History and examination

Most adults with esophageal foreign body obstruction present with symptoms, but infants, children, or mentally-impaired adults may not give a history of foreign body ingestion or complain of dysphagia. Typically, acute onset of dysphagia and inability to swallow saliva are the key symptoms of esophageal obstruction. Inability to swallow saliva indicates complete esophageal obstruction and requires urgent attention. Hypersalivation, retrosternal fullness and pain, regurgitation, hiccups, and retching may also occur. Odynophagia, or painful swallowing, or hematemesis raise the possibility of esophageal laceration or perforation. In contrast, respiratory symptoms, such as stridor, dyspnea, asthma, or cough, all resulting from tracheal compression, may predominate in young children.

Treatment

Table 20.2 highlights the seven sequential steps in treatment of esophageal foreign body obstruction [4]. The first four of these steps are implemented by the emergency room physician who assesses the patient and who, depending on the circumstances, solicits the involvement of an endoscopist, an ear, nose, and throat, or a thoracic surgeon (Fig. 20.7).

Gastrointestinal Emergencies, Third Edition. Edited by Tony C. K. Tham, John S. A. Collins, and Roy Soetikno.
© 2016 John Wiley & Sons, Ltd. Published 2016 by John Wiley & Sons, Ltd.

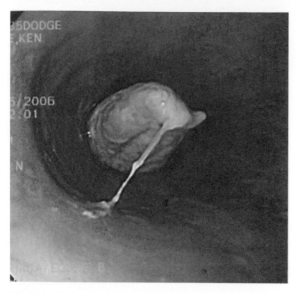

Fig. 20.1 Chicken meat bolus impacted above a distal esophageal mucosal (Schatzki's) ring (not shown). The bolus was grasped using the polypectomy snare and lifted off the distal esophageal stenosis before being removed by mouth using the Roth net. (*see insert for color representation of the figure.*)

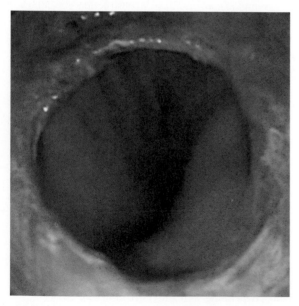

Fig. 20.2 Endoscopic appearance of a distal esophageal mucosal (Schatzki's) ring severed by the passage of the food bolus into the stomach under direct endoscopic visualization, water and air instillation, and gentle pressure by the endoscope tip. Mucosal rings account for many episodes of acute esophageal impaction, typically with a meat bolus (Steak house syndrome). (*see insert for color representation of the figure.*)

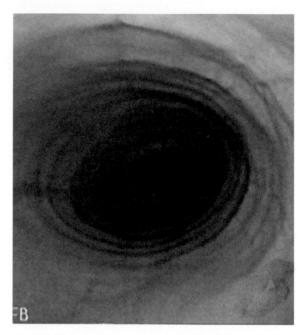

Fig. 20.3 Characteristic appearance of eosinophilic esophagitis, a clinical condition that underlies many foreign body impactions today. This endoscopic photograph, depicting multiple rings along the esophageal body, was taken upon introduction of the endoscope in the proximal esophagus and hence provided with an endoscopic clue to the etiology of impaction, which occurred more distally in this patient (not shown). (*see insert for color representation of the figure.*)

Airway evaluation

Stridor, choking, or dyspnea, suggest a compromised airway. If there is impending asphyxiation, emergency endotracheal intubation is needed. Even in the absence of respiratory symptoms, airway protection and continuous oropharyngeal suction are important to avoid pulmonary aspiration. Airway obstruction can occur during the removal of the foreign body and a laryngoscope should be immediately available.

Assessment of the urgency of removal

The appropriate timing for endoscopic retrieval varies with the type of object as well as the site and completeness of obstruction (Table 20.3) [5]. Retained or impacted esophageal foreign bodies should be promptly removed to avoid esophageal perforation or pulmonary aspiration and under no circumstances should they be allowed to remain in the esophagus beyond 24 hours after ingestion. Endoscopy should be performed

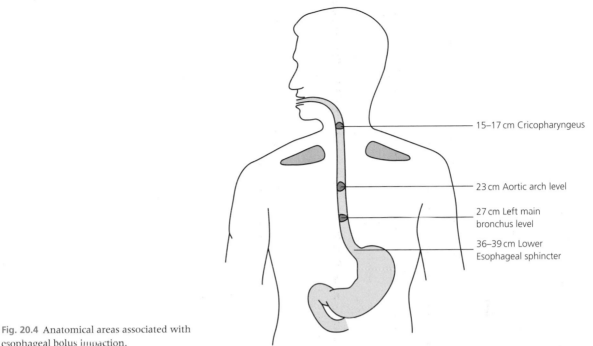

15–17 cm Cricopharyngeus

23 cm Aortic arch level

27 cm Left main bronchus level

36–39 cm Lower Esophageal sphincter

Fig. 20.4 Anatomical areas associated with esophageal bolus impaction.

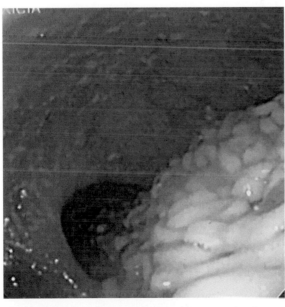

Fig. 20.5 Food impaction in a patient with severe scleroderma esophagus and secondary esophageal candidiasis. Note the dilated esophagus and the esophageal mucosal changes consistent with *Candida* infection. Careful water instillation allowed the endoscope to break up the food residue that initially appeared as a cast of the esophageal body. The repeated use of the Roth retrieval net eventually relieved the patient's impaction and associated acute dysphagia. (*see insert for color representation of the figure.*)

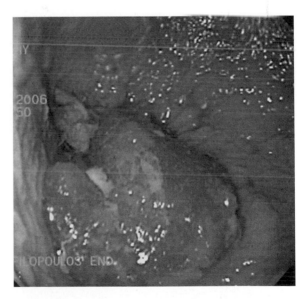

Fig. 20.6 Food impaction in a patient with esophageal achalasia. Note the distorted appearance of the distal esophageal mucosa consistent with stasis esophagitis. Because of the associated atony and dilation of the esophageal body, water instillation allowed the endoscope to bypass the impaction and break up the food residue in small particles. Using the endoscope, the food particles were then pushed into the stomach and relieved the patient's dysphagia. (*see insert for color representation of the figure.*)

Table 20.1 Underlying conditions in esophageal foreign body impaction.

Eosinophilic esophagitis
Distal esophageal (Schatzki's) ring
Esophageal carcinoma
Peptic stricture
Esophageal diverticulum
Postsurgical (fundoplication, esophago-gastrostomy)
Hiatal hernia
Achalasia
Prior esophageal atresia

Source: Triadafilopoulos et al. 2013. Reproduced with permission of Springer.

Table 20.2 Seven steps in management of esophageal foreign body obstruction.

Airway evaluation
Assessment of the urgency of removal
Radiological localization
Medical management
Endoscopic retrieval
Monitoring for complications
Endoscopic therapy and/or surgery for complications

Source: Triadafilopoulos et al. 2013. Reproduced with permission of Springer.

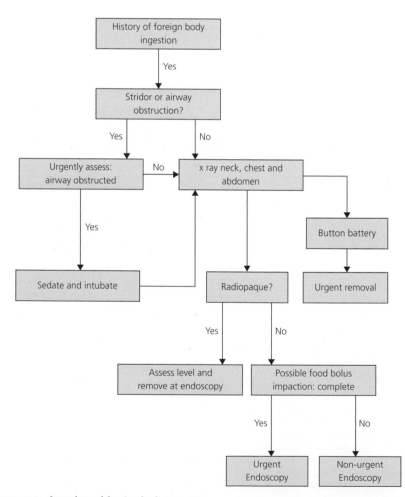

Fig. 20.7 Management of esophageal foreign body impaction.

Table 20.3 Appropriate timing for endoscopic retrieval.

Foreign body	Location	Time of endoscopy (h)
Coin	Upper	4–6
Coin	Lower	12–18
Meat	Any/complete obstruction	
Urgent		
Meat	Any/incomplete obstruction	8–10
Sharps	Any	4–6

Source: Webb and Taylor 1997.

immediately in patients who are unable to handle oral secretions or who have ingested sharp objects (pins, partial dentures, fish bones, toothpicks) that are likely to perforate the esophagus, and in patients with impacted disc or button batteries – typically ingested accidentally by children – in order to avoid caustic injury and perforation.

Radiological evaluation

Depending on the reliability of the clinical history and the clinical presentation, plain neck, chest, and abdominal X-rays are required and they may reveal a radioopaque foreign body, or mediastinal, subdiaphragmatic, or subcutaneous air or pleural effusion, all suggestive of esophageal perforation. If possible, radiographic localization and identification of esophageal foreign bodies is important prior to any attempt at extraction. In particular, identification of airway landmarks on posterior–anterior and lateral chest radiographs is important to differentiate between tracheobronchial and esophageal foreign bodies. Flat objects, such as coins, usually orient themselves in the coronal plane when lodged in the esophagus, and are best seen on anteroposterior projections. Tracheal foreign bodies align in the sagittal plane and are best seen on a lateral projection. Disc batteries may be seen as a double shadow or a stack of coins. Toothpicks or fish bones may not be seen on radiographs; thus, failure to locate an object on radiographic examination does not preclude its presence. Food or meat bolus impaction will not be evident radiologically unless bony tissue is present. Computerized tomography (CT) is superior to plain radiographs for the detection of pharyngoesophageal foreign bodies and provides additional crucial information for the

management of complicated cases, especially related to sharp, pointed, or perforating ingested foreign bodies. Barium swallow should not be performed since it may impair subsequent endoscopic visualization and increase aspiration risk.

Medical management

No treatment is needed if a patient with a history of foreign body ingestion is asymptomatic and has negative plain radiographs, since the foreign body may have passed out of the esophagus. With food boluses, 1 mg of glucagon IV may relax the esophagus and allow spontaneous bolus passage into the stomach.

Endoscopic retrieval

Sharp objects impacted above the cricopharyngeus should be removed with a laryngoscope. If endoscopic visualization distal to the impaction is feasible, gentle pushing of the bolus into the stomach using the tip of the endoscope may be attempted (Figs 20.1, 20.5, and 20.6).

If an esophageal stricture or ring is identified after clearing a food bolus, dilation should be performed during the same session. Esophageal biopsy and esophageal motility should be considered in order to rule out underlying esophageal structural or motor abnormality, such as eosinophilic esophagitis or achalasia (Figs 20.3, 20.5, and 20.6). If eosinophilic esophagitis is suspected, dilation should be performed with extreme caution because of the risk of perforation (Fig. 20.3).

Endoscopy, using a flexible forward-viewing endoscope under conscious sedation, is the procedure of choice and is successful in >90% of cases with <5% complication rate. Rigid esophagoscopy requires general anesthesia and carries a 10% complication rate but it is preferable in children with impacted sharp foreign bodies. The endoscopic tools used to remove obstructing esophageal bodies vary and a full-range of retrieval accessories should always be readily available (Table 20.4) [4]. Coins are best retrieved with a rattooth or alligator forceps, or the retrieval net. Round objects such as disc or button batteries are best captured using the retrieval net. If there is no distal obstruction, blunt objects (i.e. meat bolus) <2 cm in diameter may be gently pushed into the stomach. Sometimes breaking a food bolus into smaller particles facilitates either its endoscopic retrieval using a retrieval net or its gentle advancement into the stomach using the endoscope.

Table 20.4 Useful endoscopic accessories for esophageal foreign body removal.

Alligator forceps (strong toothed forceps with a double clamp)
Rat-tooth forceps, rat-tooth alligator jaw (tissue forceps that have one or two fine teeth on the tip of the beak; ideal for soft objects, such as food bolus and flat objects, such as coins)
Shark tooth forceps (features a shark tooth grasping jaw for accurate foreign body retrieval; ideal for flat objects, such as coins or dentures)
Rubber tip forceps (ideal for retrieval of sharp objects, such as nails, needles, blades)
Stent removal forceps (strong grasping forceps that combines rat tooth and alligator jaw for firm grip)
V-shaped grasping forceps (features two flat arms for capture and retrieval of flat objects)
Tripod, Talon grasping device (ideal for removal of meat bolus)
Stone (Dormia) baskets; Falcon rotatable retrieval device (ideal for round slippery objects)
Roth retrieval net (large capacity net for object retrieval)
Polyp retrieval snare (a soft, more pliable, twisted wire that requires less force to open and close the loop designed to snag the meat bolus preventing slippage)
Nakao snare system (a snare and a retrieving net that is specially designed to slide up and down the snare, gently cradling the bolus)
Overtube (with a tapered tip design to protect against mucosal damage)
Latex-protector hood (to protect against sharp-pointed foreign bodies)
Endoscopic clips (to close mucosal tears)
Esophageal stents (to seal esophageal perforation)

Source: Triadafilopoulos et al. 2013. Reproduced with permission of Springer.

For removal of sharp objects (i.e. safety pins), a protector hood should be placed at the tip of the endoscope or an overtube should be inserted. The protector hood maintains its bell portion inverted during insertion of the endoscope; the bell portion then flips back to its original shape as it crosses the gastroesophageal junction during withdrawal, thereby protecting the esophageal and pharyngeal walls from injury. It is important to grasp the object so that its sharp end is trailing upon withdrawal. The overtube is also useful in the removal of objects that are difficult to grasp securely or when multiple passes of the endoscope are needed [6].

Blunt objects <2 cm that have already entered the stomach can usually be managed conservatively, since most of them will pass within several days. Surgical removal should be considered if the object remains in the same location for more than one week, or in patients who develop fever, vomiting, or abdominal pain, suggestive of perforation. Long objects (>5 cm), such as toothbrushes and spoons, are unlikely to pass and should be removed. Such objects may be grasped with a snare or basket and drawn into an overtube and withdrawn [7].

Sharp objects (i.e. chicken or fish bones, paper clips, toothpicks, needles, and dental bridges) should be urgently removed endoscopically to avoid perforation. Using a retrieval basket or net, disk batteries should be removed promptly, since their contact with the esophageal wall may rapidly result in necrosis and perforation. If drug smuggling with cocaine body stuffing is suspected, particular attention needs to be taken not to rupture the bag and thus abort acute drug overdose. Drug packets should not be removed endoscopically because of the risk of rupture. Urgent surgery is needed when packages fail to advance or if there are signs of intestinal obstruction or rupture.

Monitoring for complications

Although endoscopic retrieval is associated with high probability for success and quite frequently leads to an expedited discharge from the emergency room soon after the patient has recovered from conscious sedation, it is important to monitor the patient for the development of complications that were not recognized early, prior to disimpaction, or occurred iatrogenically. Complications of foreign body ingestion or food impaction include esophageal ulcer formation, laceration, perforation, intestinal obstruction, aortoesophageal or tracheoesophageal fistula formation, and bacteremia. Perforation of the oropharynx or proximal esophagus may lead to neck swelling, tenderness, erythema, or crepitus. Perforation in the mid or distal esophagus may result in retrosternal chest and/or upper abdominal pain, dyspnea, fever, and shock. Perforation of the stomach, small bowel, or colon may present with signs of peritonitis, such as abdominal pain, rebound, guarding, tachycardia, hypotension, and fever. Depending on the nature and magnitude of these complications, medical therapy (i.e. proton pump inhibition, antibiotics), endoscopic therapy, or surgery may be needed.

Endoscopic management and/or surgery

Some patients with esophageal perforations that are immediately recognized at the time of endoscopy may be treated with removable plastic or covered metal esophageal stents [8]. Stents are particularly suitable for patients with an underlying esophageal neoplasm or for those who are unlikely to tolerate surgery. Endoscopic clips may be used to treat patients who have acute esophageal perforations as long as there is no evidence of mediastinal contamination.

Surgery should be performed in patients with foreign body-induced esophageal perforation, particularly when it is recognized late. The surgical approach depends on the location of perforation, the nature of the foreign body, underlying esophageal disease or other comorbidity, and the severity of mediastinal necrotic or inflammatory response assessed by CT scan. Primary esophageal repair is preferable for perforations that are recognized early, but exclusion-diversion of the esophagus and thorough drainage may be needed. Rarely, non-operative, conservative management may be adequate for small, contained perforations.

References

1. Eisen GM, Baron TH, Dominitz JA, et al. Guideline for the management of ingested foreign bodies. *Gastrointest. Endosc.* 2002;**55**:802–6.
2. Sperry SL, Crockett SD, Miller CB, Shaheen NJ, Dellon ES. Esophageal foreign-body impactions: epidemiology, time trends, and the impact of the increasing prevalence of eosinophilic esophagitis. *Gastrointest. Endosc.* 2011;**74**(5): 985–91.
3. Diniz LO, Towbin AJ. Causes of esophageal food bolus impaction in the pediatric population. *Dig. Dis. Sci.* 2012;**57**: 690–3.
4. Triadafilopoulos G, Roorda A, Akiyama J. Update on foreign bodies in the esophagus: diagnosis and management. *Curr. Gastroenterol. Rep.* 2013;**15**(4):317.
5. Webb, WA, Taylor MB. Foreign bodies of the upper gastrointestinal tract. In Gastrointestinal Emergencies, 2nd edition, Taylor MB (ed.). Lippincott Williams & Wilkins, Philadelphia, 1997: 3–18.
6. Li Z-S, Sun Z-X, Zou D-W, Xu G-M, Wu R-P, Liao Z. Endoscopic management of foreign bodies in the upper-GI tract: experience with 1088 cases in China. *Gastrointest. Endosc.* 2006;**64**:485–92.
7. Leopard D, Fishpool S, Winter S. The management of oesophageal soft food bolus obstruction: a systematic review. *Ann. R. Coll. Surg. Engl.* 2011;**93**(6):441–4.
8. van Heel NC, Haringsma J, Spaander MC, Bruno MJ, Kuipers EJ. Short-term esophageal stenting in the management of benign perforations. *Am. J. Gastroenterol.* 2010;**105**:1515–20.

CHAPTER 21

Esophageal perforation

Ioannis S. Papanikolaou[1] and Peter D. Siersema[2]

[1] *"Attikon" University General Hospital, University of Athens, Greece*
[2] *University Medical Center, Utrecht, The Netherlands*

Introduction

Esophageal perforation is a life-threatening condition caused by a great variety of disorders. Among them, iatrogenic perforation during endoscopic instrumentation or complicating surgery is the most common cause. Perforation may also occur spontaneously during vomiting (Boerhaave's syndrome). Finally, esophageal leaks can be found in the context of a fistula as a consequence of radiation therapy or invasive malignancy, involving the esophagus [1].

The successful management of esophageal perforation depends on early diagnosis and prompt treatment. However, its diagnosis is often difficult to establish and warrants the alertness of the physician. Surgery is the classic treatment. However, surgery is not always feasible in patients with delayed referral, with a coexistent esophageal malignancy, or those who develop an anastomotic dehiscence after esophageal surgery. Moreover, a substantial number of patients are old, fragile, or are in a debilitated state, which may result in increased morbidity and a less favorable outcome following surgical management [2].

Repair of an esophageal perforation can also be accomplished by the use of endoscopic techniques and tools [3]. The aim is to close or seal an esophageal perforation from the luminal site. In addition, it is important to adequately drain the mediastinum, pleural and/or peritoneal cavity, administer broad-spectrum antibiotics and analgesics, and routinely start nutritional support, preferably by the enteral route.

The aim of this chapter is to provide an overview of the endoscopic management of esophageal perforations. The management of esophageal fistulae, either benign or malignant, will not be discussed.

Etiology

In a series of 559 patients with esophageal perforation from the USA, iatrogenic injury to the esophagus was the most common cause of perforation with instrumentation accounting for 59% of patients [4] (Table 21.1). Other causes included Boerhaave's syndrome (15%), foreign body ingestion (12%), trauma (9%), operative injury (2%), tumor (1%), and other causes (2%).

Clinical presentation

A high index of suspicion is critical to establish the diagnosis of esophageal perforation given that the presentation is not always typical.

Clinical symptoms depend on the location of the perforation in the esophagus, and can be subdivided as follows [3]:

1 Cervical esophagus: neck pain, tachycardia, "early" dysphagia, symptoms of coughing following drinking or eating, dysphonia, bloody regurgitation, and cervical crepitus.
2 Thoracic esophagus: chest pain, tachycardia, tachypnea, fever, pleural effusion, cardiac effusion, low blood pressure, sepsis, and shock.

Table 21.1 Causes of esophageal perforation [1].

Causes of perforation	(%)
Instrumentation	59
Boerhaave's syndrome	15
Foreign body	12
Trauma	9
Operative injury	2
Tumor	1
Other	2

Source: Walker 1985. Reproduced with permission of Wiley.

3 Esophagus around the gastroesophageal junction: epigastric pain, back pain, inability to remain in a supine position, acute abdomen, sepsis, and shock.

Examination

Physical examination is often not conclusive. A diagnosis of esophageal perforation should however be suspected if a patient presents with cervical crepitus, pleural fluid, sepsis, or shock in the presence of chest pain. In addition, esophageal perforation should be suspected if a patient has undergone esophageal surgery or esophagoscopy and develops fever one or more days after the procedure.

Investigations

If a patient presents with symptoms suggestive of an esophageal perforation, the initial investigation is a chest radiograph, both posteroanterior and lateral. If this shows no signs of perforation, for example the presence of free air, pleural fluid or pneumonia, a gastrografin swallow should then follow. Gastrografin should be preferred, instead of barium, as the former is water-soluble, whereas barium is not (Fig. 21.1).

In cases with a high index of suspicion, a computerized tomography (CT) scan is the preferred investigation. This CT should include a scan of the neck, the chest, and, if indicated, the upper abdomen. This can be followed by upper endoscopy to establish the exact location of the perforation and ideally perform therapeutic interventions.

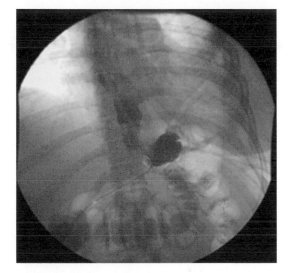

Fig. 21.1 Gastrografin swallow showing leakage of contrast outside the esophagus.

Diagnosis

As discussed above, the diagnosis of esophageal perforation is established if the clinical symptoms are suggestive and the radiological and/or endoscopic investigations reveal the esophageal wall defect.

Management

Surgery
Generally, surgery is indicated if the patient remains unstable following perforation, if recognition of the perforation is late (more than 24 hours), if free perforation and/or significant fluid is accumulated in the mediastinum and/or pleural cavities, in centers lacking endoscopic expertise and in cases endoscopy fails to close the defect.

The aim of surgery is the prevention of further contamination, elimination of the infectious tissue, restoration of the integrity of the esophagus, and establishing the intake of nutrients. Surgical treatment options include surgical repair, esophageal diversion and exclusion, or esophagectomy.

Primary surgical closure and mediastinal drainage, particularly if performed within 24 hours of the injury, has been shown to improve survival [5]. Repair of the perforation requires extensive mobilization of the esophagus to identify the perforation and to allow a tension-free repair. In addition, extensive drainage of the mediastinum with one or more chest tubes is required.

If primary repair is not possible, because of the extent of the paraesophageal inflammation, mediastinal drainage with diversion and exclusion (cervical esophagostomy for diversion, a gastrostomy for decompression and a jejunostomy for enteral feeding) or creation of a controlled esophagocutaneous fistula with T-tube drainage of the perforation can be performed [6]. This is a rather safe and uncomplicated approach as a first step but needs to be followed by reconstruction 6 months later. Esophagectomy is indicated for patients with perforation in a carcinoma, but also in cases where extensive necrosis is present or when the esophageal stricture is already difficult to manage (e.g. in cases with repeat dilation for caustic injury).

The mortality of a surgical procedure for esophageal perforation has been reported to vary between 10 and 20%. This mainly depends on the cause and location of the perforation, the interval between the perforation and initiation of therapy, the extent of contamination of the mediastinum, the type of surgery and the age and condition of the patient. A delay in diagnosis and therapy for more than 24 hours after the perforation can substantially increase mortality [7].

Endoscopy

An endoscopic approach to esophageal perforation has several advantages over surgery, as:
- Closure of the perforation can be performed under direct observation.
- Endoscopy can be performed under conscious sedation, which avoids the disadvantages of general anesthesia.
- Trauma associated with a surgical approach by performing thoracotomy, mediastinal exploration or extensive dissection can be avoided.

In the last few years, various reports in the literature, including an increasing number of case reports and case series have reported on the endoscopic treatment of esophageal perforation. Experience has been gained with the following endoscopic techniques and tools (8,9):
- Sealants (glue or graft) used to plug a defect.
- Endoclips, which approximate the edges of a perforation.

- Endoscopic vacuum therapy, which favors healing by secondary intention.
- Stents, which are used to seal a perforation.

Factors influencing the final outcome of an esophageal perforation treated endoscopically include comorbidities, time to intervention (ideally within 24 hours) and location (cervical leaks have a better prognosis compared to thoracic and abdominal ones).

An endoscopic option should always be combined with drainage of the mediastinal cavity and/or pleural cavity. Drainage tubes can be placed percutaneously, or CT- or endoscopic ultrasound (EUS)-guided. Active lavage, irrigation and drainage of the abscess cavity are of importance. In selected cases, endoscopic debridement of the abscess can be performed [10,11]. This should be supported by the administration of intravenous broad-spectrum antibiotics. Administration of intravenous proton pump inhibitors and agents for pain management according to the patient's needs is crucial. Fasting is maintained until a gastrografin swallow demonstrates that the perforation is adequately closed (in the case of sealants or clips) or sealed (when using stents). Finally, nutritional support should be initiated at an early stage. Enteral feeding by an endoscopically placed feeding tube in the distal duodenum is preferable. Total parental nutrition is indicated in case enteral feeding is not possible.

Endoscopic sealants

Sealants include fibrin glue, cyanoacrylates and tissue grafts [12,13]. Sealants are produced by different manufacturers (Table 21.2).

Most experience has been gained with fibrin glue, which has been reported to be successful in closure of esophageal perforations, but mainly in all kinds of esophageal fistulae and anastomotic leaks [14,15]. Cyanoacrylate has been used in a few case reports to close esophageal fistulae but no experience has been reported regarding acute esophageal perforations [16,17]. Endoscopic insertion of tissue grafts, an acellular matrix derived from porcine submucosa, is a relatively new method. It has successfully been reported in the closure of 12 of 17 refractory esophagogastric fistulae that had developed after bariatric surgery [18].

Technically, prior to injecting fibrin glue into a fistulous opening, it is recommended to brush the fistulous tract or anastomotic leak. Subsequently, the catheter with fibrin glue is placed inside the orifice. Once fibrin is applied, it is important to avoid contact of the catheter

Table 21.2 Endoscopic accessories used for esophageal perforations (including manufacturer and product name).

Endoscopic sealants
a. Fibrin glue
• Tisseel (Baxter Westlake Village, CA)
• Hemaseel (Hemacure, Sarasota, FL)
b. Cyanoacrylates
• Histoacryl (B. Braun, Melsungen, Germany)
• Glubran (GEM, Viareggio, Italy)
• Dermabond (Ethocon, Somerville, NJ)
c. Tissue grafts
• Surgisis (Wilson-Cook, Winston-Salem, NC)
Endoclips
• Endosclip or Quickclip (Olympus, Tokyo, Japan)
• Triclip (Wilson-Cook, Winston-Salem, NC)
• Resolution Clip (Boston Scientific, Natick, MA)
• Over-the-scope-clip (Ovesco Endoscopy, Tubingen, Germany)
Stents
a. Metal (fully covered)
• Wallflex (Boston Scientific)
• Niti-S (Taewoong Medical)
• Evolution (Cook Medical)
• Ella HV (Ella CS)
• Alimaxx-ES (Merit Medical Endotek)
b. Plastic (fully covered)
• Polyflex (Boston Scientific)

with the fistulous tract. Repeat application, for example every 48 hours, for some weeks, is sometimes required to close a fistula or anastomotic leak. Regarding tissue grafts, although insertion seems promising, it is often difficult to apply them into a fistula or leak by endoscopic means, as no specific delivery system (e.g. catheter, etc.) for this purpose is commercially available yet.

Closing a fistula or leak is most successful if the diameter of the defect is not larger than 8–10 mm. Successful outcome of endoscopic closure is also dependent on the length and number of branches of the fistulous tract, the absence of active inflammation around the fistula or leak, and the absence of cancer or obstruction in the fistulous tract.

Endoclips
Through-the-scope clips (TTS clips)
Three types of TTS clip devices are commercially available: Endoclip or Quickclip (Olympus, Tokyo, Japan), Triclip (Wilson-Cook), and Resolution clip (Boston Scientific, Natick, MA) (Table 21.2). So far, the only published data that are available refer to the use of the Quickclip in the treatment of esophageal perforations [3]. However, it seems most likely that with the other available types of clips, comparable results can be obtained.

TTS clip application has been shown to be successful in the closure of esophageal perforations from Boerhaave's syndrome, foreign body ingestion, and following dilation of esophageal strictures, achalasia, and anastomotic strictures. In addition, TTS clips have been shown to be highly successful in treating postoperative or post-EMR esophageal leakages. In a systematic review of TTS clip closure for esophageal perforations in 17 patients (7 acute perforations, 6 chronic perforations, and 4 perforations between 2 and 10 days), TTS clips were used with success to close perforations ranging from 3 to 25 mm (median size: 10 mm and interquartile range 8–12 mm) [19].

In our experience, endoclips are particularly successful for the closure of acute perforations varying from a few millimeters to 1.5–2 cm, with the latter sizes always requiring multiple endoclips. In the case of a larger perforation, it is advisable to start clipping at the middle part of the perforation, and then work towards both lateral ends of the perforation.

Closure of acute perforations occurs within 3–7 days; however, a longer time (up to 2–4 weeks) may be required for more chronic perforations, or those that are associated with paraesophageal inflammation.

No complications have been reported with the use of endoclips. The placement of endoclips in the esophagus can be technically demanding, as it may be difficult to approach the defect under direct view. In these situations, it is helpful to have a cap at the end of the endoscope.

Over-the-scope clips (OTSC)
As stated, TTS clips are unable to close large defects due to their limited wingspan. Inflammation or scarring of the perforation edges in case of late intervention, also reduce their efficacy. On that basis, over-the-scope clips (OTSC, Ovesco Endoscopy, Tubingen, Germany) have been developed to treat large defects in the gastrointestinal tract, including the esophagus. OTSC are fitted over a cap on the endoscope tip and are deployed in a fashion similar to that of the endoscopic variceal ligation technique. Eventually, OTSC creates a full-thickness closure at the perforation site, that may size up to 3 cm in diameter.

With respect to esophageal wall defects, OTSC have been already successfully used in the management of acute iatrogenic perforations as well as Boerhaave's syndrome and postoperative esophageal leaks [20–25]. Appropriate endoscopist training is definitely needed to ensure correct handling and placement of this type of endoclip.

Endoscopic vacuum therapy (EVT)

EVT reduces bacterial contamination, secretions, and edema and therefore enhances the formation of granulation tissue and healing by secondary intention. EVT is performed by placing a sponge attached to the tip of a nasogastric tube at the site of perforation under endoscopic vision. The nasogastric tube is connected to a vacuum system with continuous controlled suction. Ideally, the sponges should be changed initially every third day and then, twice a week after the first seven days [26].

Stents

Apart from numerous case reports, several retrospective and prospective studies have been published, regarding the use of stents to seal esophageal perforations resulting from postoperative complications (anastomotic or post-resection leaks), endoscopic procedures, Boerhaave's syndrome, and dilation of post-radiation strictures and foreign body ingestion [8,27–52] (Table 21.3).

The stent types that are used in the treatment of esophageal perforations include preferably fully covered

Table 21.3 Summary of previous studies on the use of stents in the management of oesophageal perforation.

First author, year	Patients, no.	Stent type	Technical success, %	Complications, %
Lee, 2000 [27]	2	SEMS	100	0
Chung, 2001 [28]	3	SEMS	100	33
Wadhwa, 2003 [29]	5	SEMS	60	20
Siersema, 2003 [30]	11	SEMS	100	18
Doniec, 2003 [31]	21	SEMS	100	62
Evrard, 2004 [32]	4	SEPS	100	75
Gelbmann, 2004 [33]	9	SEPS	100	33
Hünerbein, 2004 [34]	9	SEPS	100	22
Langer, 2005 [35]	24	SEPS	75	55
Radecke, 2005 [36]	5	SEPS	100	N/A
Schubert, 2005 [10]	12	SEPS	100	17
Peters, 2006 [37]	3	SEMS	100	33
Eroglu, 2009 [38]	4	SEMS	100	0
Freeman, 2009 [39]	19	SEPS	100	24
Salminen, 2009 [40]	8	SEMS	100	25
Amrani, 2009 [41]	2	SEMS	100	0
Leers, 2009 [42]	9	SEMS	100	N/A
Kiernan, 2010 [43]	8	SEMS	100	N/A
Vallböhmer, 2010 [44]	12	SEMS	100	8
Van Heel, 2010 [45]	31	SEMS/SEPS	100	33
Swinnen, 2011 [46]	23	SEMS	100	N/A
Dai, 2011 [47]	5	SEPS	N/A	N/A
D'Cunha, 2011 [48]	15	SEMS/SEPS	95	13
Van Boeckel, 2012 [52]	52	SEMS/SEPS	100	46
Wilson, 2013 [50]	7	SEMS	100	N/A
Schweigert, 2013 [51]	13	SEMS/SEPS	100	85
Lin, 2014 [49]	9	Mesh-covered	100	4

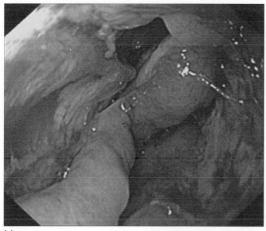

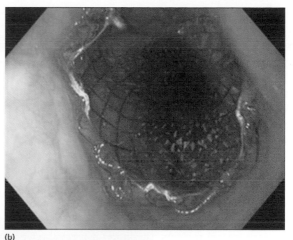

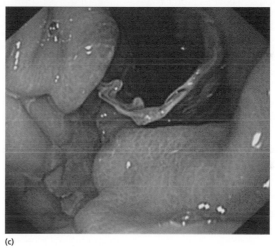

Fig. 21.2 Patient presenting with a perforation due to Boerhaave's syndrome (a). A fully covered Wallflex stent was placed (b), which was extending just below the gastroesophageal junction (c). (*see insert for color representation of the figure.*)

self-expandable metal stents (SEMS) and a fully covered self-expandable plastic stent (SEPS) named Polyflex (Boston Scientific). Of note, esophageal perforations may necessitate combined treatment with both stents and endoclips [53,54].

In the reported series, stents were placed within 83 days following perforation, but best results are obtained when placed within a few hours to days of a perforation (Fig. 21.2). If some time has elapsed following perforation, the paraesophageal tissues (i.e. the mediastinum, the pleural cavity, and the peritoneal cavity), in selected cases, should be considered to be severely contaminated. In such cases, apart from placing a stent in the esophagus, drainage tubes in the mediastinum and/or pleural cavity and drains in abscesses in the peritoneum are necessary. Some authors have added traditional surgical principles to their treatment algorithm, including endoscopic cleansing of fistulae and paraesophageal collections [10,11]. It remains to be established through randomized multicenter studies whether endoscopic cleaning is indeed needed or whether adequate drainage of the mediastinum and/or pleural cavity in combination with immediate stent placement suffices.

Complications associated with stent placement include chest pain, fever, bleeding, perforation, gastroesophageal reflux disease, stent occlusion, and stent migration.

The latter represents the most common complication occurring at a frequency of 7–75% and may take place either during the early (within 2–4 weeks) or the late post-procedural period. To note, the migration risk is greater for the fully-covered stents as compared to the partially covered ones. To minimize migration risk Gelbmann et al. suggested stent fixation with an endoclip [33].

In recent studies stents are removed after 2–4 weeks and only replaced if a perforation is still endoscopically present. In the studies using Polyflex stents, no difficulties were reported in stent retrieval. In contrast, partially covered metal stents may be difficult to extract in case the uncovered portions are too firmly embedded in the esophageal mucosa. Therefore, it seems preferable to use stents that are completely covered and easily removable despite the higher migration risk. It remains to be established what type of stent material (metal, polyester, silicone, etc.) is most suitable for these benign indications.

Summary

Based on this overview, it can be concluded that endoscopic therapy is an attractive modality for the treatment of esophageal perforation in the majority of patients with this complication. In our opinion, surgery should only be the first choice in patients who develop a perforation during instrumentation. Examples of this include patients with a perforation that:
- develops during the work-up of esophageal carcinoma, particularly if no evidence of metastatic disease is present;
- develops after dilation of a refractory esophageal stricture, such as those following caustic ingestion;
- develops after pneumatic dilation of achalasia;
- persists under endoscopic therapy; or
- is larger than 50–70% of the circumference.

The remainder of esophageal perforation can be treated with an endoscopic technique or tool. In summary, in patients with small leaks (2 cm or less than 25% of the circumference), it is recommended to use an endoscopic sealant (1 cm), or endoclips (2 cm). However, if a stricture is also present it is preferable to use a (fully covered, i.e. Polyflex) stent. When the perforation is larger than 2 cm or between 25% and 50–70% of the circumference, a stent or OTSC should be placed. If the perforation is larger than 50–70% of the circumference, for example in the case of an anastomotic dehiscence, a surgical procedure is often required.

Future developments

Is there anything new in the horizon of endoscopic therapy? It would be a real step forward if we could endoscopically suture an esophageal perforation as our surgeon colleagues do. Recently, a case was reported on a persistent esophagopleural fistula treated by endoscopic suturing [55]. Additionally, endoscopic suturing was effective in the treatment of iatrogenic esophageal perforations according to a randomized trial in a porcine model [56]. As suturing is one of the most demanding endoscopic procedures, it would be a real challenge to develop easy-to-apply suturing devices that can also be used in the esophagus. Experience gained from closure techniques used during natural orifice transluminal endoscopic surgery (NOTES) [57] might help us produce ideas that would lead to improvements in this field.

Covered biodegradable stents have are already been used with promising results in the management of benign esophageal perforations, although large trials are needed in order to advocate their widespread application [58]. An alternative could be the use of biodegradable formulations that can be used to cover fistulous tracts, cavities, etc. These formulations have been shown not to cause abnormal growth behavior, morphological changes or inhibition of metabolic activity. In addition, they may stimulate connective tissue and vascular growth [59].

It can be envisioned that, in time, such accessories will become available to interventional endoscopists in the effort to optimize the minimally invasive management of esophageal perforation.

References

1. Walker WS, Cameron EWS, Walbaum PR. Diagnosis and management of spontaneous transmural rupture of the oesophagus. *Br. J. Surg.* 1985;**72**:204–7.
2. Sawyer R, Philips C, Vakil N. Short- and long-term outcome of esophageal perforation. *Gastrointest. Endosc.* 1995;**41**:130–4.
3. Raju GS, Thompson C, Zwischenberger JB. Emerging endoscopic options in the management of esophageal leaks. *Gastrointest. Endosc.* 2005;**62**:278–86.

4. Brinster CJ, Singhal S, Lee L, et al. Evolving options in the management of esophageal perforation. *Ann. Thorac. Surg.* 2004;**77**:1475–83.

5. Zwischenberger JB, Savage C, Bidani A. Surgical aspects of esophageal disease. Perforation and caustic injury. *Am. J. Respir. Crit. Care Med.* 2001;**164**:1037–40.

6. Bufkin BL, Miller JI jr, Mansour KA. Esophageal perforation: emphasis on management. *Ann. Thorac. Surg.* 1996;**61**:1447–51.

7. Tilanus HW, Bossuyt P, Schattenkerk ME, et al. Treatment of oesophageal perforation: a multivariate analysis. *Br. J. Surg.* 1991;**78**:582–5.

8. Paspatis GA, Dumonceau JM, Barthet M, et al. Diagnosis and management of iatrogenic endoscopic perforations: European Society of Gastrointestinal Endoscopy (ESGE) Position Statement. *Endoscopy* 2014;**46**(8):693–711.

9. Gomez-Esquivel R, Raju GS. Endoscopic closure of acute esophageal perforations. *Curr. Gastroenterol. Rep.* 2013;**15**:321.

10. Schubert D, Scheidbach H, Kuhn R, et al. Endoscopic treatment of thoracic esophageal leaks by using silicone-covered, self-expanding polyester stents. *Gastrointest. Endosc.* 2005;**61**:891–6.

11. Wehrmann T, Stergiou N, Vogel B, et al. Endoscopic debridement of paraesophageal, mediastinal abscesses: a prospective case series. *Gastrointest. Endosc.* 2005;**62**:344–9.

12. Petersen B, Barkun A, Caroenter S, et al. Tissue adhesives and fibrin glues. *Gastrointest. Endosc.* 2004;**60**:327–33.

13. ASGE Technology Committee, Bhat YM, Banerjee S, et al. Tissue adhesives: cyanoacrylate glue and fibrin sealant. *Gastrointest. Endosc.* 2013;**78**:209–15.

14. Fernandez FF, Richter A, Freudenberg S, et al. Treatment of endoscopic esophageal perforation. *Surg. Endosc.* 1999;**13**:962–6.

15. Rábago LR, Castro JL, Joya D, et al. Esophageal perforation and postoperative fistulae of the upper digestive tract treated endoscopically with the application of Tissucol. *Gastroenterol. Hepatol.* 2000;**23**:82–6.

16. Devière JP, Quarre JP, Love J, et al. Self-expandable stent and injection of tissue adhesive for malignant broncho-esophageal fistula. *Gastrointest. Endosc.* 1994;**40**:508–10.

17. Yellapu RK, Gorthi JR, Kiranmayi Y, et al. Endoscopic occlusion of idiopathic benign esophago-bronchial fistula. *J. Postgrad. Med.* 2010;**56**:284–6.

18. Maluf-Filho F, Moura E, Sakai P, et al. Endoscopic treatment of esophagogastric fistulae with an acellular matrix (abstract). *Gastrointest. Endosc.* 2004;**59**:AB151.

19. Qadeer MA, Dumot JA, Vargo JJ, et al. Endoscopic clips for closing esophageal perforations: case report and pooled analysis. *Gastrointest. Endosc.* 2007;**66**:605–11.

20. Voermans RP, Le Moine O, von Renteln D, et al. Efficacy of endoscopic closure of acute perforations of the gastrointestinal tract. *Clin. Gastroenterol. Hepatol.* 2012;**10**:603–8.

21. Baron TH, Song LM, Ross A, et al. Use of an over-the-scope clipping device: multicenter retrospective results of the first US experience (with videos). Use of an over-the-scope clipping device: multicenter retrospective results of the first US experience (with videos). Gastrointest. *Endosc.* 2012;**76**:202–8.

22. Hadj Amor WB, Bonin EA, Vitton V, et al. Successful endoscopic management of large upper gastrointestinal perforations following EMR using over-the-scope clipping combined with stenting. *Endoscopy* 2012;**44**(Suppl 2 UCTN):E277–823.

23. Ramhamadany E, Mohamed S, Jaunoo S, et al. A delayed presentation of Boerhaave's syndrome with mediastinitis managed using the over-the-scope clip. *J. Surg. Case Rep.* 2013;**2013**(5)pii:rjt020. doi: 10.1093/jscr/rjt020

24. Markar SR, Koehler R, Low DE, et al. Novel multimodality endoscopic closure of postoperative esophageal fistula. *Int. J. Surg. Case Rep.* 2012;**3**:577–9.

25. Pohl J, Borgulya M, Lorenz D, et al. Endoscopic closure of postoperative esophageal leaks with a novel over-the-scope clip system. *Endoscopy* 2010;**42**:757–9.

26. Loske G, Schorsch T, Muller C. Intraluminal and intracavitary vacuum therapy for esophageal leakage: a new endoscopic minimally invasive approach. *Endoscopy* 2011;**43**:540–4.

27. Lee JG, Hsu R, Leung JW. Are self-expanding metal mesh stents useful in the treatment of benign esophageal stenoses and fistulas? An experience in four cases. *Am. J. Gastroenterol.* 2000;**95**:1920–5.

28. Chung MG, Kang DH, Park DK, et al. Successful treatment of Boerhave's syndrome with endoscopic insertion of a self-expandable metallic stent: report of three cases and a review of the literature. *Endoscopy* 2001;**33**:894–7.

29. Wadhwa RP, Kozarek RA, France RE, et al. Use of self-expandable metallic stents in benign GI diseases. *Gastrointest. Endosc.* 2003;**58**:207–12.

30. Siersema PD, Homs MYV, Haringsma J, et al. Use of large-diameter metallic stents to seal traumatic nonmalignant perforations of the esophagus. *Gastrointest. Endosc.* 2003;**58**:356–61.

31. Doniec JM, Schniewind B, Kahlke V, et al. Therapy of anastomotic leaks by means of covered metallic stents after esophagogastrectomy. *Endoscopy* 2003;**35**:652–8.

32. Evrard S, le Moine O, Lazaraki G, et al. Self-expanding plastic stents for benign esophageal lesions. *Gastrointest. Endosc.* 2004;**60**:894–900.

33. Gelbmann CM, Ratiu, NL, Rath HC, et al. Use of self-expandable plastic stents for the treatment of esophageal perforations and symptomatic anastomotic leaks. *Endoscopy* 2004;**36**:695–9.

34. Hünerbein M, Stroszcynski C, Moesta KT, et al. Treatment of thoracic anastomotic leaks after esophagectomy with self-expanding plastic stents. *Ann. Surg.* 2004;**240**:801–7.

35. Langer FB, Wenzl E, Prager G, et al. Management of postoperative esophageal leaks with the Polyflex self-expanding covered plastic stent. *Ann. Thorac. Surg.* 2005;**79**:398–403.

36. Radecke K, Gerken G, Treichel U. Impact of a self-expanding plastic esophageal stent on various esophageal stenoses, fistulas and leakages. *Gastrointest. Endosc.* 2005;**61**:812–18.

37. Peters JH, Craanen ME, van der Peet DL, et al. Self-expanding metal stents for the treatment of intrathoracic esophageal anastomotic leaks following esophagectomy. *Am. J. Gastroenterol.* 2006;**101**:1393–5.

38. Eroglu A, Turkyilmaz A, Aydin Y, et al. Current management of esophageal perforation: 20 years experience. *Dis. Esoph.* 2009;**22**:374–80.

39. Freeman RK, Van Woerkom JM, Vyverberg A, et al. Esophageal stent placement for the treatment of spontaneous esophageal perforations. *Ann. Thorac. Surg.* 2009;**88**:194–8.

40. Salminen P, Gullichsen R, Laine S. Use of self-expandable metal stents for the treatment of esophageal perforations and anastomotic leaks. *Surg. Endosc.* 2009;**23**:1526–30.

41. Amrani L, Menard C, Berdah S, et al. From iatrogenic digestive perforation to complete anastomotic disunion: endoscopic stenting as a new concept of "stent-guided regeneration and re-epithelialization". *Gastrointest. Endosc.* 2009;**69**:1282–7.

42. Leers JM, Vivaldi C, Schäfer H, et al. Endoscopic therapy for esophageal perforation or anastomic leak with a self-expandable metallic stent. *Surg. Endosc.* 2009;**10**:2258–62.

43. Kiernan PD, Khandhar SJ, Fortes DL, et al. Thoracic esophageal perforations. *Am. Surg.* 2010;**76**:1355–62.

44. van Heel NC, Haringsma J, Spaander MC, et al. Short-term esophageal stenting in the management of benign perforations. *Am. J. Gastroenterol.* 2010;**105**:1515–20.

45. Vallböhmer D, Holscher AH, Holscher M, et al. Options in the management of esophageal perforation: analysis over a 12-year period. *Dis. Esoph.* 2010;**23**:185–90.

46. Swinnen J, Eisendrath P, Rigaux J, et al. Self-expandable metal stents for the treatment of benign upper GI leaks and perforations. *Gastrointest. Endosc.* 2011;**73**:890–9.

47. Dai Y, Chopra SS, Kneif S, et al. Management of esophageal anastomotic leaks, perforations, and fistulae with self-expanding plastic stents. *J. Thorac. Cardiovasc. Surg.* 2011;**141**:1213–17.

48. D'Cunha J, Rueth NM, Groth SS, et al. Esophageal stents for anastomic leaks and perforations. *J. Thorac. Cardiovasc. Surg.* 2011;**142**:39–46.

49. Lin Y, Jiang G, Liu L, et al. Management of thoracic esophageal perforation. *World J. Surg.* 2014;**38**:1093–9.

50. Wilson JL, Louie BE, Farivar AS, et al. Fully covered self-expanding metal stents are effective for benign esophagogastric disruptions and strictures. *J. Gastrointest. Surg.* 2013;**17**:2045–50.

51. Schweigert M, Beattie R, Solymosi N, et al. Endoscopic stent insertion versus primary operative management for spontaneous rupture of the esophagus (Boerhaave's syndrome): an international study comparing the outcome. *Am. Surg.* 2013;**79**:634–40.

52. van Boeckel PG, Dua KS, Weusten BL, et al. Fully covered self-expandable metal stents (SEMS), partially covered SEMS and self-expandable plastic stents for the treatment of benign esophageal ruptures and anastomotic leaks. *BMC Gastroenterol.* 2012;**12**:19.

53. Schmidt SC, Strauch S, Rosch T, et al. Management of esophageal perforations. *Surg. Endosc.* 2010;**24**:2809–13.

54. Biancari F, Saarnio J, Mennander A, et al. Outcome of patients with esophageal perforations: a multicenter study. *World J. Surg.* 2014;**38**:902–9.

55. Bonin EA, Wong Kee Song LM, Gostout ZS, et al. Closure of a persistent esophagopleural fistula assisted by a novel endoscopic suturing system. *Endoscopy* 2012;**44**:E8–E9.

56. Fritscher-Ravens A, Hampe J, Grange P, et al. Clip closure versus endoscopic suturing versus thoracoscopic repair of an iatrogenic esophageal perforation: a randomized, comparative, long-term survival study in a porcine model (with videos). *Gastrointest. Endosc.* 2010;**72**:1020–6.

57. Rolanda C, Silva D, Branco C, et al. Peroral esophageal segmentectomy and anastomosis with single transthoracic trocar: a step forward in thoracic NOTES. *Endoscopy* 2011;**43**:14–20.

58. Černá M, Köcher M, Válek V, et al. Covered biodegradable stent: new therapeutic option for the management of esophageal perforation or anastomotic leak. *Cardiovasc. Intervent. Radiol.* 2011;**34**:1267–71.

59. van Minnen B, Leeuwen MB, Stegenga B, et al. Short-term in vitro and in vivo biocompatibility of a biodegradable polyurethane foam based on 1,4-butanediisocyanate. *J. Mater. Sci. Mater. Med.* 2005;**16**:221–7.

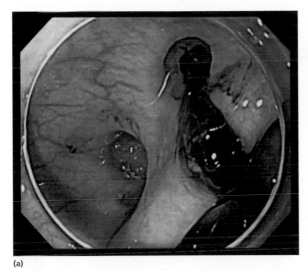 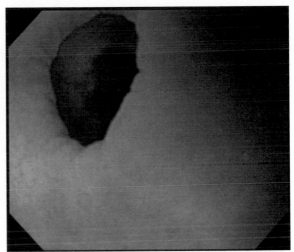

(a) (b)

Fig. 6.2 Diverticular bleed with stigmata of an adherent clot.

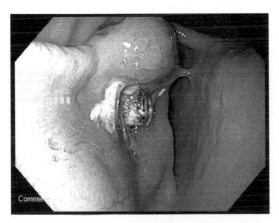

Fig. 9.1 Endoscopic appearance of a buried bumper at endoscopy.

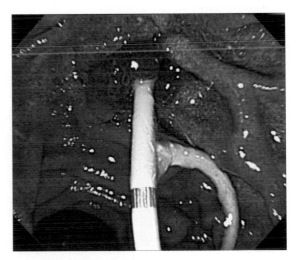

Fig. 11.1 Temporary pancreatic duct stent with single external pigtail, inserted for post-ERCP pancreatitis prophylaxis in a high-risk patient.

Gastrointestinal Emergencies, Third Edition. Edited by Tony C. K. Tham, John S. A. Collins, and Roy Soetikno.
© 2016 John Wiley & Sons, Ltd. Published 2016 by John Wiley & Sons, Ltd.

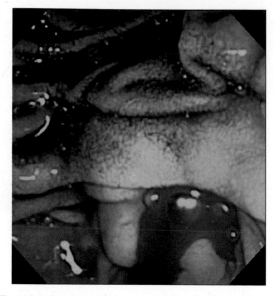

Fig. 11.2 Delayed post-sphincterotomy bleeding in a patient who had to start full anticoagulation therapy soon after ERCP with sphincterotomy.

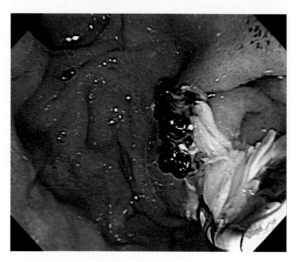

Fig. 11.3 Cholangitis with immediate release of intraductal stones and pus from the bile duct after biliary sphincterotomy.

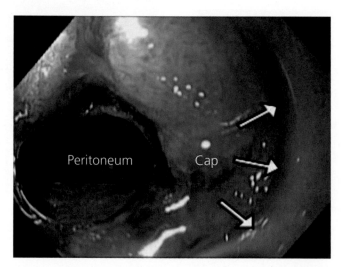

Fig. 11.4 Perforation of the afferent enteral limb with a duodenoscope in a patient with Billroth II anatomy. After obtaining an emergent surgical consultation in the endoscopy unit, the defect was immediately managed endoscopically with a cap-fitted, forward-viewing gastroscope with complete clip-closure of the perforation. The ERCP was then able to be completed in the same session with the cap-fitted, forward-viewing instrument.

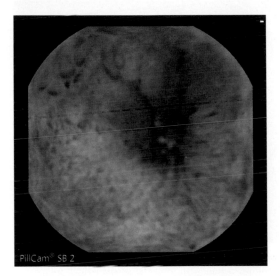

Fig. 15.1 Small bowel tumor causing capsule retention.

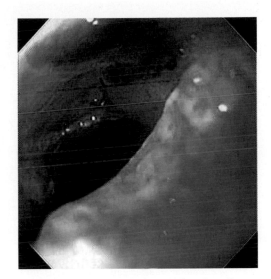

Fig. 16.3 Esophageal tear after passage of the echoendoscope.

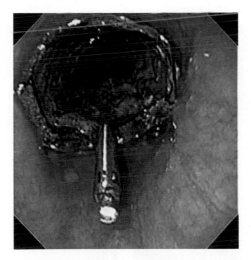

Fig. 16.4 Esophageal stent placed over the site of perforation.

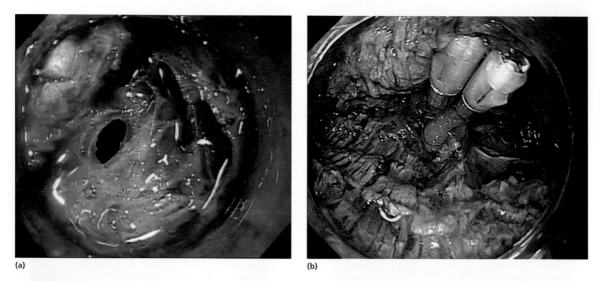

Fig. 17.1 (a) Perforation occurred during gastric ESD. (b) Perforation closed successfully with "omental-patch method" using endoclips.

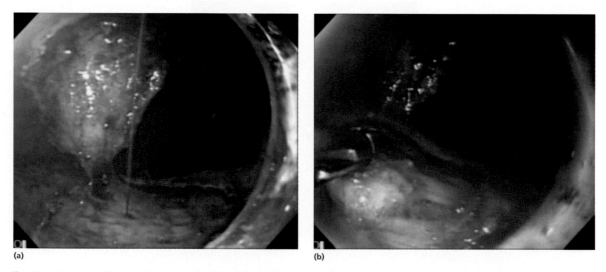

Fig. 17.2 (a) Arterial bleeding during gastric ESD. (b) Arterial bleeding managed by electrocautery using hemostatic forceps.

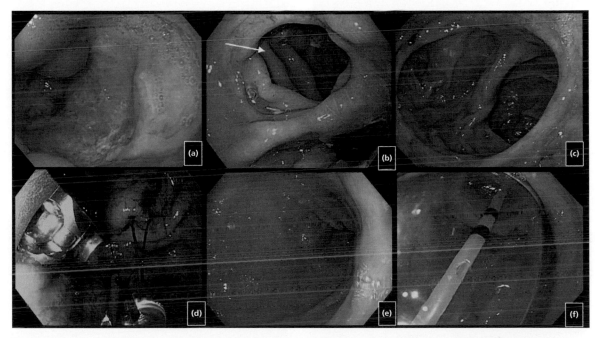

Fig. 18.2 Endoscopic examples of complications and/or treatments including marginal ulceration (a), gastro-gastric fistula (b), dilated gastrojejunal anastamosis (c) and an endoscopic suturing procedure to decrease stoma size (d) following Roux-en-Y gastric bypass, and gastric outlet obstruction at the incisura angularis (e) with subsequent endoscopic balloon dilation (f) following sleeve gastrectomy.

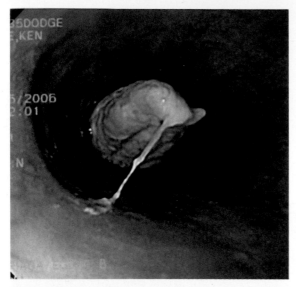

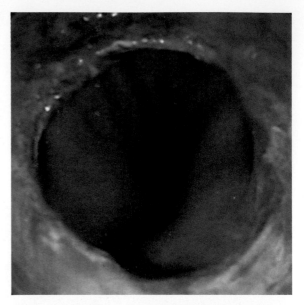

Fig. 20.1 Chicken meat bolus impacted above a distal esophageal mucosal (Schatzki's) ring (not shown). The bolus was grasped using the polypectomy snare and lifted off the distal esophageal stenosis before being removed by mouth using the Roth net.

Fig. 20.2 Endoscopic appearance of a distal esophageal mucosal (Schatzki's) ring severed by the passage of the food bolus into the stomach under direct endoscopic visualization, water and air instillation, and gentle pressure by the endoscope tip. Mucosal rings account for many episodes of acute esophageal impaction, typically with a meat bolus (Steak house syndrome).

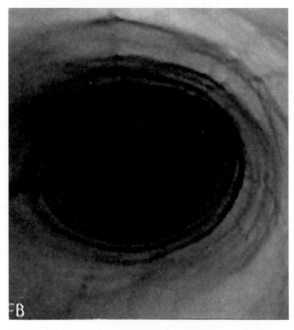

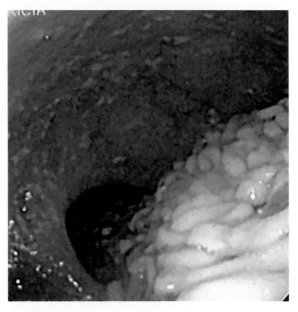

Fig. 20.3 Characteristic appearance of eosinophilic esophagitis, a clinical condition that underlies many foreign body impactions today. This endoscopic photograph, depicting multiple rings along the esophageal body, was taken upon introduction of the endoscope in the proximal esophagus and hence provided with an endoscopic clue to the etiology of impaction, which occurred more distally in this patient (not shown).

Fig. 20.5 Food impaction in a patient with severe scleroderma esophagus and secondary esophageal Candidiasis. Note the dilated esophagus and the esophageal mucosal changes consistent with Candida infection. Careful water instillation allowed the endoscope to break up the food residue that initially appeared as a cast of the esophageal body. The repeated use of the Roth retrieval net eventually relieved the patient's impaction and associated acute dysphagia.

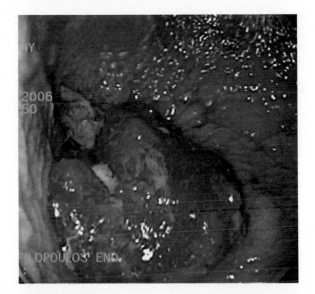

Fig. 20.6 Food impaction in a patient with esophageal achalasia. Note the distorted appearance of the distal esophageal mucosa consistent with stasis esophagitis. Because of the associated atony and dilation of the esophageal body, water instillation allowed the endoscope to bypass the impaction and break up the food residue in small particles. Using the endoscope, the food particles were then pushed into the stomach and relieved the patient's dysphagia.

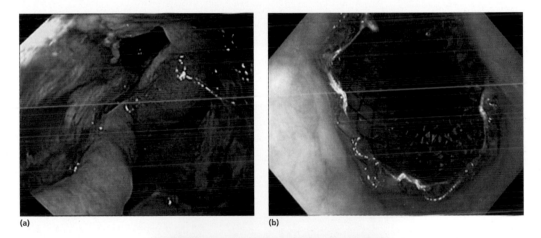

(a)

(b)

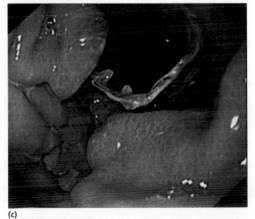

(c)

Fig. 21.2 Patient presenting with a perforation due to Boerhaave's syndrome (a). A fully covered Wallflex stent was placed (b), which was extending just below the gastroesophageal junction (c).

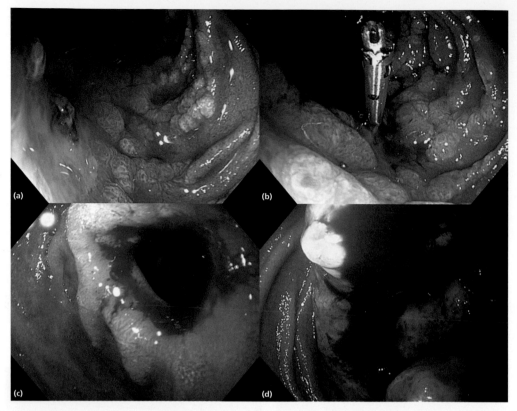

Fig. 32.1 Deep enteroscopy images. (a) Duodenal ulcer with a visible vessel. (b) Duodenal ulcer with visible vessel after endoscopic clipping. (c) Same under NBI. (d) Jejunal tumor.

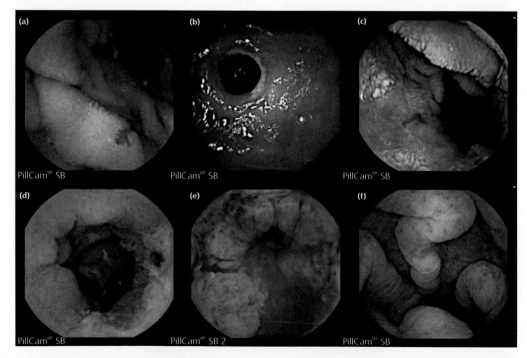

Fig. 32.2 Capsule endoscopy images. (a) Intestinal AVM. (b) Meckel's diverticulum opening. (c) Duodenal ulcer with bleeding visible vessel. (d) NSAID enteropathy with a visible clot. (e) Bleeding ileal tumor. (f) Active gastric bleeding in a patient with portal hypertensive gastropathy.

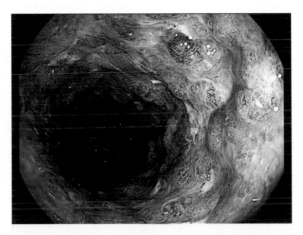

Fig. 34.4 Endoscopic appearance of severe colitis despite treatment with infliximab for 7 days. The patient underwent colectomy.

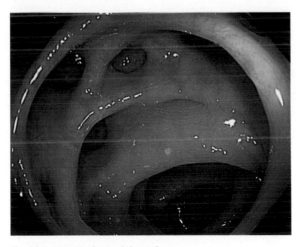

Fig. 36.1 Diverticulosis of the Colon.

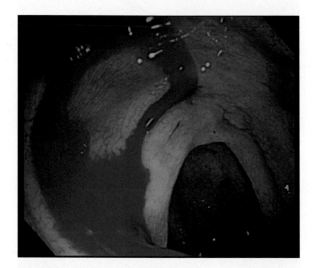

Fig. 36.2 Active Diverticular Bleed.

CHAPTER 22

Acute upper non-variceal gastrointestinal hemorrhage

Kelvin Palmer

Western General Hospital, Edinburgh, UK

Introduction

The mortality of patients admitted to hospital for acute gastrointestinal bleeding is about 7%, rising to more than 25% in patients who bleed as inpatients. Crude mortality has only marginally over 60 years although the case mix has changed greatly over this time, and patients are now older and have greater medical disability than was the case 50 years ago [1].

The incidence of acute upper gastrointestinal haemorrhage in the United Kingdom ranges between 50–190/10 000/year and is highest in areas of social deprivation. The number of admissions for bleeding is stable or slightly increasing in elderly patients in the UK. The prevalence of *Helicobacter pylori*, use of non-steroidal anti-inflammatory drugs (NSAIDs) and prevalence of liver disease are important factors [2].

See also Chapter 3 on Approach to Upper Gastrointestinal Bleeding.

Risk assessment

At the time of first assessment it is important to identify patients who have significant liver disease. Patients with liver disease are best managed at presentation by gastroenterologists (or hepatologists). Most patients will have a history of alcohol abuse or chronic viral hepatitis, have clinical evidence of liver disease, and abnormal serum liver function tests.

Death following admission to hospital for gastrointestinal bleeding is almost invariably a consequence of

decompensated comorbidity; it is seldom caused by exsanguination. Sudden blood loss and circulatory collapse may result in fatal cardiac or cerebrovascular events in patients with underlying vascular disease, and postoperative complications following emergency surgery are more likely in the presence of medical comorbidity. Therefore, risk assessment is based on the severity of the hemorrhage and medical comorbidity.

When patients present with acute upper gastrointestinal hemorrhage, it is crucial to define factors with prognostic value. Those at high risk of continuing bleeding or rebleeding need intensive monitoring and early endoscopic intervention, whereas low-risk patients should be "fast-tracked" towards early hospital discharge.

Rebleeding is associated with a 10-fold increase in hospital mortality. In clinical trials, it is often used as an end-point for defining success or failure of putative treatments. Mortality is particularly high in patients who bleed during a hospital stay for another serious disease (25% in the recent UK audit).

The Blatchford score [3] (Table 22.1) can be easily calculated at the time of presentation on the basis of basic clinical investigations and laboratory blood tests and predicts the need for intervention (principally urgent endoscopy). It also reliably identifies low risk patients who do not need hospital admission and can be referred for outpatient endoscopy (Table 22.2).

The Rockall score [4] (Table 22.3) is a well-validated risk assessment tool that was developed from a large audit of patients admitted to hospitals in England for acute upper gastrointestinal bleeding. Multi-variant analysis identified age, shock, comorbidity and specific

Gastrointestinal Emergencies, Third Edition. Edited by Tony C. K. Tham, John S. A. Collins, and Roy Soetikno.
© 2016 John Wiley & Sons, Ltd. Published 2016 by John Wiley & Sons, Ltd.

Table 22.1 The Blatchford Scoring system.

Variable		Score
Urea (mmol/L)		
	>6.5 < 8.0	2
	>8 < 10	3
	>10 <25	4
	>25	6
Hemoglobin (g/dL)		
Men	Women	
>12 <13	>10 <12	1
>10 <12		3
<10	<10	6
Systolic BP (mmHg)		
	100–109	1
	90–99	2
	<90	3
Pulse >100		1
Melena		1
Syncope		2
Liver disease		2
Cardiac failure		2

Source: Blatchford 2000. Reproduced with permission of Elsevier.

Table 22.2 Total Blatchford Score and need for Intervention (i.e. transfusion, endoscopic therapy, surgery).

Total score	Need for intervention (approximate %)
<3	<10
4	25
5	40
6	50
7–9	75
>10	95

Table 22.3 The Rockall scoring system.

Variable	Score 0	Score 1	Score 2	Score 3
• Age (years)	<60	60–79	>80	–
• Shock	None	Pulse >100 beats/minute	Blood pressure <100 mmHg	–
• Comorbidity	None		Cardiac or other major disease;	Renal or liver failure; advanced malignancy
• Diagnosis	None	–	Esophagogastric malignancy	–
	No stigmata of recent hemorrhage Mallory–Weiss tear			
•	Major stigmata of recent hemorrhage	None	–	–
	Black spots	Clot		
	Non-bleeding visible vessel		Blood in lumen Spurting hemorrhage	

The total score is calculated by simple addition of each variable.
Source: Rockall 1996. Reproduced with permission from the BMJ.

endoscopic findings as independent variables predicting re-bleeding and death (Table 22.4).

Endoscopy provides important prognostic information (Tables 22.5 and 22.6). The presence of blood in the upper gastrointestinal tract, active spurting hemorrhage, and a "non-bleeding visible vessel" are signs of poor prognosis. Active ulcer bleeding implies an 80–90% risk of continuing hemorrhage or rebleeding. A visible vessel (representing adherent blood clot or a pseudoaneurysm over the arterial defect) is associated with a 50% risk of rebleeding during that hospital stay [5]. Therapeutic endoscopists attempt to wash the bleeding point vigorously to display these major endoscopic stigmata of recent hemorrhage, using washing catheters and snares to remove blood clot. These maneuvers risk provoking further bleeding, but this can usually be managed by one of the techniques described in subsequent sections. Sometimes, the clot cannot be

Table 22.4 Mortality and rebleeding of patients with peptic ulceration and esophageal varices according to complete Rockall Score.

Total Rockall Score							
	0	1	2	3	4	5	6
Bleeding peptic ulcers (Total 162 patients)							
Rebled (%)	0	0	14	6.7	8	26.7	30.4
Mortality (%)	0	0	0	0	8	13	13
Oesophageal varices (Total 196 patients)							
Rebled (%)	0	0	0	0	3.8	17	31
Mortality (%)	0	0	0	3.8	0	10.6	4

Source: Villanueva 2013.

Table 22.5 Causes of hematemesis and melena.

Cause	Proportion of patients (%)
Peptic ulcer (duodenal, gastric and stomal)	30–35
Varices	5–10
Esophagitis	10–15
Mallory–Weiss tear	5
Erosions (gastric and duodenal)	10–15
Tumors (benign and malignant)	2–4
Vascular malformations	1–3
Small bowel and colonic	5
None found	20–22

Table 22.6 Endoscopic stigmata and the risk of rebleeding.

Endoscopic finding	Risk of rebleeding (%)
Clean base	3
Flat spots	7
Oozing only	10
Adherent clot	33
Non-bleeding visible vessel	50
Active bleeding	90

removed, and the presence of non-adherent blood clot carries an intermediate risk of further bleeding.

Diagnosis and etiology

See Table 22.5 for causes of acute non-variceal gastrointestinal hemorrhage.

Management

An algorithm for management is shown in Fig. 22.1.

The principles of "airway, breathing, and circulation" apply in resuscitation. Patients presenting with major bleeding are often elderly and have significant cardiorespiratory, renal, and cerebrovascular comorbidity. It is vital that these conditions are recognized and supported. In critically ill patients it is wise to enlist the services of specialists in critical care and to support the patient in a high dependency unit.

Intravenous fluid replacement to maintain blood pressure and urine output is the first step in management, coupled with appropriate management of cardiac and

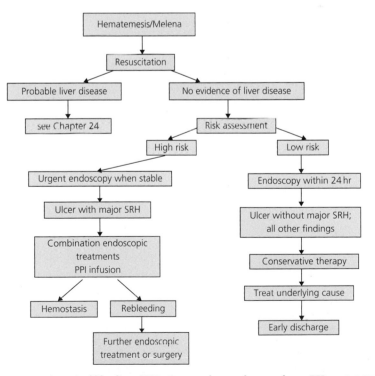

Fig. 22.1 Algorithm for acute gastrointestinal bleeding. SRH, stigmata of recent haemorrhage; PPI, proton pump inhibitors.

respiratory disease. Central venous pressure (CVP) monitoring is useful in the elderly and in many patients with cardiac disease, to optimize decisions concerning volume of fluid replacement. Intravenous fluids should be given through a large cannula inserted in an antecubital vein. Crystalloids (principally normal saline) are used to normalize blood pressure and urine output; colloids (e.g. Gelofusine) are often used in the presence of major hypotension, but there is no evidence that they have advantages over crystalloids.

Blood transfusion is administered to patients who are shocked and bleeding actively. The threshold for blood transfusion in stable patients is controversial. Whilst a hemoglobin concentration of 10 g/dL is conventionally used to trigger blood transfusion, the evidence base for this is poor and there is increasing evidence that blood transfusion is associated with an increased rebleeding rate compared to that in patients of comparable severity who have not received blood products [6]. A recent prospective randomized trial showed that restricting transfusion to a Hb of <10 g/dL is associated with decrease in rebleeding and better outcomes [7].

Patients presenting with acute upper gastrointestinal bleeding whilst taking aspirin or clopidogrel present a clinical dilemma. Stopping these drugs may reduce the risk of continuing bleeding but risks vascular events that can prove fatal. Both aspirin and clopidogrel bind irreversibly to platelet receptors, thereby impairing platelet function for 7–10 days. The rationale for discontinuing their use following the onset of bleeding is therefore ill founded, and for patients in whom there is a good indication for their use, it is wise to continue aspirin and clopidogrel despite upper gastrointestinal hemorrhage.

Monitoring includes measurement of pulse, blood pressure, urine output (through an indwelling catheter), and (in selected patients) CVP. Actively bleeding patients with evidence of shock (defined as pulse > 100 beats/minute and/or systolic blood pressure <100 mmHg) are best managed in a high-dependency environment.

Endoscopy is the primary diagnostic investigation and is undertaken after optimum resuscitation has been achieved. In most cases, it is best performed within 24 hours of admission, on the first available elective list. Out-of-hours emergency endoscopy is occasionally required in actively bleeding, shocked patients.

Endoscopy has three purposes:

1 To provide an accurate diagnosis. Certain diagnoses greatly influence management; for example, esophageal varices and active bleeding from peptic ulcers require specific endoscopic and pharmacological interventions.
2 Prognostic information. Stigmata of recent hemorrhage (Table 22.6) and variceal appearances – or their absence – help direct the patient to the high-dependency unit, the general ward or, in some very low-risk cases, to immediate hospital discharge. Most importantly, endoscopy facilitates application of specific therapies to high-risk bleeding lesions.
3 Endoscopic therapy: At least 80% of patients admitted to hospital for hematemesis and melena have an excellent prognosis; bleeding stops spontaneously and supportive therapy is all that is required.

Endoscopic therapy is indicated in the following situations:

- Bleeding esophageal varices.
- Peptic ulcer with major stigmata of recent hemorrhage (active spurting bleeding, a non-bleeding visible vessel, and non-adherent clot).
- Vascular malformations: including actively bleeding arteriovenous malformations (AVMs), gastric antral vascular ectasia, and Dieulafoy's lesion.
- Active bleeding from a Mallory–Weiss tear (rarely).

Management of peptic ulcer bleeding

Peptic ulcer is the most frequent cause of major, life-threatening acute gastrointestinal bleeding. Significant hemorrhage results from erosion of an underlying artery and the magnitude of bleeding is related to the size of the arterial defect and the diameter of the artery. Consequently, bleeding may be particularly severe from large, posterior duodenal ulcers, which erode the gastroduodenal artery, and high, lesser curve gastric ulcers involving branches of the left gastric artery. Most patients present with little or no history of dyspepsia. A history of aspirin or NSAID use is common.

The evidence supporting endoscopy for non-variceal therapy is principally based on clinical trials for peptic ulcer hemorrhage. Three categories of direct endoscopic treatment have been evaluated; each attempts to seal the arterial defect created by the ulcer.

- Injection – direct injection of fluids into the bleeding ulcer using disposable needles is technically straightforward. The most widely used injection fluid is 1:10 000 epinephrine. This stops active bleeding in more than 90% of patients, but 15–20% rebleed [8]. Epinephrine injection is extremely safe and has no significant complications. It cannot be recommended as sole treatment and should be used in combination with other endoscopic treatments. Thrombin is probably a more effective injection material; it carries a low risk of complications rate but is not freely available.

- Heat energy – in this method, devices are applied directly to the bleeding point at to cause coagulation and thrombosis. The heater probe is pushed firmly onto the bleeding lesion to apply tamponade, and defined pulses of heat energy are then given to coagulate the vessel. Clinical trials have shown the device to be as effective and as safe as injection therapy. Multipolar coagulation, in which electrical energy is conducted between multiple probes on the tip of an endoscopically positioned catheter, is as effective as the heater probe. The argon plasma coagulator also appears to be effective in arresting bleeding in limited clinical trials. Thermal treatments can cause perforations but this risk is very low.
- Mechanical devices – "endoclips" can be applied to visible vessels. They can be difficult to deploy on awkwardly positioned ulcers, but may be the best option for treatment of major bleeding ulcers and for the Deulafoy lesion. Arterial defects of more than 1 mm diameter do not usually respond to injection therapy, but an adequately positioned clip can stop bleeding from relatively large arteries. The major hazard is exacerbation of bleeding should application prove unsuccessful.
- Combinations of endoscopic therapy – although the exact modes of action of these endoscopic therapies are largely speculative, it is clear that each achieves hemostasis by a different mechanism. A meta-analysis of published trials shows that combination of injection and thermal treatments is superior to single modality treatment [10].

Endoscopy should be repeated within 12–36 hours in patients undergoing endoscopic haemostasis if there is uncertainty about the efficacy of the index procedure. Those with residual bleeding or persisting major stigmata are subjected to further therapy.

Endoscopic therapy can achieve primary hemostasis in most bleeding ulcer patients. However, rebleeding occurs in 15–20% of cases, usually within the first 24 hours. It is most common when the initial bleeding episode was severe; thus, shocked patients presenting with active, spurting hemorrhage from large, posterior duodenal ulcers are the group most likely to rebleed.

Management following rebleeding is often difficult and is largely based on clinical judgement and local expertise. Discussion between endoscopist, interventional radiologist and gastrointestinal surgeon is vital. In most patients, it is appropriate to repeat the endoscopy and re-treat the bleeding lesion. A trial from Hong Kong showed that the mortality and blood transfusion requirements of patients who rebled after initially successful endoscopic therapy were similar whether they were treated with urgent surgery or repeat endoscopic therapy [11]. If unsuccessful, intra-arterial embolization of the bleeding artery represents optimal treatment in the majority of patients. Urgent surgery is still indicated in patients with major uncontrolled bleeding although carries a very high risk of death.

Drug therapy

A range of drugs have been used with the aim of reducing further bleeding once endoscopic haemostasis has been achieved. Of these, only acid suppressive therapy has a strong evidence base. The rationale is based upon the observation that the stability of blood clot is low in an acid environment. It is crucial that gastric pH does not fall below 6, and the only practical means of achieving this is constant infusion of a proton pump inhibitor. This can be achieved most readily by intravenous infusion of a proton pump inhibitor drug (e.g. omeprazole, 80 mg bolus followed by an 8 mg/hour infusion for 72 hours). Meta-analyses have demonstrated that this significantly reduces the risk of re-bleeding and need for emergency surgery, although it has not been shown to significantly reduce mortality [10].

Somatostatin and tranexamic acid are also sometimes used to reduce ulcer rebleeding although the evidence base for their use is less secure.

Secondary prophylaxis

After hemostasis has been achieved, it is important to prevent recurrent hemorrhage. For ulcer patients eradication of *H. pylori* effectively abolishes the risk of late re-bleeding. In patients who need, for good reason, to continue NSAID therapy, the following should be considered.

- Use the least toxic NSAID (usually ibuprofen) that controls the arthritic symptoms.
- Co-prescribe a proton pump inhibitor with the NSAID.
- Consider use of a cyclo-oxygenase-2-specific anti-inflammatory drug, rather than a conventional NSAID. These are associated with significantly fewer recurrent ulcer-related adverse events (both hemorrhage and perforation) although concerns concerning increased vascular events have largely precluded their use.

The management of patients with *H. pylori* who need to continue taking an NSAID remains controversial. Gastritis (an inevitable consequence of *H. pylori* infection) induces mucosal prostaglandin production, and this may protect the gastroduodenal mucosa from the harmful effects of NSAIDs. However, current studies suggest that the magnitude of prostaglandin production is unlikely to outweigh the deleterious effects of *H. pylori*, and that eradication therapy is indicated in patients with a bleeding ulcer who are *H. pylori* positive and require NSAID therapy.

Management of varices

Management of varices is discussed in Chapter 25, Variceal Hemorrhage.

Management of Mallory–Weiss tears

Mallory–Weiss tears occur at the esophagogastric junction and are due to prolonged retching. Alcohol abuse is the usual cause, but other causes of nausea and vomiting (e.g. chemotherapy, digoxin toxicity, renal failure, advanced malignancy) may be responsible. Bleeding usually stops spontaneously and active endoscopic or surgical intervention is seldom required.

Management of esophagitis

Esophagitis is common in elderly patients presenting with "coffee-ground" hematemesis. Bleeding is seldom life-threatening; in most cases, conservative supportive therapy combined with proton pump inhibitor drugs is all that is necessary. However, it is important to be aware that, in this group of patients, coffee-ground vomiting may have another cause (drug toxicity, underlying renal or cardiac failure, pancreatitis, or colon cancer), even when esophagitis is proven at endoscopy.

Although the natural history of the bleeding event may be benign, the prognosis is dependent upon underlying causes.

Management of gastritis, duodenitis, and gastroduodenal erosions

Gastritis, duodenitis, and gastroduodenal erosions are associated with NSAIDs and *H. pylori* infection. In most patients, supportive therapy and cessation of NSAID use or *H. pylori* eradication therapy achieve a favorable outcome.

Management of vascular anomalies

Vascular anomalies may present with hematemesis and melena.

- Small AVMs are often found at routine endoscopy during investigation for dyspepsia, and in this situation should be ignored. In other cases, large or multiple AVMs can cause significant bleeding. This usually leads to insidious development of iron-deficiency anemia, but occasionally major acute hemorrhage occurs. Most AVMs have no obvious cause and present in elderly patients; in younger patients, they are sometimes caused by hereditary hemorrhagic telangiectasia. Other patients have valvular heart disease or an artificial heart valve, and bleeding may be exacerbated by anticoagulant drugs.
- Gastric antral vascular ectasia is an uncommon vascular anomaly characterized by linear, readily bleeding red streaks radiating from the pylorus into the gastric antrum. It is occasionally associated with liver disease. Most patients present with iron-deficiency anemia rather than acute bleeding, and some require frequent blood transfusion.
- Portal hypertensive gastropathy results from venous congestion of the gastric mucosa; in most patients, this is caused by portal hypertension from cirrhosis.
- Dieulafoy's lesion is an unusual cause of acute bleeding, in which a superficial submucosal artery is eroded. The diagnosis can be made only when endoscopy is undertaken during active bleeding. Arterial disruption is probably caused by a small ulcer, but no mucosal lesion can be identified after bleeding has ceased. The most common site of Dieulafoy's lesion is the gastric fundus; it may also develop in the duodenum or other parts of the stomach.

Management of tumors

Esophagogastric tumors are a relatively uncommon cause of acute upper gastrointestinal hemorrhage. The most important benign type is gastrointestinal stromal cell tumor (previously termed leiomyoma), which arises from the muscle layers of the gastric or duodenal wall. Erosion through the mucosa gives a characteristic umbilicated endoscopic appearance. These tumors erode underlying arteries and may cause major bleeding. Rarely, large tumors become malignant.

Carcinomas and lymphomas of the stomach tend to present with other upper gastrointestinal symptoms and iron-deficiency anemia rather than with hematemesis and melena.

Management of fistulas

Aortoduodenal fistula should be considered in all patients presenting with major upper gastrointestinal bleeding after aortic graft insertion. Bleeding occurs from the second part of the duodenum, is massive and may recur over hours or days. All such patients should be referred to a vascular unit immediately after initial resuscitation.

Management of bleeding distal to the ligament of Treitz

See Chapter 32 on Middle Gastrointestinal Bleeding for this topic.

Small bowel or right-sided colonic disease sometimes presents with melena and rarely with hematemesis. Colonoscopy, barium radiology, capsule endoscopy, and enteroscopy are used to identify the underlying tumor or vascular anomaly when upper gastrointestinal endoscopy fails to identify a bleeding source. In young patients, a bleeding Meckel's diverticulum should be considered.

References

1. Hearnshaw S, Logan RFA, Lowe D, Travis SPL, Murphy MF. Acute upper gastrointestinal bleeding in the UK; patient characteristics, diagnosis and outcomes in the 2007 audit. *Gut* 2011;**60**(10):1327–35.
2. Church NC, Palmer KR. Non-variceal gastrointestinal haemorrhage. In *Evidence-based Gastroenterology and Hepatology*, 2nd edition, McDonald JWD, Burroughs AK, Feagan BG (eds). Blackwell Publications, Oxford, 2004: 139–59.
3. Blatchford O, Murray WR, Blatchford M. A risk score to predict need for treatment for upper gastrointestinal haemorrhage. *Lancet* 2000;**356**:1319.
4. Rockall T A, Logan R F A, Devlin H B, Northfield T C. Risk Assessment following Acute Upper Gastrointestinal Haemorrhage. *Gut* 1996;**38**:316–21.
5. Bornman PC, Theodorou N, Shuttleworth RD, et al. Importance of hypovolaemic shock and endoscopic signs in predicting recurrent haemorrhage from peptic ulceration: a prospective evaluation. *Br. Med. J.* 1985;**291**:245–7.
6. Hearnshaw S A, Logan RFA, Palmer KR, Card TR Travis SPL, Murphy MF. Outcomes following early red cell transfusion in acute upper gastrointestinal bleeding. *Aliment. Pharmacol. Ther.* 2010;**32**:215–24.
7. Villanueva C, Colomo A, Bosch A, et al. Transfusion strategies for acute upper gastrointestinal bleeding. *N. Engl. J. Med.* 2013;**368**(1):11–21.
8. Chung SCS, Leung JWC, Steele RJC. Endoscopic injection of adrenaline for actively bleeding ulcers: a randomised trial. *Br. Med. J.* 1988;**296**:1631–3.
9. Calvet X, Vergara M, Brullet E, et al . Addition of a second endoscopic treatment following epinephrine injection improves outcome in high-risk bleeding ulcers. *Gastroenterology* 2004;**126**:441–50.
10. Lau JY, Sung JJ, Lam YH, et al. Endoscopic retreatment compared with surgery in patients with recurrent bleeding after initial endoscopic control of bleeding ulcers. *N. Engl. J. Med.* 1999;**340**:751–4.
11. Leontiadis GI, Sharma VK, Howden CW. Proton pump inhibitor treatment for acute peptic ulcer bleeding Cochrane Database Syst. Rev. 2006;Issue 1:CD002094.

CHAPTER 23

Acute pancreatitis

David R. Lichtenstein

Boston University School of Medicine, Boston, MD, USA

Introduction

Acute pancreatitis is best defined as an acute inflammatory process of the pancreas that may also involve peripancreatic tissues and remote organ systems. It is the leading cause of hospitalization among gastrointestinal disorders in the United States, with more than 200 000 annual admissions. This translates into an overall incidence of 1 in 4000 for the general population. Most patients with acute pancreatitis have a mild course and recover with restoration of normal pancreatic function and gland architecture. However, 10–20% develop a more severe form of the disease manifest by systemic inflammatory response syndrome (SIRS), organ dysfunction, and pancreatic necrosis. The overall mortality is 5% with a range from less than 3% for patients with the mild form of acute pancreatitis to 15% for those with necrotizing disease.

Early intervention in patients with acute pancreatitis can decrease disease severity, morbidity, and mortality. Prevention of the septic and non-septic complications in patients with severe acute pancreatitis depends largely on monitoring, vigorous hydration, and early recognition of pancreatic necrosis and choledocholithiasis.

Clinical presentation (Table 23.1)

The hallmark of acute pancreatitis is the presence of persistent abdominal pain although in atypical cases patients may present with unexplained organ failure or postoperative ileus. Pain is usually located in the epigastric and periumbilical regions and may radiate to the back, chest, flanks, and lower abdomen. The onset of pain is typically sudden and often associated with nausea and vomiting. Patients are usually restless and the supine position may increase the intensity of pain. Patients tend to bend forward (knee-chest position) in order to alleviate the pain. Physical examination usually reveals severe upper abdominal tenderness at times associated with guarding. Ileus occurs when there is extension of the inflammatory process into the small intestinal and colonic mesentery or a chemical peritonitis occurs.

Grey Turner's sign (ecchymosis of the flank) or Cullen's sign (ecchymosis in the periumbilical region) may be seen in association with hemorrhagic pancreatitis.

Metabolic problems are common in severe disease and include hypocalcemia, hyperglycemia, and acidosis. Hypocalcemia is most commonly caused by concomitant hypoalbuminemia [1]. Local spread of inflammation leads to effects on contiguous organs that include gastritis and duodenitis, splenic vein thrombosis, colonic necrosis, and external compression of the common bile duct leading to biliary obstruction. Trypsin can activate plasminogen to plasmin and induce clot lysis. Conversely, trypsin can activate prothrombin and thrombin and produce thrombosis, leading to disseminated intravascular coagulation.

Diagnosis: clinical and imaging

The diagnosis of acute pancreatitis (Table 23.2) is based on a combination of clinical, biochemical, and radiologic factors. There is general acceptance that a diagnosis of

Gastrointestinal Emergencies, Third Edition. Edited by Tony C. K. Tham, John S. A. Collins, and Roy Soetikno.
© 2016 John Wiley & Sons, Ltd. Published 2016 by John Wiley & Sons, Ltd.

Table **23.1** Clinical manifestations of acute pancreatitis; the effects of pancreatitis are manifest at three sites.

mild ↓ severe	Pancreatic Autodigestion	• Edema, hemorrhage, necrosis, atrophy
		• Reduced exocrine function
		• Reduced endocrine function
	Local Spread	• Fat necrosis
		• Peripancreatic fluid
		✓ ascites, pseudocyst, abscess
		• Retroperitoneal hemorrhage
		• Enteric erosion or obstruction
	Systemic	• Hypovolemia, hypoalbuminemia
		• Coagulopathies
		• Pulmonary dysfunction (ARDS)
		• CNS
		• Renal

Table **23.2** Diagnostic features of acute pancreatitis.

Signs and Symptoms	Labs	Differential Diagnosis
• Abdominal pain	• ↑ WBC	• Cholecystitis
• Abdominal tenderness	• ↑ Serum amylase	• Peptic ulcer disease
		• Diverticulitis
• Nausea & vomiting	• ↑ Serum lipase	• Intestinal ischemia
• Fever		• Intestinal obstruction
• Tachycardia		• Salpingitis
		• Ectopic pregnancy

acute pancreatitis requires two of the following three features:

1 Abdominal pain characteristic of acute pancreatitis,

2 Serum amylase and/or lipase ≥3 times the upper limit of normal, and

3 Characteristic findings of acute pancreatitis on computerized tomography (CT) scan.

Elevations in amylase or lipase levels less than three times the upper limit of normal have low specificity for acute pancreatitis and are consistent with but not diagnostic of acute pancreatitis. Serum pancreatic enzyme levels can be elevated in other processes being considered in the differential diagnosis such as bowel perforation, intestinal obstruction, mesenteric ischemia, dissecting aortic aneurysm, tubo-ovarian disease, and renal failure [2]. In general, serum lipase is thought to be more sensitive and specific than serum amylase in the diagnosis of acute pancreatitis. Serum lipase may be preferable because it remains normal in some non-pancreatic conditions associated with an elevation of serum amylase including macroamylasemia, parotitis, and tubo-ovarian disease. Serum lipase remains elevated longer than serum amylase and therefore may be helpful if a patient delays seeking medical attention [2]. Repeated measurements of pancreatic enzymes have little value in assessing clinical progress of the illness or ultimate prognosis. Moreover, the magnitude of serum amylase or lipase elevation does not correlate with the severity of pancreatitis.

Transabdominal ultrasound (US) and CT are the two imaging modalities most frequently used in patients with acute pancreatitis. These techniques tend to be complementary. US is very good at detecting gallbladder stones (accuracy of 90%); however, the reported sensitivity of US for the detection of common bile duct (CBD) stones is limited and ranges from 20% to 75%, although specificity is quite high if they are identified. Dilation of the common bile duct alone is neither sensitive nor specific for the detection of common bile duct stones. Visualization of the pancreas with US in the face of ongoing acute pancreatitis tends to be poor due to overlying intestinal gas. Occasionally, the pancreas is adequately visualized by abdominal ultrasound to reveal features that are consistent with the diagnosis of acute pancreatitis including diffuse glandular enlargement, hypoechoic texture of the pancreas reflective of edema, and ascites.

Contrast enhanced CT (CECT) scan [1,2] is preferred for imaging the pancreas and should be obtained on admission when the diagnosis is in doubt. Supportive CT findings include pancreatic enlargement, peripancreatic inflammatory change, and extrapancreatic fluid collections. CT scan findings may also prove useful for assessing the severity of disease and to identify complications of pancreatic necrosis and peripancreatic fluid collections. Abnormal CT scan does not exclude the diagnosis of acute pancreatitis as the pancreas appears normal in up to 15–30% of those with mild disease. CT scanning should be performed after adequate fluid resuscitation to minimize the risk of contrast-induced nephrotoxicity. Also recognize that early CT scanning (within 72 hours of symptom onset) can underestimate the presence and extent of pancreatic necrosis.

Magnetic resonance imaging (MRI) with gadolinium enhancement [3] is as accurate as CT in imaging the pancreas and determining severity of disease and determining the degree of necrosis. However, MRI scanning is more difficult in critically ill patients and similarly carries a risk of contrast-induced renal failure [4]. MRI is also sensitive for the detection of necrosis and small neoplasms when these are under consideration. MRCP is a noninvasive means of imaging the pancreaticobiliary tree with a sensitivity of greater than 90% for detecting common bile duct stones.

Endoscopic ultrasound (EUS) is highly sensitive for the identification of common bile duct stones and sludge not seen with other imaging modalities. Small ampullary or pancreatic tumors may also be visualized.

Endoscopic retrograde cholangiopancreatography (ERCP) does not play a role in establishing the diagnosis of acute pancreatitis, with the exception of sphincter of Oddi manometry for suspected sphincter of Oddi dysfunction (SOD). Its primary role is for treatable disorders identified on noninvasive imaging (e.g. pancreas divisum, gallstone pancreatitis with biliary obstruction).

Etiology of acute pancreatitis

During the initial hospitalization for acute pancreatitis, reasonable attempts to determine etiology is appropriate, and in particular those causes that may affect acute management. The cause for acute pancreatitis is readily identified in 70% to 90% of patients after an initial evaluation consisting of history, physical examination, focused laboratory testing, and routine radiologic evaluation. Gallstones are the etiology in 45%, alcohol 35%, miscellaneous causes 10%, and idiopathic in 10–20%. Relevant historical clues include any previous diagnosis or symptoms of biliary tract disease or gallstones, acute or chronic pancreatitis or their complications, use of ethanol, medications and the timing of their initiation, recent abdominal trauma, weight loss or other symptoms suggesting a malignancy, history of autoimmune disorders, or a family history of pancreatitis. Blood tests within the first 24 h should evaluate for hypertriglyceridemia, hypercalcemia, or a three-fold or greater elevation in alanine transaminase (ALT), which is highly predictive of biliary pancreatitis. There are an extensive number of potential etiologies for acute pancreatitis as indicated below (Table 23.3).

Gallstone pancreatitis

Among patients with gallstones, the incidence of acute pancreatitis is 0.17% per year. The presence of gallstones, however, increases the relative risk of pancreatitis up to 25- to 35-fold. It is theorized that gallstone passage causes

Table 23.3 Etiology of acute pancreatitis.

Obstructive Causes
Gallstones
Tumors—ampullary or pancreatic tumors
Parasites—*Ascaris* or *Clonorchis*
Developmental anomalies—pancreas divisum, choledochocele, annular pancreas
Periampullary duodenal diverticula
Hypertensive sphincter of Oddi
Afferent duodenal loop obstruction

Toxins
Ethyl alcohol
Methyl alcohol
Scorpion venom—excessive cholinergic stimulation causes salivation, sweating, dyspnea, and cardiac arrhythmias; seen mostly in the West Indies
Organophosphorus insecticides

Drugs
Definite association (documented with rechallenges): azathioprine/6-MP, valproic acid, estrogens, tetracycline, metronidazole, nitrofurantoin, pentamidine, furosemide, sulfonamides, methyldopa, cytarabine, cimetidine, ranitidine, sulindac, dideoxycytidine
Probable association: thiazides, ethacrynic acid, phenformin, procainamide, chlorthalidone, L-asparaginase

Metabolic Causes
Hypertriglyceridemia, hypercalcemia, end-stage renal disease

Trauma
Accidental—blunt trauma to the abdomen (car accident, bicycle)
Iatrogenic—postoperative, ERCP, endoscopic sphincterotomy, sphincter of Oddi manometry

Infectious
Parasitic—ascariasis, clonorchiasis
Viral—mumps, rubella, hepatits A, hepatitis B, non-A, non-B hepatitis, coxsackievirus B, echo, adenovirus, cytomegalovirus, varicella, Epstein-Barr, human immunodeficiency virus
Bacterial—mycoplasma, *Campylobacter jejuni*, tuberculosis, *Legionella*, leptospirosis

Vascular
Ischemia—hypoperfusion (such as after cardiac surgery) or atherosclerotic emboli
Vasculitis—systemic lupus erythematosus, polyarteritis nodosa, malignant hypertension

Idiopathic
10–30% of pancreatitis; up to 60% of these patients have occult gallstone disease (biliary microlithiasis or gallbladder sludge); other less common causes include sphincter of Oddi dysfunction and mutations in the cystic fibrosis transmembrane regulator

Miscellaneous
Penetrating peptic ulcer
Crohn's disease of the duodenum
Pregnancy associated
Pediatric association—Reye's syndrome, cystic fibrosis

transient obstruction of the pancreatic duct, precipitating acute pancreatitis. Acute gallstone pancreatitis should be suspected when associated with transient elevation in liver associated enzymes and in particular ALT>150 IU [5]. Most stones pass spontaneously from the ampulla and do not require intervention.

Alcohol

Acute alcoholic pancreatitis is the second most common cause of pancreatitis in the United States. Alcohol is responsible for approximately 30% of cases of acute pancreatitis in the United States. Approximately 10% of chronic alcoholics develop attacks of pancreatitis that are indistinguishable from other forms of acute pancreatitis. Alcoholics who present with acute pancreatitis often have underlying chronic disease. However, some have true acute alcoholic pancreatitis as not all patients progress to chronic pancreatitis, even with continued alcohol abuse. The exact mechanism of pancreatic injury, the genetic and environmental factors that influence the development of pancreatitis in alcoholics, and the reason why only a small proportion of alcoholics develop pancreatitis, are unclear.

Microlithiasis

Microlithiasis may be identified in up to 30% to 65% of patients with idiopathic acute relapsing pancreatitis [6]. Bile collected from the biliary tree during ERCP or aspirated from the duodenum after administration of cholecystokinin should be examined for cholesterol monohydrate crystals or calcium bilirubinate granules under a polarizing light microscope. Several important issues limit the use of bile analysis. Many patients (29%–34%) with gallstones (who all should be expected to have microlithiasis or crystals) have a negative bile analysis. Moreover, the technique is not standardized, and in particular the quantity of crystals needed to define a positive result differs among institutions. However, most believe that the presence of even a small number of crystals is abnormal. Prospective controlled trials in patients with acute relapsing pancreatitis have demonstrated that when microlithiasis is identified, treatment with cholecystectomy, biliary sphincterotomy, or dissolution therapy can prevent recurrence of pancreatitis.

Hereditary pancreatitis

A number of studies have identified genetic mutations in patients with idiopathic pancreatitis, including mutations in the genes encoding cationic trypsinogen (*PRSS1*), pancreatic secretory trypsin inhibitor (serine protease inhibitor Kazal Type 1 or *SPINK-1*) and cystic fibrosis transmembrane conductance regulator (*CFTR*) [7]. In general, the role of genetic testing in idiopathic acute pancreatitis is controversial. Diagnosis of these genetic disorders currently contributes little to direct patient management since no specific therapy is available. Similarly, inadvertent disclosure of the results of genetic testing might have significant negative effects on the patient and the ability to obtain health insurance. On the other hand, one could argue that the identification of an underlying genetic cause may obviate the need for further testing, might allow more informed family planning, and might allow better surveillance for complications including pancreatic cancer. The decision to pursue genetic testing is one that should only be made with the advice and involvement of an experienced counselor.

Pancreas divisum

Pancreas divisum is a developmental anomaly where the duct of Wirsung drains only the ventral pancreas through the major ampulla and the duct of Santorini drains the bulk of the pancreas (dorsal pancreas) through the relatively small accessory ampulla. This common anomaly, termed *pancreas divisum* is present in 5–10% of the general population. It is estimated that fewer than 5% of patients with pancreas divisum develop pancreatic symptoms with an association noted with both acute and chronic pancreatitis. Pancreas divisum is diagnosed by pancreatography via magnetic resonance imaging of the pancreatic duct (MRCP) and ERCP is reserved for therapy (Fig. 23.1).

Caution should be exercised in the management of patients with pancreas divisum. Those with pain and no evidence of pancreatitis should not be treated; they are likely to have another etiology of their pain (e.g. irritable bowel syndrome). The greatest likelihood of a response occurs in patients with recurrent episodes of acute pancreatitis. Treatment of symptomatic pancreas divisum has traditionally been approached by a surgical sphincteroplasty to increase drainage through the accessory papilla. Similar results are obtained with endoscopic approaches including minor papilla sphincterotomy.

Hypertriglyceridemia

Hypertriglyceridemia accounts for 1–4% of acute pancreatitis cases. The breakdown products of triglycerides include toxic free fatty acids which are theorized to

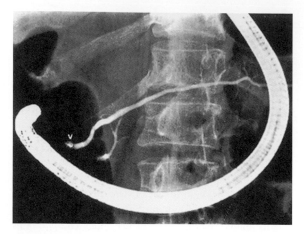

Fig. 23.1 ERCP of pancreatic ductal system in pancreas divisum. The upper duct (dorsal pancreas) was obtained by injecting contrast into the duct of Santorini. The lower duct (ventral pancreas) was obtained by injecting the duct of Wirsung.

injure the endothelial lining of the small pancreatic blood vessels. Triglyceride levels greater than 1000 mg/dL are usually required to induce acute pancreatitis. In addition to primary hyperlipidemia, hypertriglyceridemia may result from therapy with estrogens and other pharmacologic agents. Reports have suggested the use of insulin combined with heparin or apheresis for treatment. Once patients recover from the acute episode, treatment with lipid-lowering agents and diet can effectively reduce the rate of recurrence.

Post-ERCP pancreatitis

Iatrogenic pancreatitis attributed to manipulation of the major papilla during ERCP is becoming an increasingly common cause of pancreatitis. In some series this is the third most common cause following gallstones and alcohol use. Post-ERCP pancreatitis is more likely to occur following sphincter of Oddi manometry, biliary sphincterotomy, pancreatic duct manipulation, and in patients with a history of unexplained acute relapsing pancreatitis. Post-ERCP pancreatitis occurs in approximately 3–5% of patients but may be as high as 25% in those suspected to have sphincter of Oddi dysfunction. Pharmacologic intervention to prevent post-ERCP pancreatitis has been disappointing with the exception of indomethacin suppositories [8]. Prophylactic pancreatic stenting also reduces the frequency and severity of pancreatitis in selected individuals at high risk for post-ERCP pancreatitis [9].

Autoimmune pancreatitis

Autoimmune pancreatitis [10] (AIP) is a benign disease characterized by irregular narrowing of the pancreatic duct, swelling of parenchyma, lymphoplasmacytic infiltration and fibrosis, and a favorable response to corticosteroid treatment. The most common presentation is obstructive jaundice closely mimicking pancreatic cancer with focal enlargement of the pancreatic head. AIP can also present with acute pancreatitis in up to 15–30% of individuals and about 5% of patients evaluated for pancreatitis (acute and chronic) have AIP as the etiology. Most AIP patients presenting with acute pancreatitis also have biliary involvement with cholestatic liver function tests (LFTs).

Two subtypes have been identified with substantial clinical overlap but distinctive histopathologic features. Type 1 AIP is the most common form worldwide accounting for more than 80% of cases in the United States. It has a peak incidence in the sixth or seventh decades of life and tends to affect men twice as often as women. Type 1 AIP has a characteristic histology known as lymphoplasmacytic sclerosing pancreatitis (LPSP). It is characterized by a periductal lymphoplasmacytic infiltrate, storiform fibrosis, obliterative phlebitis, and abundant IgG4 immunostaining (>10/high power field IgG4-positive cells). Type 1 AIP is a multiorgan disease termed "IgG4-related disease" as more than 60% of individuals have clinical and histologic involvement of other organs including the biliary tree, retroperitoneum, lacrimal and salivary glands, lymph nodes, periorbital tissues, kidneys, thyroid, lungs, meninges, aorta, breast, prostate, pericardium, and skin. CT imaging typically demonstrates diffuse enlargement of the pancreas with delayed (rim) enhancement and a diffusely irregular, attenuated main pancreatic duct. The classic EUS feature of AIP is that of a diffusely hypoechoic gland. Type 2 patients present at a younger age (a decade earlier), do not have elevated serum IgG4 as the disease is not IgG4 mediated and do not have extra-pancreatic organ involvement. Imaging alone cannot differentiate between the two subtypes and both are steroid responsive; however, type 2 patients are unlikely to relapse following steroid therapy. At present, pancreatic histology is required for the definitive diagnosis of type 2 AIP. The histologic hallmark of type 2 AIP is the presence of the granulocyte epithelial lesion (GEL) in pancreatic ducts with scant to no IgG4-positive cells.

Patients with AIP should be treated with glucocorticoids. A common approach is to initiate treatment with prednisone at a dosage of 40 mg/day for 4 to 6 weeks followed by a taper of 5 mg/week. Most patients destined to respond demonstrate clinical and/or radiologic improvement within the first several weeks. Failure to respond in this timeframe should raise the possibility of an alternative diagnosis.

Smoking

Smoking was once thought to be a risk factor due to its association with alcohol. However, recent studies have suggested that cigarette smoking is an independent risk factor for acute and chronic pancreatitis by mechanisms that are unclear.

Idiopathic pancreatitis

Patients in whom an initial evaluation does not reveal an underlying etiology are classified as having "idiopathic" acute pancreatitis. The most common explanations which are identified with a more extensive evaluation include microlithiasis, SOD, pancreas divisum, and other congenital abnormalities, pancreatic and ampullary neoplasm, and genetic causes (Fig. 23.2) [11]. Ten to twenty percent of adults with pancreatitis are termed idiopathic, although this classification is expected to become less common as factors of genetic predisposition and environmental susceptibility are elucidated. Elevations of liver chemistries are seen most commonly in patients with acute pancreatitis due to a biliary source, such as gallstones, pancreatic or ampullary neoplasm, microlithiasis, choledochal cyst, choledochocele, and SOD. An elevation of the ALT of greater than or equal to 150 IU/L (approximately a three-fold elevation) is associated with a 95% probability of biliary pancreatitis.

Assessment of severity and outcome

The revised classification of acute pancreatitis [12] describes two phases of the disorder: early and late. During the early phase, systemic disturbances result from the host response to local pancreatic injury. Inflammatory mediators and cytokine activation may manifest as systemic inflammatory response syndrome (SIRS). When SIRS is persistent, there is an increased risk of developing organ failure. Severity is classified as mild, moderate or severe. *Mild acute pancreatitis*, the most common form, is characterized by the absence of organ failure and the absence of local or systemic complications. Mild pancreatitis usually does not require pancreatic imaging and the process usually resolves during the early phase, with discharge within a week of symptom onset. Patients with mild acute pancreatitis constitute 80% of all attacks and less than 5% of mortality. *Moderately severe pancreatitis* is defined by the presence of transient organ failure, local complications, or exacerbation of an underlying

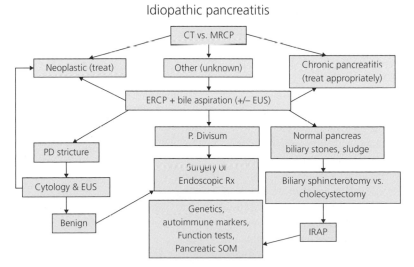

Fig. 23.2 Proposed algorithm for evaluation of patients with idiopathic pancreatitis.

comorbid illness. Mortality in these individuals is much less common than in severe pancreatitis. *Severe acute pancreatitis* is defined by persistent organ failure extending for >48 hours. Most individuals with persistent organ failure have underlying necrotizing disease. Three organ systems should be assessed to define organ failure: respiratory, cardiovascular, and renal. When organ failure affects more than one organ system it is termed multiple organ failure.

Despite the importance of recognizing severe disease early in the course, many patients initially identified as having mild disease progress to severe disease indolently over the initial 48 to 96 hours. The overall mortality rate for acute pancreatitis is 5% to 10%. Early deaths within the first 2 weeks are frequently due to multisystem organ failure caused by the release of inflammatory mediators and cytokines. Late deaths are more likely to result from local or systemic infection. The risks of infection and death correlate with severity of disease and the presence and extent of pancreatic necrosis. Therefore, patients should be stratified into severity levels of illness based on clinical assessment, scoring systems, serum markers, and CECT scanning [1,2].

Predictors of severe pancreatitis

- The development of persistent organ dysfunction as defined by the 2012 Revision of the Atlanta Classification predict severe pancreatitis.
- SIRS predisposes to multiple organ dysfunction and/or pancreatic necrosis. SIRS is defined by two or more of the following criteria for > 48 hours:

Heart rate	>90 beats/minute
Temperature	>38°C or <36°C
White blood cell count	>12 000 or <4000 cells/μL or >10% bands
Respiratory status	Respiratory rate >20/min or $PaCO_2$ < 32 mmHg

- Clinical predictors of a poor outcome include severe co-morbid illnesses, older age, and obesity.
- A pleural effusion on chest x-ray within the first 24 h correlates with severity.
- A blood urea nitrogen (BUN) level of 20 mg/dL or higher and any rise in BUN during the first 24 h of admission is associated with increased mortality.
- A serum level of creatinine >1.8 mg/dL within the first 24 h of hospitalization is associated with a 35-fold increased risk of development of pancreatic necrosis.

- Hemoconcentration from third spacing of fluids reflected by an elevated hematocrit (Hct) ≥ 44 on admission or failure of the hematocrit to decrease in the first 24–48 hours of treatment is predictive of severe pancreatitis. The absence of hemoconcentration on admission or during the initial 24 hours with rehydration is predictive of a benign clinical course.
- Individual serum markers reflecting a robust systemic inflammatory response such as C-reactive protein (CRP) > 150 mg/dL suggests severe pancreatitis (sensitivity of 80%, specificity of 76%, positive predictive value of 67%, and negative predictive value of 86%) and is strongly associated with the existence of pancreatic necrosis.
- Scoring systems such as Ranson's criteria (Table 23.4), the Acute Physiologic and Chronic Health Evaluation (APACHE II) system, or Bedside Index for Severity of Acute Pancreatitis (BISAP) scores are used by some clinicians but they have limitations.
  - ○ The APACHE II scale is calculated by assigning points based on age, heart rate, temperature, respiratory rate, MAP, P_aO_2, pH, K, Na, Cr, Hct, WBC, Glasgow Coma Scale, and previous health status. With increasing scores, the likelihood of a complicated, prolonged, and often fatal course increases.

Table 23.4 Ranson's prognostic scoring criteria.

At admission		
Age > 55 years		
WBC >16 000/mm³		
Glucose >200 mg/dL (10 mmol/L)		
LDH >350 IU/L		
AST >250 U/L		
During initial 48 hours		
Haematocrit decrease of >10		
Urea increase of >5 mg/dL		
Calcium <8 mg/dL (2 mmol/L)		
PaO_2 <60 mmHg (8 kPa)		
Base deficit >4 mEq/L		
Fluid sequestration >6 L		
Signs	**Morbidity**	**Mortality**
<2	<5%	<1%
3–5	30%	5%
>6	90%	20%

○ Ranson's 11 prognostic indicators include five that are available on admission which in general reflect the severity of the acute inflammatory process (age >55 years, white blood cells >16 000/mm³, glucose >200 mg/dL, lactate dehydrogenase >350 IU/L, aspartate aminotransferase >250 U/L) whereas the six that are measured at the end of the first 48 hours reflect the systemic effects of circulating enzymes including respiratory failure, renal failure and fluid sequestration (Hct decreased >10, BUN >5 mg/dL, PO_2 <60 mmHg, base deficit >4 mEq/L, serum calcium <8 mg/dL, and estimated fluid sequestration >6 L). In many series, mortality is approximately 10% to 20% when there are three to five signs, and >50% when there are six or more Ranson's signs.

○ The BISAP score (13) is calculated with five variables available in the initial 24 hours. A BUN greater than 25 mg/dl, impaired mental status (Glasgow Coma Score less than 15), presence of SIRS, age greater than 60 years, and pleural effusion on imaging. Each variable adds one point to the total score, and scores of 3, 4, and 5 correspond to a mortality of 5.3, 12.7, and 22.5%, respectively.

▪ Imaging stratification of pancreatitis severity.

CECT is useful for assessing severity of pancreatitis and should be performed in patients with evidence of organ failure or those with predicted severe disease after the initial 72 hours. A CT severity index (Table 23.5) grades severity of pancreatitis by the number of peripancreatic fluid collections and amount of necrosis on dynamic scanning. The distinction between interstitial and necrotizing acute pancreatitis has important prognostic implications (Fig. 23.3). Approximately 5–10% of patients with acute pancreatitis develop *necrotizing pancreatitis*, which manifests as necrosis involving both the pancreas and peripancreatic tissues and less commonly as necrosis of the pancreatic parenchyma or peripancreatic tissue alone. Necrotizing pancreatitis is characterized by disruption of the pancreatic microcirculation such that large areas do not enhance on CT following bolus administration of IV contrast material. The majority of acute pancreatitis is in the form of *interstitial pancreatitis*, defined by an intact microcirculation and uniform enhancement of the gland on contrast-enhanced CT scanning. Approximately 10% of patients with interstitial disease experience organ failure and the mortality rate is very low (<3%). The clinical significance of pancreatic necrosis is that it predicts a worse severity of pancreatitis and increased risk of infection in the necrotic pancreatic tissue termed infected necrosis.

Pancreatic infection develops in 30–40% of patients with acute necrotizing pancreatitis but rarely in those with interstitial disease (<1%). Infected necrosis is rare during the first week of illness. Translocation of bacteria from the colon is likely the most important cause of infected necrosis. Because clinical and laboratory findings are often similar in patients with either sterile or infected necrosis (i.e. fever, leukocytosis, and abdominal pain), the diagnosis of infected necrosis is made by percutaneous CT-guided needle aspiration for gram stain and culture. The overall mortality in severe acute necrotizing pancreatitis triples if there is infected necrosis (10% vs. 30%). Moreover, infected necrosis with persistent organ failure portends a worse prognosis compared to those with infected necrosis but no organ failure.

Table 23.5 CT severity index for acute pancreatitis.

Unenhanced CT finding	Grade	Score	Enhanced CT	
			Necrosis	Score
Normal	A	0		
Pancreatic enlargement	B	1	0	0
Peripancreatic stranding	C	2	<33%	2
Single peripancreatic collection	D	3	33–50%	4
Multiple peripancreatic collections	E	4	>50%	6

CT severity index equals unenhanced CT score plus necrosis score: maximum=10, greater than or equal to 6=sever disease
Adapted from Balthazar EJ. Radiology 2002;223:603

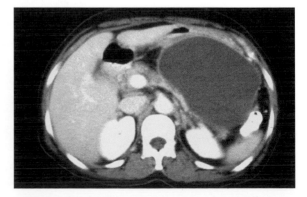

Fig. 23.3 Computed tomography scan of a patient with a large pancreatic pseudocyst.

Treatment of acute pancreatitis

The treatment of acute pancreatitis (Fig. 23.4) depends on the severity of the disease, as well as the presence of any complications. The goals of medical therapy include supportive care, limitation of systemic complications, and prevention of pancreatic infection once necrosis takes place.

Patient triage

Patients with mutiorgan dysfunction are at the greatest risk for adverse outcomes and should be managed in a critical care unit with multidisciplinary input. In addition, those individuals with predicted development of severe disease including persistent SIRS, increased hematocrit, underlying cardiopulmonary disease, and elevated BUN, Hct or renal dysfunction should be considered for management in a monitored setting.

Supportive care

Patients with mild disease are treated supportively with intravenous hydration, parenteral analgesics, and bowel rest. Supplemental oxygen is recommended initially for all patients. Nasogastric tube suction is indicated for symptomatic relief in patients with nausea, vomiting and ileus. Severe acute pancreatitis with its inherent increased morbidity and mortality requires intensive care unit monitoring, aggressive fluid and electrolyte monitoring and replacement. There are no specific treatments proven to

be effective in limiting systemic complications. Agents that put the pancreas to rest (e.g. somatostatin, calcitonin, glucagon, nasogastric suction, H_2 blockers) and enzyme inhibitors (e.g. aprotinin, Gabexate mesylate) have not been shown to lower morbidity and mortality [1,2].

Fluid management

Vigorous fluid resuscitation beginning immediately upon diagnosis in the emergency department is of importance for maintaining the mircrocirculation and perfusion of the pancreas translating into a potential benefit of reducing complications of necrosis and organ failure. There is no consensus as to the best rate, type, and volume of initial resuscitation. Crystalloid (normal saline or lactated Ringers) is recommended in most instances. In one study lactated Ringer's solution reduced the incidence of SIRS by >80% compared to saline infusion but this requires confirmatory investigation. Colloid may be considered with packed red blood cells when the hematocrit falls below 25% and albumin if the serum albumin level drops to less than 2 g/dL. Based on expert opinion and societal guidelines, patients can be given a 1–2 L fluid bolus while in the emergency room. This can be followed by an infusion based on the patient's volume status. Patients with severe volume depletion should be resuscitated with 500–1000 mL/h, patients with signs of extracellular fluid loss (not severe) should be initiated at a rate of 300 to 500 mL/h, and those without volume

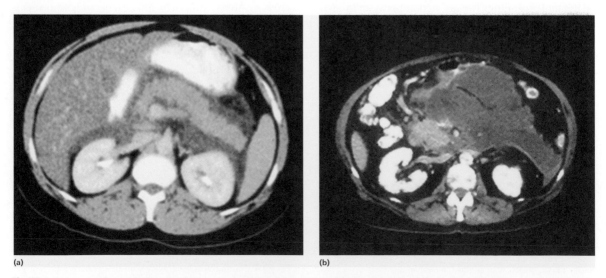

(a)   (b)

Fig. 23.4 Contrast-enhanced CT scans demonstrating interstitial pancreatitis (a) and necrotizing pancreatitis (b).

depletion at a rate of 250 to 350 mL/h. Adequate fluid resuscitation should achieve a urine output >0.5 mL/kg/h in the absence of renal failure. Adjustment of fluids is made every several hours based on hemodynamic and volume status. Caution must be used in the elderly and those with underlying cardiovascular or renal impairment.

Analgesia

Although there is a theoretical concern of sphincter of Oddi spasm from narcotics, there is no evidence to support that they should be withheld in acute pancreatitis. Consider liberal use of patient-controlled analgesia although this approach has not been compared prospectively to on-demand analgesia. There is no evidence to indicate superiority of a specific opiate. Patients administered repeated doses of narcotic analgesics should have oxygen saturation monitored due to risks of unrecognized hypoxia.

Nutritional care

Most patients with acute pancreatitis have mild disease and can resume oral feeding within several days. Patients with mild disease may initiate oral intake when pain resolves and appetite returns starting with a liquid diet and advancing as tolerated to a low-fat solid diet. For patients with predicted severe pancreatitis or those patients unlikely to start oral intake within 5–7 days, providing supplemental nutrition is important. Besides maintaining adequate caloric intake and resting the pancreas, nutritional support helps reduce infectious complications. The options for providing nutrition include total parenteral nutrition (TPN) through central venous access or preferably as enteral feeding through a nasoenteric feeding tube placed into the jejunum. In general, it is reasonable to conclude from small, prospective, randomized, nonblinded studies that enteral feeding is safer and less expensive than TPN [14,15]. A Cochrane meta-analysis of eight randomized controlled trials demonstrated a reduction in systemic infection, need for surgical intervention, multiorgan failure, and mortality in those receiving enteral compared to parenteral nutrition [16]. Recent trials support the nasogastric route as an alternative to nasojejunal for enteral nutrition [17].The optimal site for enteric feeding (nasojejunal vs. nasogastric) is the subject of current investigation (clinicaltrials.gov NCT00580749). Furthermore, enteral feeding is usually well tolerated in patients with ileus. Nevertheless, total parenteral nutrition may be necessary for patients with nasoenteric tube discomfort, those who cannot obtain sufficient calories through enteral nutrition or in whom enteral access cannot be maintained.

ERCP in gallstone pancreatitis

Urgent ERCP with identification and clearance of bile duct stones is recommended for patients with evidence of ongoing biliary obstruction, as suggested by clinical and laboratory data. ERCP may also be considered for patients with severe, acute pancreatitis within 24 to 48 hours of the onset of the attack, although this remains controversial due to conflicting data from endoscopic studies [18]. MRCP and EUS can be used when there is a lower suspicion for CBD stones.

The risk of gallstone pancreatitis recurrence is as high as 50% to 75% in patients with an intact gallbladder within the subsequent 6 months; therefore cholecystectomy is generally recommended. Biliary sphincterotomy leaving the gallbladder in situ is considered an effective alternative for those not considered to be candidates for cholecystectomy.

Definition and management of local complications

Local complications should be considered when there is persistence or recurrence of abdominal pain, organ dysfunction, or clinical signs of sepsis.

Acute peripancreatic fluid collections (APFC) are defined as peripancreatic fluid confined by normal peripancreatic fascial planes, without a definable wall encapsulating the collection. These fluid collections occur within the first 4 weeks following interstitial pancreatitis. Most remain sterile and are commonly resorbed spontaneously within the first several weeks after the onset of acute pancreatitis. When a localized APFC persists beyond 4 weeks, it is likely to develop into a pancreatic pseudocyst.

Pancreatic pseudocysts (Fig. 23.5) are encapsulated fluid collections with a well-defined inflammatory wall usually outside the pancreas with minimal or no necrosis. They occur a minimum of 4 weeks after the onset of acute pancreatitis. In symptomatic patients, if the pseudocyst is mature and encapsulated, treatment can involve endoscopic, surgical, and percutaneous drainage.

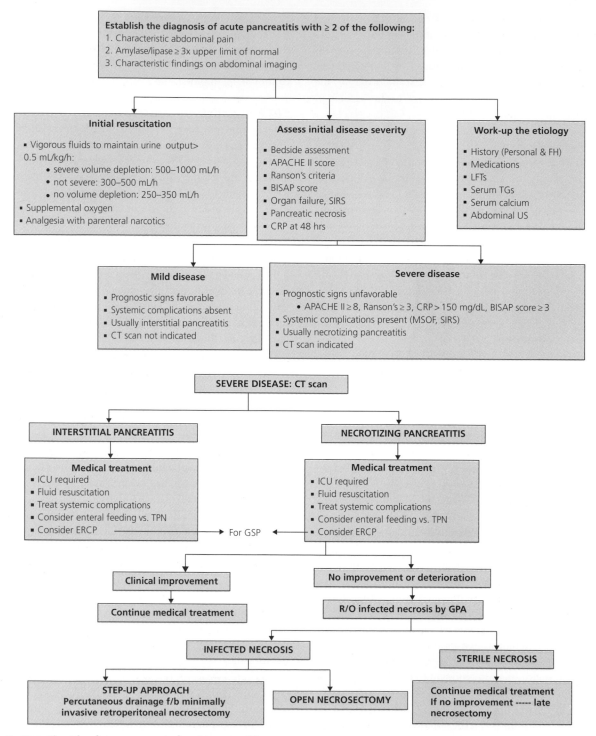

Establish the diagnosis of acute pancreatitis with ≥ 2 of the following:
1. Characteristic abdominal pain
2. Amylase/lipase ≥ 3x upper limit of normal
3. Characteristic findings on abdominal imaging

Initial resuscitation

- Vigorous fluids to maintain urine output> 0.5 mL/kg/h:
  - severe volume depletion: 500–1000 mL/h
  - not severe: 300–500 mL/h
  - no volume depletion: 250–350 mL/h
- Supplemental oxygen
- Analgesia with parenteral narcotics

Assess initial disease severity

- Bedside assessment
- APACHE II score
- Ranson's criteria
- BISAP score
- Organ failure, SIRS
- Pancreatic necrosis
- CRP at 48 hrs

Work-up the etiology

- History (Personal & FH)
- Medications
- LFTs
- Serum TGs
- Serum calcium
- Abdominal US

Mild disease

- Prognostic signs favorable
- Systemic complications absent
- Usually interstitial pancreatitis
- CT scan not indicated

Severe disease

- Prognostic signs unfavorable
  - APACHE II ≥ 8, Ranson's ≥ 3, CRP > 150 mg/dL, BISAP score ≥ 3
- Systemic complications present (MSOF, SIRS)
- Usually necrotizing pancreatitis
- CT scan indicated

SEVERE DISEASE: CT scan

INTERSTITIAL PANCREATITIS

Medical treatment
- ICU required
- Fluid resuscitation
- Treat systemic complications
- Consider enteral feeding vs. TPN
- Consider ERCP

NECROTIZING PANCREATITIS

Medical treatment
- ICU required
- Fluid resuscitation
- Treat systemic complications
- Consider enteral feeding vs. TPN
- Consider ERCP

For GSP

Clinical improvement

Continue medical treatment

No improvement or deterioration

R/O infected necrosis by GPA

INFECTED NECROSIS

STERILE NECROSIS

STEP-UP APPROACH
Percutaneous drainage f/b minimally invasive retroperitoneal necrosectomy

OPEN NECROSECTOMY

Continue medical treatment
If no improvement ----- late necrosectomy

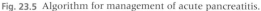

Fig. 23.5 Algorithm for management of acute pancreatitis.

While most pseudocysts remain asymptomatic, presenting symptoms may include abdominal pain, early satiety, nausea, and vomiting due to compression of the stomach or gastric outlet. Rapidly enlarging pseudocysts may rupture, hemorrhage, obstruct the extrahepatic biliary tree, erode into surrounding structures, and become infected. Indications for pseudocyst drainage include suspicion of infection or progressive enlargement with associated symptoms described above. Asymptomatic pseudocysts should be followed. Pseudocysts can be drained surgically, percutaneously, or endoscopically.

Acute necrotic collection describes a non-organized collection of heterogeneous fluid and necrotic material in the setting of necrotizing pancreatitis. The necrosis may involve the pancreatic parenchyma and peripancreatic tissue.

Walled off pancreatic necrosis (WOPN) is a mature, encapsulated collection of pancreatic and/or peripancreatic necrosis usually greater than 4 weeks after the onset of necrotizing pancreatitis

Management of sterile pancreatic necrosis

A role for prophylactic antibiotics in severe pancreatitis was initially given support by a randomized trial demonstrating that the administration of imipenem reduced infectious complications, including central-line sepsis, pulmonary infection, urinary tract infection, and infected pancreatic necrosis [19]. However, a recent meta-analysis of seven trials (467 patients) found no significant difference in mortality despite a significantly lower rate of pancreatic infection in those treated with imipenenm [20]. The most recent meta-analysis included 14 trials totaling 841 patients and no demonstrable improvement in infection or mortality with antibiotic prophylaxis [21].As a result of these findings, prophylactic antibiotics are no longer recommended in acute necrotizing pancreatitis. Moreover, there is the added concern that prolonged use of potent antibiotic agents may lead to the emergence of resistant organisms and fungal infections in the necrotic pancreas.

Sterile pancreatic necrosis is generally treated medically during the first several weeks even in the presence of multisystem organ failure. Eventually, after the acute pancreatic inflammatory process has subsided and coalesced into an encapsulated structure, frequently called WOPN, debridement may be required for intractable abdominal pain, vomiting caused by extrinsic compression of stomach or duodenum, or systemic toxicity. Debridement is delayed for at least 4–6 weeks after the onset of pancreatitis and can be performed by a combination of endoscopic, radiologic or surgical techniques [1,2,17].

Infected pancreatic necrosis

Infection is a strong determinant of the severity of illness and accounts for a large percentage of the deaths from acute pancreatitis. Infected necrosis should be suspected in patients with persistent symptoms of fever, SIRS, or organ dysfunction.

Diagnosis

The diagnosis of infected necrosis is important because of the need for antibiotic treatment and debridement. The presence of infection can be made if there is extra-lumninal gas in the pancreatic or peripancreatic tissues on CECT. Otherwise, image-guided fine needle aspiration is recommended in patients with acute necrotizing pancreatitis if they have persistent fever, SIRS or organ dysfunction despite aggressive supportive care. The technique of fine needle aspiration is safe and accurate for diagnosis of infected necrosis. Antibiotic therapy may be initiated prior to confirmatory diagnosis with the initial choice taking into consideration the pathogenic organisms and the ability of the antimicrobials to penetrate into the pancreatic tissues. Imipenem-cilastatin, meropenem, or a combination of a quinolone and metronidazole are most commonly chosen. Some centers use antifungal therapy in addition to antibacterial therapy, but this practice has not been validated by randomized trials. Once culture results are available the antibiotics can be tailored appropriately.

Treatment

Infected pancreatic necrosis is best treated with drainage and/or debridement [17]. In most cases, the diagnosis of infected necrosis is confirmed by fine-needle aspiration before intervention, but because false negative results can occur (reported sensitivity, 88%), debridement also warrants consideration when there is a high index of suspicion of infected necrosis even if infection is not documented.

There is consensus that the best outcomes are achieved when surgery is delayed for a minimum of

3–4 weeks after the onset of disease to allow for lique-faction. Patients with infected necrosis are initially treated with broad-spectrum antibiotics and medical support to allow encapsulation of the necrotic collections, which may facilitate intervention and reduce complications of bleeding and perforation. In some instances where there is dramatic clinical deterioration a delay is not feasible and early intervention is required.

Traditional management of infected pancreatic necrosis typically involved surgical debridement with open necrosectomy and closed irrigation via indwelling catheters, necrosectomy with closed drainage without irrigation, or necrosectomy and open packing. This is an invasive approach with a high morbidity (34–95%) and mortality (11–39%). A more conservative "step-up" approach has gained favor in which percutaneous drainage is the initial treatment. If this initial approach fails it is followed by a less invasive video-assisted retro-peritoneal debridement (VARD) or endoscopic transgas-tric/transduodenal approach when expertise is available [22]. The PANTER trial compared a surgical step-up approach with traditional open necrosectomy. The step-up approach reduced the combined primary end point of death and major complications (enterocutaneous fistula, perforation, new multiorgan failure or bleeding) from 69% to 40%. At 6 months follow-up, step-up patients had lower rates of incisional hernias and diabetes. Furthermore, 35% of patients in the step-up arm were treated with percutaneous drainage alone.

Other complications

These include compartment syndrome, pancreatic ductal disruption, arterial pseudoaneurysm formation, peripancreatic vascular thrombosis (splenic vein, portal vein, and superior mesenteric vein), and exocrine or endocrine insufficiency.

Pancreatic fistulae [23] occur as a result of duct disruption and are treated with parenteral nutrition, endoscopic stenting, and somatostatin analog. Surgical intervention may be needed if this conservative approach is unsuccessful.

Abdominal compartment syndrome (ACS) is diagnosed when the intra-abdominal pressure exceeds 20 mmHg and there are signs of new organ failure (i.e. respiratory, renal, or vascular). Intra-abdominal hypertension (IAH) generally occurs early and is the result of pancreatic inflammation and fluid third spacing. ACS is associated with high mortality rates of up to 50–75% [24].

Suggested treatment includes analgesics, sedation, nasogastric tube decompression, and fluid restriction. If these measures do not result in improvement, percutaneous catheter decompression followed if unsuccessful by a surgical laparotomy approach is recommended. The ability of this approach to improve outcomes is the focus of an ongoing randomized study (http:/clincaltrials.gov NCT00793715).

References

1. Forsmark CE, Baillie J. AGA Institute Technical Review on Acute Pancreatitis. *Gastroenterology* 2007;**132**:2022–44.
2. Balthazar EJ. Acute pancreatitis: Assessment of severity with clinical and CT evaluation. *Radiology* 2002;**223**: 603–13.
3. Arvvanitakis M, Delhave M, De Maertelaere VD, et al. Computed tomography and magnetic resonance imaging in the assessment of acute pancreatitis. *Gastroenterology* 2004;**126**:715–23.
4. Laissy JP, Idee JM, Fernandez P, et al. Magnetic resonance imaging in acute and chronic kidney disease: present status. *Nephron Clin. Pract.* 2006;**103**:50–7.
5. Tenner S, Dubner H, Steinberg W. Predicting gallstone pancreatitis with laboratory parameters: A meta-analysis. *Am. J. Gastroenterol.* 1994;**89**:1863–9.
6. Saraswat VA, Sharma BC, Agarwal DK, et al. Biliary microlithiasis in patients with idiopathic acute pancreatitis and unexplained biliary pain: Response to therapy. *J. Gastroenterol. Hepatol.* 2004;**19**:1206–11.
7. Witt H, Apte MV, Keim AV, Wilson JS. Chronic pancreatitis: challenges and advances in pathogenesis, genetics, diagnosis, and therapy. *Gastroenterology* 2007;**132**:1557–73.
8. Elmunzer BJ, Sceiman JM, Lehman GA, et al. A randomized trial of rectal indomethacin to prevent post-ERCP pancreatitis. *N. Engl. J. Med.* 2012;**366**:1414–22.
9. Choudhary A, Bechtold ML, Arif M, et al. Pancreatic stents for prophylaxis against post-ERCP pancreatitis: a meta-analysis and systematic review. *Gastrointest. Endosc.* 2011;**73**:275–82.
10. Kim KP, Kim MH, Song MH, et al. Autoimmune pancreatitis. *Am. J. Gastroenterol.* 2004;**99**:1605–16.
11. Dragnov P, Forsmark CE. Idiopathic pancreatitis. *Gastroenterology* 2005;**128**:756–63.
12. Banks PA, Bollen TL, Dervenis C, et al. Classification of acute pancreatitis-2012: revision of the Atlanta classification and definitions by international consensus. *Gut* 2013;**62**:102–11.
13. Singh VK, Wu BU, Bollen TL, et al. A prospective evaluation of the bedside index for severity in acute pancreatitis score in assessing mortality and intermediate markers of severity in acute pancreatitis. *Am. J. Gastroenterol.* 2009;**104**: 966–71.

14. Olah A, Pardavi G, Belagyi T, et al. Early nasojejunal feeding in acute pancreatitis is associated with a lower complication rate. *Nutrition* 2002;**18**:259–62.

15. Petrov MS, Kukosh MV, Emelyanov NV. A randomized controlled trial of enteral versus parenteral feeding in patients with predicted severe acute pancreatitis shows a significant reduction in mortality and in infected pancreatic complications with total enteral nutrition. *Dig. Surg.* 2006;**23**:336–45.

16. Al-Omran M, Albalawi ZH, Tashkandi MF, et al. Enteral versus parenteral nutrition of acute pancreatitis. Cochrane Database Syst. Rev. 2010:CD002837.

17. Kumar A, Singh N, Prakash S, et al. Early enteral nutrition in severe acute pancreatitis: a prospective randomized controlled trial comparing nasojejunal and nasogastric routes. *J. Clin. Gastroenterol.* 2006;**40**:431–4.

18. Mark DH, Lefevre F, Flamm CR, et al. Evidence-based assessment of ERCP in the treatment of pancreatitis. *Gastrointest. Endosc.* 2002;**56**(6 suppl):S249–54.

19. Pederzoli P, Bassi C, Vesentini S, et al. A randomized multi-center trial of antibiotic prophylaxis of septic complications in acute necrotizing pancreatitis with imipenem. *Surg. Obstet. Gynecol.* 1993;**176**:480–3.

20. Bai Y, Gao J, Zou D, et al. Prophylactic antibiotics cannot reduce infected pancreatic necrosis and mortality in acute necrotizing pancreatitis: evidence from a meta-analysis of randomized controlled trials. *Am. J. Gastroenterol.* 2008;**103**:104–10.

21. Wittau M, Mayer B, Scheele J, et al. Systematic review and meta-analysis of antibiotic prophylaxis in severe acute pancreatitis. *Scand. J. Gastroenterol.* 2011;**46**:261–70.

22. Van Santvoort HC, Besselink MG, Bakker OJ, et al. A step-up approach or open necrosectomy for necrotizing pancreatitis. *N. Engl. J. Med.* 2010;**362**:1491–502.

23. Telford JJ, Farrell JJ, Saltzman JR, et al. Pancreatic stent placement for duct disruption. *Gastrointest. Endosc.* 2002;**56**:18–24.

24. Mentula P, Hienonen P, Kemppainen E, et al. Surgical decompression for abdominal compartment syndrome in severe acute pancreatitis. *Arch. Surg.* 2010;**145**:764–69.

CHAPTER 24

Biliary tract emergencies

Joseph K. N. Kim[1] and David L. Carr-Locke[2]

[1] *Icahn School of Medicine, New York, USA*

[2] *Division of Digestive Diseases, Mount Sinai Beth Israel Medical Center, New York, USA*

Introduction

Biliary emergencies are the result of compromising the natural pathway of bile flow through the biliary system to and through the normal exit at the papilla. Biliary emergencies must be identified quickly and managed appropriately either medically, endoscopically, or surgically in a timely fashion to prevent poor outcomes. This chapter describes several categories of biliary emergency manifesting as gallstone pancreatitis (see also Chapter 23 Acute Pancreatitis), cholangitis, bile leaks, and acute cholecystitis.

Gallstone pancreatitis

See also, Chapter 23, Acute Pancreatitis. More than 240 000 case of acute pancreatitis are reported annually in the United States, of which gallstone disease, the most common cause, accounts for approximately 50% of cases [1]. Most patients present with mild disease and follow a benign hospital course with recovery achieved by conservative measures. However, cases of severe gallstone pancreatitis can lead to mortality and need to be identified and treated more aggressively.

Mortality may be as high as 5% in patients with acute pancreatitis in general and approaches 20–30% in cases of severe pancreatitis [2–4]. In cases of multi-organ failure, mortality reaches more than 50% [5].

The pathogenesis of gallstone pancreatitis remains unclear. The largely accepted theory states that gallstones may compress the septum of the biliary and pancreatic orifices causing obstruction of the pancreatic duct while the pancreas is secreting. Another proposed mechanism involves a gallstone residing in the common channel for long enough to allow reflux of bile into the pancreatic ductal system [6]. Whichever the mechanism, whether pancreatic duct obstruction, reflux of biliary secretions into the pancreatic system, pancreatic duct hypertension, or aberrant secretion of acinar cells, gallstone pancreatitis leads to inappropriate activation of trypsinogen, pancreatic autodigestion and an acute inflammatory response in and around the pancreas [7–10]. Gallstones have been recovered in stool from 85–95% of patients with acute pancreatitis [7]. Approximately 50% of cases of acute pancreatitis are caused by stones less than 5 mm [7].

The role and timing of ERCP in patients with acute biliary pancreatitis has been controversial. Clinical trials have been reviewed in six meta-analyses and systematic reviews. The reviews have inherent weaknesses including differences in study design and inclusion/exclusion criteria. The overall consensus is that in the absence of cholangitis and biliary obstruction, performance of early endoscopic retrograde cholangiopancreatography (ERCP), defined as 24–72 hours after admission, does not lead to reduction in mortality. The data clearly support early ERCP in patients with biliary obstruction and/or concomitant cholangitis, defined by the presence of fever, jaundice, sepsis or a conjugated bilirubin level >5 mg/dL [11–16]. Regardless of the recommendations, each patient should be individualized and certainly early interventional ERCP should be considered in patients without the above-mentioned criteria

Gastrointestinal Emergencies, Third Edition. Edited by Tony C. K. Tham, John S. A. Collins, and Roy Soetikno.

who have clinical deterioration including worsening pain, persistent leukocytosis, and vital sign instabilities [2]. The American Gastroenterological Association (AGA) published their position statement in 2007, reporting that the "role of routine ERCP in severe biliary pancreatitis remains controversial. Urgent ERCP (within 24 hours after admission) was recommended, however, in patients with cholangitis, early ERCP (within 72 hours after admission) was recommended if suspicion of persistent bile-duct stones remained high [17]." The most recent guideline, published by the American College of Gastroenterology in 2013, suggests that "urgent ERCP (within 24 hours after admission) is indicated in patients with biliary pancreatitis who have concurrent acute cholangitis, but it is not needed in most patients who do not have evidence of ongoing biliary obstruction [18]."

In patients with suspected biliary pancreatitis without jaundice or clinical deterioration, endoscopic ultrasonography and magnetic resonance cholangiopancreatography are good diagnostic tests for the detection of choledocholithiasis [19,20]. Endoscopic ultrasound (EUS) has a 95% sensitivity and 98% specificity for diagnosing choledocholithiasis [21]. Compared to magnetic resonance cholangiopancreatography (MRCP), EUS is better able to detect stones less than 5 mm in smaller-caliber bile ducts.

Medical treatment includes aggressive intravenous hydration at rates of more than 250 mL/hour at least for the initial 24 hours after admission since treatment of intravascular depletion appears to improve outcomes [22].

Endoscopic treatment includes ERCP with biliary stent placement or biliary sphincterotomy and complete removal of the stone(s) if possible. Patients with suspected biliary obstruction should receive prophylactic antibiotics, preferably a quinolone or cephalosporin, since Gram-negative bacilli are most commonly involved. If the patient demonstrates periprocedural or intraprocedural instability and the culprit is a large difficult stone requiring prolonged procedural time, a biliary stent should be placed to decompress the bile duct with plans of a two stage treatment algorithm. The stone may be addressed once the patient has stabilized with conservative medical treatment. If a stone is not identified on cholangiography and there is a strong clinical suspicion of gallstone pancreatitis, an empiric biliary sphincterotomy should be performed. Microlithiasis may result in attacks of pancreatitis just as severe as that

associated with large stones. An International Normalized Ratio (INR) below 1.5, as well as a platelet count greater than 75 000/mm^3 are preferred, but certainly exceptions on presphincterotomy parameters can be made depending on the clinical necessity.

Once the bile duct has been cleared, the patient should undergo a cholecystectomy if able. One study examined 120 patients who underwent ERCP with sphincterotomy and stone extraction, then randomized subjects to laparoscopic cholecystectomy within 6 weeks after the initial procedure, or a watchful waiting approach. The watchful waiting approach arm was associated more frequent biliary complications requiring need for repeat ERCP, increased post-operative complications and longer hospital stays [23].

Cholangitis

Fifteen to 72% of patients present with Charcot's triad, comprising fever, jaundice, and abdominal pain. Four to eight% of patients present with Reynold's pentad (Charcot's triad plus hypotension and altered mental status). The most common etiology of acute cholangitis is choledocholithiasis. The pathogenesis of cholangitis requires bile duct obstruction and bacterial growth due to stasis of bile. Malignancy rarely causes acute cholangitis in the absence of previous instrumentation. The causes of acute cholangitis are:

1 Iatrogenic (biliary instrumentation)
2 Choledocholithiasis
3 Benign biliary stricture
4 Malignant biliary obstruction (rarely)
5 Sump syndrome
6 Mirizzi syndrome
7 Sclerosing cholangitis
8 Ampullary obstruction
9 Recurrent pyogenic cholangitis.

The treatment goal of acute cholangitis is biliary decompression by re-establishing patency of the biliary system. The use of medical treatment including broad spectrum antibiotics without biliary decompression is usually inadequate. When a patient presents with acute cholangitis, the three options for biliary drainage are: endoscopic drainage (ERCP and/or EUS), percutaneous drainage, or surgery. Any of these should be performed in a timely manner to prevent sepsis and clinical deterioration but surgery (laparoscopic or open) carries the highest risk. The most recent American Society for Gastrointestinal Endoscopy (ASGE) guideline recommends antibiotic prophylaxis for ERCP in patients with biliary obstruction, in which complete drainage cannot be achieved, such as sclerosing cholangitis or hilar strictures [24], although an attempt should be made to drain all contaminated/infected ducts [25]. Pre-ERCP mapping of the level and extent of the obstruction by MRCP has become routine when possible to avoid using the cholangiogram of an ERCP to delineate the extent of the disease process. In the case of choledocholithiasis, the decision must be made to decompress the biliary system via placement of a large bore stent or proceed to stone removal. Straight large-bore stents (10Fr or greater) are more effective than smaller-bore stents because they allow for higher bile flow rates and have lower rates of stent dysfunction. The decision to place stents must be tailored to each case [26]. Generally, self-expandable metal stents (SEMS) have lower rates of occlusion than plastic stents but are significantly more expensive. Any stent, including SEMS, can cause cholangitis if migration occurs so that the stent moves out of the obstructing lesion or the distal stent is occluded by the contralateral duodenal wall.

Bile leak

Bile leaks (see Chapter 12, Complications of Laparoscopic Surgery)are most commonly the result of surgical procedures such as cholecystectomy and hepatobiliary surgery, (including biliary and hepatic resection and liver transplantation), liver biopsy and percutaneous transhepatic cholangiography [27].[57] Following cholecystectomy, the most common site of bile leak is the cystic duct reported in 78% of leak cases. The ducts of Luschka (gallbladder bed) (13%) and other sites including common hepatic duct and common bile duct (9%) comprise the other sites [28].

Types of injury
- Type A: Bile leaks from the cystic duct and ducts of Luschka (from right hepatic lobe in the gallbladder fossa connecting with the right hepatic duct)
- Type B: Occlusion or section of an aberrant right hepatic duct
- Type C: Leakage of right hepatic duct

- Type D: Lateral trauma to the main bile duct causing leakage
- Type E: Involves common and main hepatic ducts and corresponds to Bismuth classification types 1 to V.

Clinically, patients with bile leaks may present with myriad symptoms including, but not limited to, abdominal pain, fevers, jaundice, and malaise. Laboratory studies may reveal elevated transaminases with hyperbilirubinemia and low grade leukocytosis. Helpful imaging studies include computerized tomography (CT) scanning with intravenous contrast or MRCP. Imaging studies may reveal a range of findings including a small leak to an unorganized collection of bile or a well-contained "biloma." The primary goal of endoscopic treatment of bile leaks is directed at reducing biliary pressure. This is accomplished in several ways, including performing a biliary sphincterotomy and/or placement of a bile duct stent across the papilla. The theory behind this is to create a negative pressure gradient across the transpapillary orifice that will naturally divert bile flow away from the leak, allowing it to heal. The stent does not need to be placed close to the leak site unless the main duct is injured. Collections will resorb over time if small or may need to be drained percutaneously.

Acute cholecystitis

Gallstones have been identified back to the ancient Egyptian mummies from at least 3500 years ago [29]. More than 700 000 cholecystectomies are performed annually in the United States alone, costing approximately 6.5 billion dollars, making gallbladder disease the most expensive digestive disorder [30]. Twenty to twenty-five million Americans have gallstones and most are asymptomatic [31,32]. One percent of patients with cholelithiasis develop complications including acute cholecystitis, gallstone pancreatitis, and choledocholithiasis [33].

Risk factors include advancing age, female gender, and obesity. A study a study in the United Kingdom reported an incidence of cholelithiasis in 24% in women 50–59 years old increasing to 30% in the ninth decade, whereas in men, the rates are 18% in the 50–59-year-old range, increasing to 29% in the ninth decade [34]. Women are at increased risk due to the effects of estrogen on the development of gallstones. Obesity has been associated with increased hepatic secretion of cholesterol. Obese women have a seven-fold increase risk in developing gallstones compared to their normal weight counterparts. Interestingly, bariatric surgery and rapid weight loss have also been associated with development of gallstones [31].

There are two types of gallstones: cholesterol and pigmented (brown/black). Most gallstones in developed countries are of the cholesterol type. Gallstone development is dependent on cholesterol supersaturation in bile, crystal nucleation, and gallbladder dysmotility.

Acute cholecystitis is most often the result of inflammation of the gallbladder caused by obstruction of the cystic duct although acalculous cholecystitis is possible. Once the cystic duct is obstructed, the gallbladder mucosa continues to produce mucus, yet has no outlet. This leads to increased gallbladder pressure and ensuing venous and arterial stasis. Eventually, gallbladder ischemia and necrosis occur ultimately leading to empyema formation or perforation. Acute cholecystitis accounts for 14–30% of cholecystectomies [35–37].

Patients with acute cholecystitis frequently present with right upper quadrant abdominal or epigastric pain with radiation to the back or right shoulder. Other general symptoms include nausea, vomiting and fever. Approximately 32–53% of patients present with fever and 51–53% demonstrate leukocytosis [38,39]. The pain associated with acute cholecystitis is differentiated from biliary 'colic' in that the pain is longer in duration and more intense in severity. Examination may demonstrate Murphy's sign which is cessation of inspiration during palpation of the gallbladder region. The differential diagnosis of acute cholecystitis is:

- Biliary "colic"
- Acute appendicitis
- Acute pancreatitis
- Hepatitis
- Peptic ulcer disease
- Renal disease
- Right sided pneumonia
- Fitz-Hugh–Curtis syndrome (ascending pelvic infection and inflammation of the liver capsule or diaphragm)
- Coronary artery disease
- Intrabdominal abscess.

Diagnostic modalities include transabdominal ultrasonography (US) and cholescintigraphy. Ultrasound may reveal a thickened gallbladder wall greater than 4 mm and pericholecystic fluid/edema. Ultrasound is inexpensive, non-invasive, and readily available. Cholescintigraphy uses technietium-labeled hepatic 2,6-dimethyl-iminodiacetic acid (HIDA) which is injected intravenously and is taken up by the liver. The HIDA is excreted in bile. If the cystic duct is obstructed, typically found in acute cholecystitis, the gallbladder is not visualized. A comparison study, comprising 11 studies, showed that cholescintigraphy was significantly superior to ultrasound with a sensitivity of 94% compared with 80% for ultrasound.

Treatment of acute cholecystitis is surgical resection of the gallbladder. The first cholecystectomy was performed in 1882 by Carl Langenbuch of Berlin and for the next century, open cholecystectomy was the standard of care. In 1987, a French surgeon introduced laparoscopic cholecystectomy and since then the laparoscopic approach has become the gold standard for treatment of cholecystitis.

The timing of cholecystectomy has been debated in the surgical literature for many years. The 'early cholecystectomy' school supports operative intervention during the index hospital stay with goals to reduce hospital stay and prevent readmissions related to gallbladder disease. The "delayed cholecystectomy" school endorses conservative treatment with antibiotics during the index hospitalization with plans to perform cholecystectomy 4–8 weeks after discharge. Most surgical data indicate that early cholecystectomy is safe and results in shorter overall hospital stay. The theory that delayed cholecystectomy reduces complications and conversion rates has not been strongly validated by existing studies.

References

1. Attasaranya S, Fogel EL, Lehman GA. Choledocholithiasis, ascending cholangitis and gallstone pancreatitis. *Med. Clin. N. Am.* 2008;**92**:925–60.
2. Banks PA, Freeman ML. Practice guidelines in acute pancreatitis. *Am. J. Gastroenterol.* 2006;**101**:2379–400.
3. Pitchumoni CS, Patel NM, Shah P. Factors influencing mortality in acute pancreatitis: can we alter them? *J. Clin. Gastroenterol.* 2005;**39**:798–814.
4. Howard TJ, Patel JB, Zyromski N, et al. Declining morbidity and mortality rates in the surgical management of pancreatic necrosis. *J. Gastrointest. Surg.* 2007;**11**:43–9.
5. Buter A, Imrie CW, Carter CR, Evans S, McKay CJ. Dynamic nature of early organ dysfunction determines outcome in acute pancreatitis. *Br. J. Surg.* 2002;**89**:298–302.

6. Fogel EL, Sherman S. ERCP for Gallstone Pancreatitis. *N. Engl. J. Med.* 2014;**370**:150–7.

7. Acosta JM, Ledesma CL. Gallstone migration as a cause of acute pancreatitis. *N. Engl. J. Med.* 1974;**290**:484–7.

8. Acosta JM, Pellegrini CA, Skinner DB. Etiology and pathogenesis of acute biliary pancreatitis. *Surgery* 1980;**88**:118–25.

9. Wang GJ, Gao CF, Wei D, Wang C, Ding SQ. Acute pancreatitis: etiology and common pathogenesis. *World J. Gastroenterol.* 2009;**15**:1427–30.

10. Lightner AM, Kirkwood KS. Pathophysiology of gallstone pancreatitis. *Front. Biosci.* 2001;**6**:E66–76.

11. Tse F, Yuan Y. Early routine endoscopic retrograde cholangiopancreatography strategy versus early conservative management strategy in acute gallstone pancreatitis. *Cochrane Database Syst Rev* 2012;**5**:CD009779–CD009779.

12. Sharma VK, Howden CW. Metaanalysis of randomized controlled trials of endoscopic retrograde cholangiography and endoscopic sphincterotomy for the treatment of acute biliary pancreatitis. *Am. J. Gastroenterol.* 1999;**94**:3211–14.

13. Ayub K, Imada R, Slavin J. Endoscopic retrograde cholangiopancreatography in gallstone-associated acute pancreatitis. *Cochrane Database Syst. Rev.* 2004;**4**:CD003630–CD003630.

14. Moretti A, Papi C, Aratari A, et al. Is early endoscopic retrograde cholangiopancreatography useful in the management of acute biliary pancreatitis? A meta-analysis of randomized controlled trials. *Dig. Liver Dis.* 2008;**40**:379–85.

15. Petrov MS, van Santvoort HC, Besselink MGH, van der Heijden GJ, van Erpecum KJ,Gooszen HG. Early endoscopic retrograde cholangiopancreatography versus conservative management in acute biliary pancreatitis without cholangitis: a meta-analysis of randomized trials. *Ann. Surg.* 2008;**247**:250–7.

16. Uy MC, Daez MLO, Sy PP, Banez VP, Espinosa WZ, Talingdan-Te MC. Early ERCP in acute gallstone pancreatitis without cholangitis: a meta-analysis. *JOP* 2009;**10**:299–305.

17. Forsmark CE, Baillie J. AGA Institute technical review on acute pancreatitis. *Gastroenterology* 2007;**132**:2022–44.

18. Tenner S, Baillie J, DeWitt J, Vege SS. American College of Gastroenterology guideline: management of acute pancreatitis. *Am. J. Gastroenterol.* 2013;**108**:1400–15.

19. Zhan X, Guo X, Chen Y, et al. EUS in exploring the etiology of mild acute biliary pancreatitis with a negative finding of biliary origin by conventional radiological methods. *J. Gastroenterol. Hepatol.* 2011;**26**:1500–3.

20. Stabuc B, Drobne D, Ferkolj I, et al. Acute biliary pancreatitis: detection of common bile duct stones with endoscopic ultrasound. *Eur. J. Gastroenterol. Hepatol.* 2008;**20**:1171–5.

21. Fan S-T, Lai ECS, Mok FPT, Lo CML, Zheng SS, Wong J. Early treatment of acute biliary pancreatitis by endoscopic papillotomy. *N. Engl. J. Med.* 1993;**328**:228–32.

22. Wall I, Badalov N, Baradarian R, Iswara K, Li JJ, Tenner S. Decreased mortality in acute pancreatitis related to early aggressive hydration. *Pancreas* 2011;**40**:547–50.

23. Boerma D, Rauws EA, Keulemans YC, et al. Wait-and-see policy or laparoscopic cholecystectomy after endoscopic sphincterotomy for bile-duct stones: a randomised trial. *Lancet* 2002;**360**:761–5.

24. ASGE Standards of Practice Committee, Banerjee S, Shen B, Baron TH, Nelson DB, Anderson MA, et al. Antibiotic prophylaxis for GI endoscopy. *Gastrointest. Endosc.* 2008;**67**:791–8.

25. De Palma GD, Pezzullo A, Rega M, et al. Unilateral placement of metallic stents for malignant hilar obstruction: a prospective study. *Gastrointest. Endosc.* 2003;**58**:50–3.

26. Carr-Locke DL, Ball TJ, Connors PJ, Cotton PB, Geenen JE, Hawes RH. Multi center randomized trial of Wallstent biliary endoprosthesis versus plastic stents. *Gastrointest. Endosc.* 1993;**39**:A310.

27. Ferreira LE, Baron TH. Acute Biliary Conditions. *Best Practice & Research Clinical Gastroenterology* 2013;**27**:745–56.

28. Sandha GS, Bourke MJ, Haber GB, Kortan PP. Endoscopic therapy for bile leak based on a new classification: results in 207 patients. *Gastrointest. Endosc.* 2004;**60**:567–74.

29. Stinton LM, Myers RP, Shaffer EA. Epidemiology of gallstones. *Gastroenterol. Clin. N. Am.* 2010;**39**(2):157–69.

30. Kehr H. Die in neiner klinik geubte technik de gallenstein operationen, mit einen hinweis auf die indikationen und die dauerersolge. Munchen: JF Lehman; 1905.

31. Shaffer EA. Gallstone disease: epidemiology of gallbladder stone disease. *Best Pract. Res. Clin. Gastroenterol.* 2006;**20**(6):981–96.

32. Halldestam I, Enell EL, Kullman E, et al. Development of symptoms and compli- cations in individuals with asymptomatic gallstones. *Br. J. Surg.* 2004;**91**(6):734–8.

33. Riall TS, Zhang D, Townsend CM Jr, et al. Failure to perform cholecystectomy for acute cholecystitis in elderly patients is associated with increased morbidity, mortality, and cost. *J. Am. Coll. Surg.* 2010;**210**(5):668–77, 677–9.

34. Bates T, Harrison M, Lowe D, et al. Longitudinal study of gall stone prevalence at necropsy. *Gut* 1992;**33**(1):103–7.

35. Steiner CA, Bass EB, Talamini MA, et al. Surgical rates and operative mortality for open and laparoscopic cholecystectomy in Maryland. *N. Engl. J. Med.* 1994;**330**(6):403 8.

36. Orlando R 3rd, Russell JC, Lynch J, et al. Laparoscopic cholecystectomy. A statewide experience. The Connecticut Laparoscopic Cholecystectomy Registry. *Arch. Surg.* 1993;**128**(5):494–8.

37. Pulvirenti E, Toro A, Gagner M, et al. Increased rate of cholecystectomies per- formed with doubtful or no indications after laparoscopy introduction: a single center experience. *BMC Surg.* 2013;**13**:17.

38. Raine PA, Gunn AA. Acute cholecystitis. *Br. J. Surg.* 1975;**62**(9):697–700.

39. Hafif A, Gutman M, Kaplan O, et al. The management of acute cholecystitis in elderly patients. *Am. Surg.* 1991;**57**(10):648–52.

CHAPTER 25

Variceal hemorrhage

Roy Soetikno[1,2] and Andres Sanchez-Yague[3,4]

[1] Stanford University, Stanford, CA, USA
[2] Veterans Affairs Palo Alto Health Care System, Palo Alto, CA, USA
[3] Vithas Xanit International Hospital, Benalmadena, Spain
[4] Hospital Costa del Sol, Marbella, Spain

Introduction

Variceal hemorrhage is a significant cause of morbidity and mortality, with varices found in half of patients screened endoscopically. Those with Child Class B and C not only have a higher incidence of varices (around 70%) but also face higher mortality rates from variceal bleeds. The incidence of a first bleed is about 12–15% per year [1, 2]. Management of varices includes primary prevention, treatment of acute variceal hemorrhage and secondary prevention.

Clinical presentation

Patients presenting with upper gastrointestinal bleeds can have hematemesis, hematochezia, or melena, or a combination of these. In patients with cirrhosis, it is important to consider causes of gastrointestinal bleeding other than varices, such as peptic ulcer disease, gastritis, Mallory–Weiss tears, and arteriovenous malformations (AVMs), as treatment modalities vary for the respective disease processes. Key elements of the history to obtain include prior episodes of gastrointestinal bleeding, prior episodes of spontaneous bacterial peritonitis, documented varices or peptic ulcer disease, use of non-steroidal anti-inflammatory drugs (NSAIDs), history of severe vomiting, mental status changes, abdominal pain and fever. Physical exam findings in patients with varices are indicative of the formation of portosystemic collaterals: visible veins around the umbilicus (caput Medusae), hemorrhoids and ascites. Signs of liver disease include scleral icterus, fetor hepaticus, jaundice, spider angiomas, gynecomastia, ascites, muscle wasting, telangiectasias, palmar erythema, asterixis, splenomegaly, and testicular atrophy.

Prevention of variceal hemorrhage

Primary prevention of variceal hemorrhage involves risk stratification to determine which patients will derive benefit. High-risk features for predicting first variceal hemorrhage include variceal size, red wale marks on varices (longitudinal dilated venules resembling whip marks), and advanced disease (Child B/C). Size appears to be most important in predicting first bleed [2, 3]. Esophagogastroduodenoscopy (EGD) is currently the most widely used and accurate method in characterizing varices. Diagnosis of variceal hemorrhage on EGD is made by the presence of active bleeding from a varix, "white nipple" overlying a varix, clots overlying a varix or varices with no other potential source of bleeding. Less-invasive methods such as capsule endoscopy and ratio of platelet count to spleen size are being investigated, but accuracy has yet to be validated. The degree of portal hypertension also helps risk-stratify patients. The most accurate method for measurement of portal hypertension is the hepatic venous pressure gradient (HVPG), which is obtained by deploying a balloon catheter through the jugular or femoral vein into the hepatic vein. This wedged pressure is corrected for intra-abdominal pressure by subtracting the free hepatic vein pressure or the IVC pressure. An HVPG greater than

Gastrointestinal Emergencies, Third Edition. Edited by Tony C. K. Tham, John S. A. Collins, and Roy Soetikno.
© 2016 John Wiley & Sons, Ltd. Published 2016 by John Wiley & Sons, Ltd.

10 mmHg denotes clinically significant portal hypertension and greater than 20 mmHg predicts a poor outcome. If the HVPG is reduced to less than 12 mmHg or 20% from baseline, there is a decreased risk of variceal hemorrhage and improved survival [4]. Measurement of HVPG is rarely done in the United States. Many non-invasive techniques to measure portal pressure are being investigated but are not widely adopted due to lack of validation, inability to grade portal pressure or inability to directly visualize varices. These techniques include transient elastography, ARFI (acoustic radiation force impulse elastography), 2D-SWE (two-dimensional shear wave elastography), strain elastography, duplex Doppler sonography, contrast-enhanced sonography, MRE (magnetic resonance elastography), fibrotest, HOMA-IR (fasting insulin, × fasting glucose/22.5), platelet count and combined test (liver stiffness × platelet count to spleen diameter ratio) [5].

Patients with cirrhosis should all be screened for the presence of varices at the time of diagnosis (Table 25.1). Those without varices should not be treated prophylactically with non-selective beta-blockers because of potential side effects without demonstrated benefit. Instead, treatment should focus on the underlying liver disease (Table 25.1). Approach to prevention of the first bleeding episode depends on the size of known varices. Small varices (<5 mm diameter) with low risk features (no red wale marks, Child class A) may be treated with non-selective beta blockers, though benefit has yet to be determined. Alternatively, these patients may be screened periodically for surveillance of variceal progression. Small varices with high-risk features (red wale marks or Child class B/C) should be treated with non-selective beta blockers. Endoscopic band ligation is not recommended for small varices for prophylaxis. For large varices, either non-selective beta blockers or band ligation can be used, depending on resources and patient preference/contraindications. There is a lack of data for prophylaxis of gastric varices, but the recommendation is to treat with non-selective beta blockers [6].

Traditional choices for therapy include propranolol (20 mg po BID) and nadolol (40 mg po daily) that are titrated to a target heart rate of 55 beats per minute. Non-selective beta-blockers are thought to both decrease

Table 25.1 Screening and treatment guidelines.

Disease state	Beta-blocker therapy	Endoscopy
Newly diagnosed cirrhosis		EGD at diagnosis for all patients
Small varices • no prior bleeding • no high risk features	+/−	EGD at diagnosis • if on beta-blocker: no follow up EGD needed • if not on beta-blocker: f/u EGD at 2 years
Small varices • no prior bleeding • with high risk features	+	EGD at diagnosis • no follow up EGD needed
Large varices • no prior bleeding • no high risk features	+ (preferred to EVL unless contraindications)	• if on beta-blocker, no follow up EGD needed • if intolerant to beta-blocker, EVL for prophylaxis • banding every 1–2 weeks until obliteration • first surveillance EGD in 1–3 months • subsequent surveillance: EGDs every 6–12 months
Large varices • no prior bleeding • with high risk features	+ (or EVL)	EVL (or beta-blockers)
Varices that have bled	+	EVL • banding every 1–2 weeks until obliteration • first surveillance EGD in 1–3 months • subsequent surveillance: EGDs every 6–12 months

Adapted from 2007 AASLD practice guidelines.
*Small <5 mm, large >5 mm.
*High risk = Child Class B or C or red wale marks on endoscopy.
*EVL=endoscopic variceal ligation.

portal pressure as well as bacterial translocation. Carvedilol has been investigated as an alternative to propranolol and nadolol, owing to its alpha-1-blocking effect that has the potential to decrease hepatic vascular resistance (in addition to decreasing cardiac output via beta-1 blockade and causing splanchnic vasoconstriction via beta-2 blockade, as do propanolol and nadolol). However, it also has the potential to cause hypotension from the alpha-1-blocking effects. A recent randomized trial showed lower rates of first variceal bleed with carvedilol 12.5 mg daily compared to band ligation, with no difference in overall or bleeding-associated mortality [7]. More studies are needed to determine whether carvedilol is superior to non-selective beta blockers or band ligation. Band ligation is performed every 1 to 2 weeks until varices are eradicated with surveillance endoscopy to follow 1–3 months after eradication and every 6–12 months thereafter [4, 8].

Secondary prevention of variceal hemorrhage

Secondary prevention is aimed at preventing rebleeding. It is not targeted at specific risk groups. Patients should be treated with a combination of non-selective beta-blockers and band ligation. Patients who are not candidates for band ligation should be treated with a combination of non-selective beta-blockers and nitrates. (isosorbide mononitrate 10 mg qhs titrated to maintain SBP >95 mmHg). If these therapies are unsuccessful at preventing rebleeding, patients should be considered for placement of a transjugular intrahepatic portosystemic shunt (TIPSS) or surgical shunt [4].

Initial emergency management of bleeding varices

As in any emergency situation, the initial priorities include focusing on achieving hemodynamic stability and airway protection. Management of acute variceal bleeds typically occurs in the intensive care unit (ICU) setting. Patients who are alert with an intact gag reflex do not need prophylactic intubation, especially given the increased risk of aspiration with prophylactic intubation [9]. However, those who have altered levels of consciousness or have massive bleeding in need of emergent endoscopy require intubation. Patients should have two large-bore (14 to18 gauge) IV catheters placed and have at least a complete blood count and type and cross sent. It is possible that in the very early stages of variceal bleed that the hemoglobin does not reflect the magnitude of acute blood loss, so it should be re-measured in a few hours to assess the degree of anemia. Resuscitation in variceal hemorrhage is unique in that excessive replacement with crystalloid and blood carries the risk of increasing portal pressure, and subsequently worsening the acute bleed. Hemoglobin targets have been the source of debate and a recent study favors the use of restrictive transfusion strategy with goal hemoglobin of 7 in upper gastrointestinal bleeds. This randomized trial showed a survival benefit in patients with an upper gastrointestinal bleed transfused to a goal hemoglobin of 7 instead of 9. Subgroup analysis indicated a survival benefit in cirrhotic patients with Child class A or B but not Child class C. In addition, rate of rebleed, length of hospital stay and frequency of need for rescue therapy with TIPSS or balloon tamponade were all reduced in the restrictive-strategy group [10]. Routine use of fresh frozen plasma (FFP) to normalize International Normalized Ratio (INR) is not recommended since INR does not necessarily correlate with bleeding risk in cirrhotics and the excess volume from FFP may contribute to worsening portal pressure. A trial comparing the use of Factor VII to placebo did not show a significant decrease in rebleeding and, thus, the routine use of Factor VII is not recommended. However, it is possible that a subgroup of patients with severe bleeding may benefit [11, 12].

Pharmacotherapy

Vasoactive medications should be started as soon as possible while preparing for more definitive endoscopic intervention. These medications reduce portal blood flow and cause splanchnic vasoconstriction. Octreotide and vasopressin are the only vasoactive medications approved in the US. Octreotide is more efficacious and has fewer side effects than vasopression, but if it is unavailable then vasopressin can be used in conjunction with IV or transdermal nitroglycerin. Octreotide is dosed as an initial 50 µg IV bolus followed by 50 µg/h continuous infusion for 48 hours to 5 days. Terlipressin, which is not approved in the US, is a vasopressin analog without as many side effects. It is dosed 2 mg IV q4h for the first 48 hours then 1 mg q4h. In addition to vasoactive drugs that directly decrease bleeding, antibiotics have been shown to improve survival and prevent rebleeding risk. Norfloxacin 400 mg po q12h is traditionally used, but a recent study shows benefit of infection prevention with ceftriaxone 1 g IV for 7 days over norfloxacin, possibly owing to increasing antibiotic resistance to fluoroquinolones [12, 13].

Balloon tamponade

Balloon tamponade is generally used in situations when endoscopy is not available, when endoscopy fails to control bleeding, or when bleeding is so profound that there is not sufficient time to wait for endoscopy. In the latter situation, tamponade is used as a temporizing measure until definitive TIPSS, surgical, or endoscopic treatment can be undertaken. Types of tubes are the Sengstaken–Blakemore tube (SBT) and the Minnesota tube and they have both an esophageal and gastric balloon. Usually only the gastric balloon is used at the gastroesophageal junction (GEJ) and the esophageal balloon is used only if the gastric balloon was ineffective. Risks of balloon tamponade include aspiration pneumonia, esophageal tears, and esophageal rupture. Esophageal necrosis can also occur if the esophageal balloon is inflated for too long, so it should periodically be deflated every 12 hours. GEJ necrosis can occur if the gastric balloon is inflated for more than 48 hours [12].

The use of balloon tamponade requires some precautions, in order to prevent complications (Fig. 25.1):

1 Ensure the placement of the gastric balloon in the stomach radiologically prior to inflating the gastric balloon of the SBT with at least 150 mL air or water (400 mL for the Linton–Nachlas balloon).

2 Put the tube under gentle external traction before inflating the esophageal balloon with maximum 80 mL air or water. The Linton–Nachlas balloon is first inflated with 150 mL air or water, and then filled up to 400 mL under gentle traction. External traction is maintained during the entire application.

Placement of the SBT in the case of endoscopically uncontrolled esophageal variceal bleeding may be cumbersome or even impossible. Additionally, patients treated with balloon tamponade are at high risk of aspiration, and therefore usually require tracheal intubation. In such cases, the use of a newly designed removable covered self-expandable metal stent (SX-Ella-Danis stent, Ella-CS s.r.o. Czech Republic) has been recommended, as it is easier to insert and does not

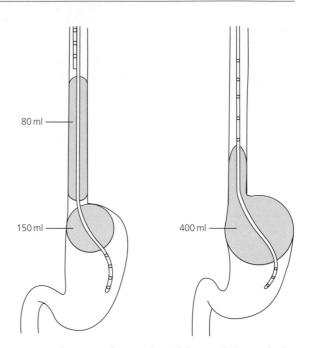

Fig. 25.1 Placement of Sengstaken–Blakemore balloon tube for esophageal variceal bleeding (left), Linton–Nachlas balloon tube for variceal bleeding from the cardia and fundus (right).

obstruct the esophagus. The stent has a length of 135 mm and a diameter of 25 mm). A balloon attached at the distal end of the delivery catheter allows for precise stent placement without fluoroscopic monitor. The stent is introduced over an endoscopically placed guide-wire. Once the tip is deeply advanced into the stomach, the balloon is inflated, and the delivery catheter is slowly withdrawn until the inflated balloon comes across the cardia. The stent can then be deployed under gentle traction in the usual manner. In the preliminary report of Hubmann et al. the stent was left for 5–7 days [14]. As for balloon tamponade, it is advisable to remove the stent as early as possible because of the potential risk of damaging the esophageal wall. Endoscopic treatment should immediately follow to eradicate the varices.

Endoscopy

Multiple endoscopic techniques can be employed in the management of an acute variceal bleed, including sclerotherapy, band ligation, and cyanoacrylate obliteration. Band ligation is the preferred form of endoscopic therapy and is superior to sclerotherapy in the prevention of rebleeding [15]. Due to higher rates of complications, rebleeding and mortality with sclerotherapy, band ligation is preferred to sclerotherapy unless there is a contraindication or it is unavailable [12]. A meta-analysis of band ligation plus sclerotherapy compared to band ligation alone showed that there was no difference in esophageal variceal rebleeding, mortality or number of sessions required for obliteration but higher rates of esophageal stricture formation in combination therapy than band ligation alone [16]. Band ligation is typically undertaken within 12 hours and usually preceded by the initiation of vasoactive drugs such as octreotide or terlipressin. In the case of emergent endoscopy, erythromycin can be used to facilitate gastric emptying and reduce the risk of aspiration of gastric contents.

Cyanoacrylate obliteration

Cyanoacrylate obliteration is the most effective at preventing rebleeding from gastric varices. Endoscopic variceal obliteration using N-butyl-2-cyanoacrylate (Histoacryl®, Braun-Melsungen, Germany, Glubran®, GEM, Italy) is undoubtedly more effective than other treatment modality for massive esophageal and fundic variceal hemorrhage. It represents the only endoscopic option to effectively control bleeding from sclerotherapy or endoscopic variceal ligation (EVL)-induced ulcers. Cyanoacrylate obliteration is also widely accepted as the currently best treatment modality for controlling acute hemorrhage from huge fundic varices N-butyl-2-cyanoacrylate is not available in the US but off-label use of 2-octyl-cyanoacrylate is used by experienced practitioners.

The tissue glue N-butyl-2-cyanoacrylate is a watery solution, which polymerizes and hardens within 20 seconds in a physiological milieu, and almost instantaneously upon contact with blood. To prevent cyanoacrylate from solidifying too quickly, it is necessary to dilute it with the oily contrast agent Lipiodol® (Guerbert Villepinte, France) in a ratio of 0.5:0.8. Lipiodol is not only compatible with the tissue adhesive but also allows fluoroscopic monitoring of the glue injection. N-butyl-2-cyanoacrylate is injected strictly into the lumen of the varix.

The most serious potential risk of intravariceal injection of N-butyl-2-cyanoacrylate is embolism. There have been several case reports on embolization of the glue from the varices into the lung, spleen, brain, and pelvic region [17]. These serious complications are rare. Usually, N-butyl-2-cyanoacrylate polymerizes and solidifies in the vessel instantaneously, so that an embolism

Table 25.2 Technique for endoscopic variceal obliteration using N-butyl-2 cyanoacrylate.

- Mix Histoacryl® with Lipiodol® in 0.5:0.8 ratio
- Inject directly into the varix
- Lubricate the injector with Lipiodol
- Measure the dead space of the injector
- Use distilled water of the same volume to flush out cyanoacrylate
- Continue flushing the injector after injection to maintain the injector patency
- Apply not more than 0.5 mL of glue per injection to avoid embolization in esophagus, and 1.0 mL in fundus, respectively
- Obliterate all visible fundic varices in one session to prevent rebleeding

is very unlikely. In the case of patent foramen ovale or other right-to-left shunting in the mediastinum, this rare, serious complication may occur. To prevent such complications, the amount of N-butyl-2-cyanoacrylate per injection should be limited to a maximum of 0.5 mL for esophageal varices and 1 mL for large fundic varices. If greater amounts are needed due to the large size of the varices, injection should be performed in succession. The details of the cyanoacrylate injection technique are described in Table 25.2.

Rescue therapy

When band ligation and cyanoacrylate obliteration are unable to control bleeding, TIPSS or surgical shunting are considered. TIPSS involves bypassing the liver by placing a shunt between the portal and hepatic veins. It is highly effective but a significant side effect is encephalopathy. TIPSS is especially effective for patients with severe bleeding and has been shown to be more effective than obturation in the treatment of gastric varices [18]. Surgical shunting is rarely done owing to side effects and the efficacy of TIPSS as definitive therapy.

Acknowledgments

We would like to acknowledge the contribution of the authors of this chapter in the second edition of this book: Drs Yan Zhong, Stefan Seewald, and Nib Soehendra. We have utilized their sections on balloon tamponade and cyanoacrylate obliteration for this chapter.

References

1. Kovalak M, Lake J, Mattek N, Eisen G, Lieberman D, Zaman A. Endoscopic screening for varices in cirrhotic patients: data from a national endoscopic database. *Gastrointest. Endosc.* 2007;**65**:82–8.

2. Brocchi E, Caletti G, Brambilla G, Mantia LL, Lupinacci G, Pisano G. Prediction of the first variceal hemorrhage in patients with cirrhosis of the liver and esophageal varices. A prospective multicenter study. N. Engl. J. *Med.* 1988;**319**:983–9.

3. Merkel C, Zoli M, Siringo S, et al. Prognostic indicators of risk for first variceal bleeding in cirrhosis: a multicenter study in 711 patients to validate and improve the North Italian Endoscopic Club (NIEC) index. *Am. J. Gastroenterol.* 2000;**95**:2915–20.

4. Garcia-Tsao G, Bosch J. Management of varices and variceal hemorrhage in cirrhosis. *N. Engl. J. Med.* 2010;**362**:823–32.

5. Zardi EM, Di Matteo FM, Pacella CM, Sanyal AJ. Invasive and non-invasive techniques for detecting portal hypertension and predicting variceal bleeding in cirrhosis: A review. *Ann. Med.* 2014;**46**:8–17.

6. de Franchis R. Revising consensus in portal hypertension: report of the Baveno V consensus workshop on methodology of diagnosis and therapy in portal hypertension. *J. Hepatol.* 2010;**53**:762–8.

7. Tripathi D, Ferguson JW, Kochar N, et al. Randomized controlled trial of carvedilol versus variceal band ligation for the prevention of the first variceal bleed. *Hepatology* 2009;**50**:825–33.

8. Giannelli V, Lattanzi B, Thalheimer U, Merli M. Beta-blockers in liver cirrhosis. *Ann. Gastroenterol.* 2014;**27**:20.

9. Koch DG, Arguedas MR, Fallon MB. Risk of aspiration pneumonia in suspected variceal hemorrhage: the value of prophylactic endotracheal intubation prior to endoscopy. *Dig. Dis. Sci.* 2007;**52**:2225–8.

10. Villanueva C, Colomo A, Bosch A, et al. Transfusion strategies for acute upper gastrointestinal bleeding. *N. Engl. J. Med.* 2013;**368**:11–21.

11. Bosch J, Thabut D, Albillos A, et al. Recombinant factor VIIa for variceal bleeding in patients with advanced cirrhosis: a randomized, controlled trial. *Hepatology* 2008;**47**:1604–14.

12. Herrera JL. Management of acute variceal bleeding. *Clin. Liver Dis.* 2014;**18**:347–57.

13. Fernández J, del Arbol LR, Gómez C, et al. Norfloxacin vs ceftriaxone in the prophylaxis of infections in patients with advanced cirrhosis and hemorrhage. *Gastroenterology* 2006;**131**:1049–56.

14. Hubmann R, Bodlaj G, Czompo M, et al. The use of self-expanding metal stents to treat acute esophageal variceal bleeding. *Endoscopy* 2006;**38**:896–901.

15. Garcia-Tsao G, Sanyal AJ, Grace ND, Carey W. Prevention and management of gastroesophageal varices and variceal hemorrhage in cirrhosis. *Hepatology* 2007;**46**:922–38.

16. Karsan HA, Morton SC, Shekelle PG, et al. Combination endoscopic band ligation and sclerotherapy compared with endoscopic band ligation alone for the secondary prophylaxis of esophageal variceal hemorrhage: a meta-analysis. *Dig. Dis. Sci.* 2005;**50**:399–406.

17. Wahl P, Lammer F, Conen D, Schlumpf R, Bock A. Septic complications after injection of N-butyl-2-cyanoacrylate: report of two cases and review. *Gastrointest. Endosc.* 2004; **59**:911–6.

18. Lo GH, Liang HL, Chen WC, et al. A prospective, randomized controlled trial of transjugular intrahepatic portosystemic shunt versus cyanoacrylate injection in the prevention of gastric variceal rebleeding. *Endoscopy* 2007;**39**:679–85.

CHAPTER 26

Acute liver failure

Philip S. J. Hall[1] and W. Johnny Cash[2]

[1] *Altnagelvin Hospital, Londonderry, UK*
[2] *Royal Victoria Hospital, Belfast, UK*

Introduction

Acute liver failure results from a rapid loss of hepatocyte function over a period of days to weeks. This causes a syndrome of progressive jaundice, coagulopathy, encephalopathy and finally cerebral oedema and death [1]. It can be the result of a multitude of etiologies, the commonest of which are drug related (particularly acetaminophen/paracetamol) and viral hepatitis. Regardless of the underlying disease, the majority of patients present with non-specific constitutional symptoms which can progress rapidly to the alteration of mental status and coma. This is accompanied by classical biochemical abnormalities, including elevated serum transaminases, hyperbilirubinemia, and a raised prothrombin time.

Patients with acute liver failure require early recognition and the prompt instigation of supportive treatment in an intensive care unit whilst a diagnosis is being sought. Aggressive supportive care may buy time and allow for hepatic recovery in some cases, but clinicians need to be aware of the adverse prognostic features that necessitate timely liver transplantation.

Definitions

A variety of definitions have been given to the syndrome of acute liver failure. The differences reflect an evolving understanding of the condition over time and attempts to classify patients into groups that will allow prognostication both before and after liver transplantation. No one definition has yet been universally adopted and usage depends largely on location and transplant practices.

Fulminant, sub-fulminant, and late onset hepatic failure

Trey and Davidson first used the term "fulminant hepatic failure" to describe patients with coagulopathy (International Normalized Ratio (INR) ≥1.5) who developed encephalopathy within 8 weeks of the onset of *illness*, with no prior evidence of liver disease [2]. "Late onset hepatic failure" has since been used to describe the development of encephalopathy between 8 weeks and 6 months after the onset of symptoms [3].

Bernuau and colleagues at the Hôpital Beaujon proposed that the term fulminant hepatic failure should be applied to patients who develop hepatic encephalopathy within 2 weeks of the onset of *jaundice* rather than the more nondescript "illness." They considered another group of patients who developed encephalopathy between 2 weeks and 3 months of the onset of jaundice to have "sub-fulminant hepatic failure" [4].

Hyperacute, acute, and subacute hepatic failure

O'Grady and colleagues from Kings College Hospital, London divided patients with acute liver failure into three subgroups based on a retrospective analysis of over 500 patients. They proposed a distinction between three separate syndromes, dependent on the time between onset of jaundice and encephalopathy: hyperacute (encephalopathy within 7 days), acute (8–28 days),

Gastrointestinal Emergencies, Third Edition. Edited by Tony C. K. Tham, John S. A. Collins, and Roy Soetikno.
© 2016 John Wiley & Sons, Ltd. Published 2016 by John Wiley & Sons, Ltd.

and subacute (29 days to 12 weeks). These group-ings reflect differences in patient survival, particularly after liver transplantation. The best prognosis was found to be in those with hyper-acute liver failure [5]. The definitions of acute liver failure are compared in Fig. 26.1.

Acute liver injury

This term refers to patients with acute liver disease and coagulopathy (INR ≥1.5) but without evidence of hepatic encephalopathy. As before the patient must have no clinical or radiological evidence of cirrhosis. The diagnosis of acute liver failure rather than acute liver injury therefore depends solely on the development of hepatic encephalopathy [6].

Epidemiology

The actual incidence of acute liver failure remains unknown, but is estimated to be fewer than 5 per million population per year in the developed world [6]. Approximately 2000 individuals develop acute liver failure annually in the United States, with 200 to 300 undergoing liver transplantation [7]. It is suspected that referral bias influences the reported etiology and out-comes of acute liver failure.

Etiology

The causes of acute liver failure are diverse and the distri-bution varies according to geographic region. The most common causes of acute liver failure are drug-induced liver injury and viral hepatitis. These account for 80% to 85% of all cases for which a cause can be determined (Table 26.1). In the pre-transplant era, hepatitis B accounted for as many as 40–50% of US cases of acute liver failure, however current data from the Acute Liver Failure Study Group (ALFSG) demonstrates that drug-induced liver injury is now much more prevalent. Acute liver failure due to acetaminophen has risen from 20% of cases in 1994–1996 to 51% of cases in 2004 [1]. Acute hepatitis B accounted for only 7% of US cases.

While this dramatic rise in acetaminophen toxicity was mirrored in most western societies during the 1990s, in developing nations different patterns of disease prevail. Data from India shows a higher proportion of patients with acute viral hepatitis, whereas drug-induced liver injury is more likely to be due to isoniazid [8].

Recent data from the King's College group demon-strates the changing patterns of acute liver failure etiology over time. Acetaminophen related acute liver failure admissions rose 400% between 1973–1978 and 1994–1998. Following the introduction of sales restrictions on acetaminophen in the United Kingdom

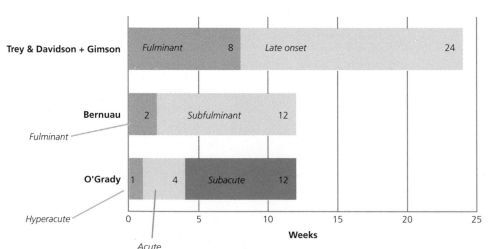

Fig. 26.1 Definitions of acute liver failure.

Table 26.1 Causes of acute liver failure.

Drug-induced liver injury (DILI)
    Acetaminophen overdose
    Idiosyncratic drug reaction
Viral hepatitis
    Hepatitis A, B, C, D and E
    Herpesviruses
    Epstein–Barr virus
    Cytomegalovirus
Vascular
    Systemic hypotension
    Budd–Chiari syndrome
    Hepatic venous/arterial occlusion
Toxins
    Amanita phalloides
    Organic solvents
Metabolic
    Acute fatty liver of pregnancy
    Reye syndrome
Miscellaneous
    Autoimmune hepatitis
    Wilson disease
    Liver transplant graft failure
    Liver neoplastic infiltration
    Iatrogenic loss of liver parenchyma (surgical resection/embolic
        therapy)

in 1998, the group found a dramatic drop in acute liver failure admissions, initial INR on presentation and acetaminophen related deaths. In Germany, acetaminophen is available by prescription only and accounts for only 9% of acute liver failure cases [6].

Other unusual etiologies of acute liver failure include toxins, metabolic diseases, vascular events, tumors, and allograft rejection [9] (Table 26.1).

Drugs

Drug-induced liver injury is the leading cause of acute liver failure in the developed world. It accounts for more than 50% of all cases of acute liver failure in the US and the UK. It can occur in as many as 20% of cases of drug-induced hepatitis. It is estimated that more than 50 000 emergency room visits and nearly 500 deaths in the US occur annually as a result of acetaminophen-related hepatotoxicity. Drug-induced liver injury is more prevalent in women and individuals older than 40 years of age. Drug-related hepatotoxicity has been divided into two groups, namely dose-dependent and idiosyncratic. Dose-dependent hepatotoxicity is predictable and presents with a typical pattern. In contrast, idiosyncratic hepatotoxicity affects less than 1% of users of an individual drug and lacks a characteristic pattern. Idiosyncratic drug reactions account for 10–15% of cases of acute liver failure, but are associated with high mortality rate.

Acetaminophen-induced hepatotoxicity occurs in a dose-dependent, predictable fashion. Acetaminophen is generally safe within the recommended dosage of 3–4 g/day, and its sulfate or glucuronide metabolites are not hepatotoxic. A minor fraction of an acetaminophen dose is metabolized by P-450 enzymes to the reactive and potentially harmful metabolite *N*-acetyl-*p*-benzoquinone imine (NAPQI) that is normally conjugated by glutathione to a nontoxic compound. Acetaminophen hepatotoxicity consistently results in hyperacute liver failure. Serum aminotransferase levels are markedly elevated in patients with acetaminophen hepatotoxicity, with values typically exceeding 3000–4000 IU/L. Acute liver failure is triggered by acetaminophen overdose when more than 10 g is ingested or with use of high therapeutic doses by alcoholics who have induced cytochrome P-450 enzymes. In addition, alcoholics may have reduced glutathione stores due to poor nutrition, leaving more toxic intermediates available to cause cell injury. These toxic intermediate metabolites accumulate and bind to cytoplasmic proteins within hepatocytes leading to cell death. Acetaminophen overdose can be associated with up to 50% mortality, whereas excessive ingestion of acetaminophen by alcoholics is associated with an approximate 20% mortality rate.

Examples of drugs that may be associated with idiosyncratic hepatotoxicity resulting in acute liver failure include halothane, isoniazid, disulfiram, valproate, phenytoin, sulfonamides, methyldopa, propylthiouracil, non-steroidal anti-inflammatory drugs, bromfenac, and troglitazone. In most cases, presumed idiosyncratic abnormalities in hepatic drug metabolism are the main underlying mechanisms of this type of injury. In patients with idiosyncratic drug-induced hepatotoxicity, eosinophilia and/or the presence of a rash are indicative of hypersensitivity reaction, although these findings are uncommon.

Viral hepatitis

All five hepatotropic viruses have been associated with acute liver failure. However, acute hepatitis C is more likely to result in chronic liver disease rather than cause fulminant hepatitis. In the past, patients with fulminant hepatic failure of no clear etiology were labeled as non-A, non-B hepatitis. It was suspected that hepatitis C virus, or some other viral agent, was the likely etiology. Subsequently, hepatitis C virus RNA and/or antibody to hepatitis C virus were found to be undetectable in the majority of patients labeled as cryptogenic fulminant hepatic failure. It is important to know that less than 1% of patients with acute viral hepatitis will develop fulminant liver failure. Patients who develop fulminant hepatic failure secondary to acute hepatitis A and acute hepatitis B present with a hyperacute course. Typically, jaundice is rapidly followed within 1 week by hepatic encephalopathy. Acute hepatitis A causes fulminant hepatic failure in 0.1 to 0.5% of cases and is common in intravenous drug users. Patients with fulminant hepatitis A usually fare well with a survival rate of 60%. Fulminant hepatitis A is more severe in older patients and individuals with pre-existing chronic liver disease. Acute hepatitis B is the most common viral cause of fulminant hepatic failure. Rapid clearance of hepatitis B virus has been reported in 30 to 50% of patients with acute hepatitis B-related fulminant hepatic failure as a result of major immunological attack on infected hepatocytes. These patients may have undetectable levels of HBsAg within a few days of onset of illness and have been wrongly labeled as cryptogenic liver disease. Hepatitis D virus is a rare cause of acute liver failure, is more prevalent in injection drug users, and typically presents in the setting of fulminant hepatitis B. Acute coinfection with hepatitis B and hepatitis D virus or superinfection with hepatitis D virus in a patient with chronic hepatitis B may precipitate fulminant hepatic failure, and coinfected patients are at higher risk for fulminant hepatic failure than patients with acute hepatitis B monoinfection [10]. Fulminant hepatic failure is infrequently associated with hepatitis E infection, but hepatitis E virus-related epidemics have been associated with fulminant hepatic failure in pregnant women. The mortality rate is approximately 40% in pregnant patients with hepatitis E-induced fulminant hepatic failure. Hepatitis caused by other viruses, including herpes viruses 1, 2, and 6, adenovirus, Epstein–Barr virus, and cytomegalovirus rarely results in acute liver failure (Table 26.1).

Toxins

Several toxins have been implicated in patients with acute hepatic failure. Organic solvents, such as fluorinated hydrocarbons, trichloroethylene, and tetrachloroethane, can induce hepatotoxicity and acute liver failure.

Metabolic conditions

Metabolic conditions associated with acute liver failure include acute fatty liver of pregnancy and Reye's syndrome. Both of these conditions present with liver biopsy findings of microvesicular fatty infiltration as compared to massive hepatic necrosis that is uniformly noted in other causes of fulminant hepatic failure. Typically, acute fatty liver of pregnancy presents in the third trimester with rapid onset of jaundice, hypoglycemia, coagulopathy, and hepatic encephalopathy. Serum aminotransferase levels are usually below 1000 IU/L. Emergent delivery of the fetus is recommended. Wilson's disease is a rare cause of acute liver failure. It should be considered in young patients, particularly those with high levels of bilirubin and low levels of alkaline phosphatase (ALP) so that bilirubin:ALP ratio exceeds 2:0 [11].

Miscellaneous

Vascular complications can also lead to the development of acute liver failure (Table 26.1). Myocardial infarction or cardiomyopathy with acute circulatory failure can precipitate acute liver failure. Rarely, hepatic venous outflow obstruction following acute Budd–Chiari syndrome or veno-occlusive disease can result in acute liver failure. Heat exhaustion-related reversible liver failure can develop in high-risk population, such as miners and long-distance runners. Metastatic tumor, causing massive hepatic infiltration, characterized by intrasinusoidal invasion can precipitate acute liver failure. Primary allograft non-function within a few days following liver transplantation can present as acute liver failure necessitating retransplantation.

The above-mentioned causes of acute liver failure may be characterized by a fulminant or sub-fulminant course of hepatic failure (Table 26.2). Fulminant hepatic failure (hyperacute or acute) is the usual presentation of liver failure in patients with acute hepatitis (types A, B, D, and E), *Amanita phalloides* poisoning, acetaminophen overdose, and acute fatty liver of pregnancy. In contrast, patients with cryptogenic acute liver failure, drug-induced liver injury, hepatic venous outflow obstruction, Wilson disease, and autoimmune hepatitis typically present with subfulminant hepatic failure. The survival rate in patients affected by fulminant hepatic failure (40–60%) is significantly better than that in patients with subfulminant hepatic failure (10–30%).

In around 15% of patients with acute liver failure, no precipitant can be found. Studies measuring acetaminophen adducts have shown that as many as 20% of these may be due to unrecognised acetaminophen overdose [1]. Liver biopsy should be considered in these cases as it may reveal a fulminant presentation of autoimmune hepatitis.

Clinical manifestations

The classic presentation of acute liver failure is a triad of jaundice, hepatic encephalopathy, and coagulopathy. The progression of acute liver failure is characterized by metabolic irregularities, renal dysfunction (50% of patients), cardiopulmonary failure, and sepsis. Patients are susceptible to bacterial infections (80% of patients)

Table 26.2 Course of acute liver failure.

Predominantly hyperacute hepatic failure:
Acetaminophen overdose
Hepatitis A, B, D and E
Ischemic liver injury
Acute fatty liver of pregnancy
Amanita phalloides
Predominantly subacute hepatic failure:
Drug-induced liver injury (DILI)
Budd–Chiari syndrome
Veno-occlusive disease
Wilson disease
Autoimmune hepatitis

or fungal infections (30% of patients). As the syndrome progresses, patients typically develop hypotension, systemic vasodilation, and have a low systemic vascular resistance. Features of chronic liver disease including portal hypertension, esophageal varices, and ascites are usually absent, except in subacute cases [1].

Symptoms and signs

Non-specific constitutional symptoms such as malaise and nausea often precede the onset of jaundice and hence early cases can be missed without biochemical analysis and a thorough assessment. Findings during physical examination depend on the time of presentation but can include jaundice, bruising, and altered mental status.

Encephalopathy is the cardinal sign that a patient with acute liver injury has developed acute liver failure. Its severity is divided into four grades in the West Haven criteria (Table 26.3). The diagnosis of grade 1 hepatic encephalopathy requires a high index of suspicion. Patients who develop grade 4 hepatic encephalopathy have a less than 20% survival rate and are at high risk of cerebral edema.

Laboratory findings

Laboratory findings noted in patients with acute liver failure vary with the severity of underlying liver disease. They include marked elevation in serum aminotransferase levels, hyperbilirubinemia, hypoprothrombinemia, hypoglycemia, and respiratory alkalosis

Table 26.3 West Haven classification for grading hepatic encephalopathy.

Grade	Level of consciousness	Personality and intellect	Neurologic signs	Electroencephalographic abnormalities
0	Normal	None	None	None
Subclinical	Normal	Forgetfulness, mild confusion, agitation and irritability	Abnormalities only on psychometric analysis	None
1	Inverted sleep pattern, restlessness	Tremor, apraxia, incoordination and impaired handwriting	Tremor, apraxia, incoordination and impaired handwriting	Triphasic waves (5 cycles/s)
2	Lethargy, slow responses		Asterixis, dysarthria, ataxia and hypoactive reflexes	Triphasic waves (5 cycles/s)
3	Somnolence but rousable, confusion	Disorientation as regards place; amnesia; disinhibited; and inappropriate behaviour	Asterixis, hyperactive reflexes, Babinski's sign and muscle rigidity	Triphasic waves (5 cycles/s)
4	Coma	None		Delta waves

Source: Cash, 2010 [21]. Reproduced with permission of OUP.

preceding metabolic acidosis. Coagulopathy in acute liver failure is characterized by a prolonged prothrombin time and a factor V level of less than 50% of normal. Other electrolyte abnormalities that are common and may require correction include hyponatremia, hypophosphatemia, hypocalcemia, and/or hypomagnesemia.

Recent data suggests that the measurement of arterial ammonia can predict the neurological sequelae to follow. An arterial ammonia concentration of <75 µM on admission indicates that a patient is unlikely to develop intracranial hypertension. A level greater than 100 µM indicates a risk of high grade hepatic encephalopathy. Levels >200 µM are associated with intracranial hypertension [12].

The measurement of serum acetaminophen levels should not be relied upon. In cases of overdose resulting in acute liver failure, the vast proportion of the drug will already have been metabolised. Patients with staggered or accidental chronic overdosing may not have toxic levels in serum.

Treatment

Successful management of acute liver failure depends upon prompt recognition and then instigation of management. All of these approaches must happen simultaneously:

- Condition-specific "antidotes"
- Meticulous supportive management and dealing with complications
- Prognostication and timely transplant.

Data from the King's College group has shown that survival from acute liver failure has improved from 17% in 1973–1978 to 62% in 2004–2008 [6]. They concluded that this improvement was largely due to earlier recognition of the condition, improvements in intensive care methods and the use of emergency liver transplantation.

Condition-specific treatment

N-acetylcysteine should be commenced where there is a suspicion of acetaminophen overdose and steroids can be commenced for a confirmed diagnosis of autoimmune hepatitis. In cases of liver failure induced by pregnancy, the fetus should be delivered without delay. It is vital not to delay transfer of the ill patient to intensive care and subsequently to a transplant centre while waiting for a diagnosis or for a specific treatment to have an effect.

Supportive management and dealing with complications

Patients with acute liver failure should be admitted to the intensive care unit and transferred to a hospital with a liver transplant program [13]. Patients may need placement of Swan–Ganz and intra-arterial catheters, a urinary catheter, and a nasogastric tube. Invasive measurement of intracerebral pressure and prompt treatment of cerebral edema may be required to prevent permanent neurological damage. Mechanical ventilation is recommended in patients with grade 3 or grade 4 hepatic encephalopathy.

Hepatic encephalopathy and cerebral edema

Liver transplantation is contraindicated in at least 30% of patients with acute liver failure as a result of neurological complications (Table 26.3). The underlying pathogenetic mechanisms for hepatic encephalopathy and cerebral edema are different. Hepatic encephalopathy is triggered by the accumulation of toxic substances in the central nervous system. The toxic agents implicated include ammonia and endogenous benzodiazepine agonists. Patients with grade 1 and grade 2 hepatic encephalopathy have a favorable outcome. Grade 3 and grade 4 hepatic encephalopathy are associated with poor prognosis. Cerebral edema is usually fatal following uncal herniation. The underlying mechanism for cerebral edema in the setting of acute liver failure remains unclear. Grade 4 hepatic encephalopathy is complicated by cerebral edema in approximately three-quarters of patients. Cerebral edema is the most common cause of death in patients with grade 4 hepatic encephalopathy. The blood–brain barrier is disrupted by cerebral edema. Cerebral ischemia develops if cerebral perfusion pressure (mean arterial pressure minus intracerebral pressure) drops below 40 mmHg.

Hepatic encephalopathy associated with fulminant hepatic failure should be managed in an intensive care unit. It is recommended that the patient head be elevated at 20–30°. Lactulose is not as effective in patients with fulminant hepatic failure but should be instituted by nasogastric tube or by rectal enema. The dose of lactulose should be titrated with a goal of two to four loose bowel movements per day. The role of antibiotics in hepatic encephalopathy secondary to fulminant hepatic failure is not well defined. Hepatic encephalopathy can deteriorate following gastrointestinal bleeding, hypokalemia, or sepsis. These aggravating conditions should be promptly diagnosed and immediately treated.

The clinical features of cerebral edema include hypertension, bradycardia, abnormal pupillary reflexes, decerebrate rigidity and posturing, and brainstem respiratory patterns and apnea. The clinical manifestations occur late and indicate poor prognosis. Computerized tomography (CT) scan of the head may be needed to exclude other intracerebral complications such as hemorrhage or other structural lesions to assess candidacy for liver transplantation. CT scan and/or magnetic resonance imaging of the head are unreliable in predicting the intracerebral pressures.

Intracranial pressure (ICP) monitoring remains a controversial issue. A retrospective study suggested that the practice is centre and operator dependant. Whilst the ICP-monitored group were more likely to receive mannitol therapy and make it to liver transplantation, there were no differences in overall outcomes between this group and those without monitoring [14].

ICP may be monitored with subdural or epidural transducers. Epidural transducers have lower sensitivity than subdural monitors but are safer to place. The transducer measurements should be closely monitored to maintain ICP below 20 mmHg and cerebral perfusion pressure above 50 mmHg. Patients with a persistently elevated ICP greater than 40 mmHg despite aggressive therapy are poor candidates for orthotopic liver transplantation.

Mannitol is the drug of choice to treat cerebral edema. It is used intravenously at a dose of 0.5–1 g/kg over 5 minutes and the same dose can be reinstituted to maintain the intracerebral pressure. Mannitol use is contraindicated if serum osmolality rises above 320 mosm/L. It should be used in conjunction with hemodialysis or continuous arteriovenous hemofiltration in patients with renal failure. In patients who are refractory to mannitol, pentobarbital can be used with boluses of 100–150 mg intravenously every 15 minutes for 1 hour followed by a continuous infusion of 1–3 mg/kg/h. Other measures to prevent increases in intracerebral pressure include: minimizing disturbance; controlling agitation; elevating the head 20–30° above the horizontal; provide moderate hyperventilation to a partial carbon dioxide pressure of 25–30 mmHg; and phenytoin use for subclinical seizures detectable by electroencephalography.

In patients with a high risk of developing cerebral oedema (e.g. hyperacute failure, elevated arterial ammonia level), the risk can be reduced by infusion of hypertonic saline to raise the serum sodium to 145–155 mmol/L. All of these treatments should be used as a bridge to transplantation as little recovery can otherwise be expected. Some centers have had success using therapeutic hypothermia as a bridge to transplantation; however, this carries with it the risk of reducing the likelihood of hepatic recovery [15].

Coagulopathy

The coagulation abnormalities noted in acute liver failure include decreased levels of factors II, V, VII, IX, and X resulting in prolonged prothrombin time and partial thromboplastin time. The coagulation studies are closely and serially monitored as a prognostic indicator. Patients with coagulopathy in the setting of fulminant hepatic failure are at increased risk for bleeding from the gastrointestinal tract and arteriovenous access sites. Therefore, use of fresh frozen plasma to correct coagulopathy is only indicated for a bleeding complication or prior to invasive procedures. Thrombocytopenia is commonly associated with fulminant hepatic failure as a result of bone marrow suppression and disseminated intravascular coagulation. Platelet counts should be monitored closely. Platelet transfusion is indicated if the platelets count drops below 50 000/μL in a patient with a bleeding complication.

Some recent studies suggest that the risk of bleeding in patients with acute liver failure may be overestimated. They suggest that because of a proportional reduction in both procoagulant *and* anticoagulant factors normally produced in the liver, that patients with acute liver failure may have blood that is hypocoagulable, hypercoagulable, or normal [16].

Cardiovascular and renal failure

Patients with acute liver failure are typically vasodilated, initially volume depleted, and will require fluid resuscitation and usually vasopressor support to maintain an adequate blood pressure and cerebral perfusion pressure in the setting of imminent cerebral edema. Vasopressors such as norepinephrine should be commenced and the mean arterial pressure titrated to 75 mmHg. Controversy exists regarding the adjunctive use of vasopressin and its analogue terlipressin, but recent data suggests that its use in this setting is safe [15].

Renal failure complicates 50% of cases and indicates a poor prognosis. Patients are typically oliguric as a result of a functional hepatorenal syndrome. Nephrotoxic drugs, such as aminoglycosides, nonsteroidal anti-inflammatory agents, or contrast agents, should be avoided and mean arterial pressure maintained as above with fluids and vasopressors. The indications for hemodialysis or continuous arteriovenous hemofiltration include severe metabolic acidosis, hyperkalemia, or fluid overload. Patients who have taken an acetaminophen overdose may show signs of acute kidney injury relating directly to the toxic effects of the drug and may require early continuous hemodialysis [1].

Hypoglycemia

Hypoglycemia in the setting of fulminant hepatic failure is not uncommon and is caused by impaired hepatic glucose production, impaired hepatic gluconeogenesis and elevated serum insulin levels. Patients with fulminant hepatic failure should be placed on continuous intravenous infusion of 10% dextrose. Infusion of hypertonic glucose may be needed to maintain blood glucose levels between 60–200 mg/dL. Caloric intake should be maintained at 35–50 kcal/kg to meet resting metabolic need. Blood glucose levels should be monitored every 4 hours following the onset of hepatic encephalopathy

Infection

The risk of bacterial and fungal infections is significantly higher in patients with fulminant hepatic failure. Sepsis is one of the leading contraindications for liver transplantation in the setting of fulminant hepatic failure. Bacteremia is a common problem in patients with altered mental status and indwelling catheters. Up to 80% of patients with fulminant hepatic failure have clinical evidence of an underlying infection. The most common sites of infection are respiratory and urinary tract systems. The most prevalent infectious organisms include Gram-positive streptococci, *Staphylococcus aureus*, and Gram-negative organisms. Approximately one-third of patients with fulminant hepatic failure develop fungal infections, of which *Candida albicans* is the most common. Broad-spectrum, intravenous antibiotic and antifungal therapy should be initiated based on presumed or documented infection. Surveillance cultures should also be performed.

Prognostication and transplantation

After making the diagnosis of acute liver failure it is important to apply prognostic criteria to identify those patients most likely to deteriorate and require consideration of liver transplantation. This allows the patient to be transferred early to the correct facility while still stable and before irreversible complications occur. Early identification of these patients is essential to allow time to find a suitable donor organ to give the best possible long-term outcome for the patient.

The etiology of acute liver failure is a major determinant of likelihood of recovery with supportive management and without the need for liver transplantation. Patients with acetaminophen hepatotoxicity, fulminant hepatitis A, and pregnancy-related liver disease demonstrate much the best survival rates (>50–90%), whereas patients with non-A, non-B hepatitis, idiosyncratic drug reactions, or Wilson's having the worst survival rates (<10–20%) [7]. The grade of hepatic encephalopathy is an important predictor of outcome, with poor survival rates associated with grade 3 and grade 4 hepatic encephalopathy. Contraindications to liver transplantation are listed in Table 26.4.

The most widely used prognostic tool is the King's College Criteria (Table 26.5), first introduced in 1989 [17]. Subsequent meta-analyses have shown these criteria to have a specificity of 82–92%, but sensitivity of 68–69% [15]. It is important therefore that all patients with a deteriorating clinical picture have the possibility of transplant considered. Further markers of a poor clinical outcome including the addition of serum lactate to Kings criteria, the Model for End-Stage Liver Disease (MELD score), and other clinical algorithms have not as yet been shown to be superior to the Kings criteria in the identification of patients for transplantation.

Liver transplantation is a proven therapy for patients with fulminant hepatic failure. In a retrospective study from the US of 295 patients with acute liver failure, 41% underwent liver transplantation, 25% recovered with

Table 26.4 Relative and complete contraindications to liver transplantation.

Advanced cardiopulmonary disease or other significant comorbid conditions
Substance abuse (chronic alcohol or drug use)
Uncontrolled sepsis
Widespread thrombosis of portal and mesenteric veins
Irreversible brain damage
Improving hepatic function
Poorly controlled psychiatric disease
Inadequate patient home/family support network

Source: Adapted from Lee et al. 2012 [15].

Table 26.5 Criteria of king's college, london.

Acetaminophen patients
pH <7.30
or
Prothrombin time >100s (INR>6.5) and serum creatinine >300 µmol/L (>3.4 mg/dL) in patients with encephalopathy
(Patients with arterial lactate >3.0 mmol/L after fluid resuscitation should be considered for transplant)
Non-acetaminophen patients
Prothrombin time >100s (INR>6.5)
or
Any 3 of the following variables:
Etiology: non-A, non-B hepatitis or drug reaction
Age <10 or >40 years
Duration of jaundice before encephalopathy >7 days
Serum bilirubin >300 µmol/L (>17 mg/dL)
Prothrombin time >50 s (INR>3.5)

Source: O'Grady et al. 1989 [17]. Reproduced with permission of Elsevier Health Science.

supportive therapy and 34% did not survive. The 1-year survival rate following liver transplantation was 76%. Survival following emergency liver transplantation has increased due to improvements in surgical procedures, more effective immunosuppressive drugs, and a multidisciplinary approach to the intensive care management.

Given the shortage of organ donors in some societies, marginal donors may be considered for emergency liver transplants and alternative procedures considered:

- *Steatotic livers* – Livers with a degree of fat content that would not normally be considered ideal.
- *Non-heart beating donors* – Increased risk of anastamotic vascular and biliary strictures in organs with prolonged ischemia.
- *ABO Incompatible livers* – Can be used in emergencies but data shows that graft survival is only 32% at one year compared with 49% for unmatched compatible grafts and 54% for matched grafts [18].
- *Living donor liver transplants* – Increasingly being used in western societies. Data from Japan where the procedure is commonplace suggest a 10 year survival of 73% [19].
- *Auxiliary orthotopic liver transplant* – This new concept involves the replacement of a patient's right lobe while leaving their own left lobe *in situ*. The native left lobe can hypertrophy in time, regaining enough function to allow immunosuppression to cease and the transplanted right lobe to atrophy. Initial studies

suggest that this procedure will benefit those patients with hyperacute liver injury such as acetaminophen-induced liver failure, where recovery of the damaged liver is expected. Diseases with subacute presentations are more likely to heal with fibrosis and are not good candidates for auxiliary transplantation.

- *Two stage liver transplantation* – In cases of fulminant liver failure with severe perioperative instability, the decision may be made to render the patient anhepatic and form a portocaval shunt. Once the patient has been stabilized and a suitable donor found then the completion of the transplant can occur. This procedure has been reported in isolated case reports and case series [20].
- *Liver support devices* – Over the last 20 years there has been much research into developing models for artificial (albumin/sorbent based) or bioartificial (pig liver cells) liver support devices. At present there is little hard evidence to suggest that these devices can be used as a bridge to recovery, or that they affect patient outcomes. Their main use at present is as a bridge to liver transplantation [15].

The use of corticosteroids, insulin, glucagon, prostaglandin analogs, repeated exchange transfusions, plasmapheresis, total body washout, and hemoperfusion through isolated primate livers remains experimental, with no proven clinical benefit in patients with fulminant hepatic failure. Future considerations must focus on developing prognostic scores and/or biomarkers that will more accurately select those patients who will benefit from a liver transplant from those that will be able to make a transplant free recovery with adequate supportive therapy.

In managing patients with acute liver failure it is important to closely monitor serial changes in the prognostic predictors and overall clinical status. It is crucial to establish the need for liver transplantation prior to the onset of grade 4 hepatic encephalopathy, cerebral edema, and multiorgan failure. In the era of donor shortage and increasing demand for liver transplantation, prudent utilization of liver transplantation in the setting of acute liver failure is necessary.

Acknowledgment

We are grateful to the previous authors of this chapter Aijaz Ahmed and Emmet B. Keeffe.

References

1. Lee WM. Recent developments in acute liver failure. Best Pract. Res. Clin. Gastroenterol. 2012;**26**(1):3–16.

2. Trey C, Davidson CS. The management of fulminant hepatic failure. Prog. Liver Dis. 1970;**3**:282–98.

3. Gimson AE, White YS, Eddleston AL, Williams R. Clinical and prognostic differences in fulminant hepatitis type A, B and non-A non-B. Gut 1983;**24**(12):1194–8.

4. Bernuau J, Rueff B, Benhamou JP. Fulminant and subfulminant liver failure: definitions and causes. Semin. Liver Dis. 1986;**6**(2):97–106.

5. O'Grady JG, Schalm SW, Williams R. Acute liver failure: redefining the syndromes. Lancet 1993;**342**(8866):273–5.

6. Bernal W, Hyyrylainen A, Gera A, et al. Lessons from lookback in acute liver failure? A single centre experience of 3300 patients. J Hepatol. 2013;**59**(1):74–80.

7. Lee WM. Acute liver failure. N. Engl. J. Med. 1993;**329**(25):1862–72.

8. Acharya SK, Dasarathy S, Kumer TL, et al. Fulminant hepatitis in a tropical population: clinical course, cause, and early predictors of outcome. Hepatology 1996;**23**(6):1448–55.

9. Keeffe EB. Acute liver failure. In *Current Diagnosis and Treatment in Gastroenterology*, F.S. McQuaid KR, Grendell JH (eds). Large Medical Books/McGraw-Hill: New York, 2003: 536–45.

10. Keeffe EB. Acute hepatitis A and B in patients with chronic liver disease: prevention through vaccination. Am. J. Med. 2005;**118**(Suppl 10A):21S–27S.

11. Korman JD, Volenberg I, Balko J, et al. liver failure: a comparison of currently available diagnostic tests. Hepatology 2008;**48**(4):1167–74.

12. Bernal W, Hall C, Karvellas CJ, Auzinger G, Sizer E, Wendon J. Arterial ammonia and clinical risk factors for encephalopathy and intracranial hypertension in acute liver failure. Hepatology 2007;**46**(6):1844–52.

13. Bernal W, Wendon J. Liver transplantation in adults with acute liver failure. J. Hepatol. 2004;**40**(2):192–7.

14. Vaquero J, Fontana RJ, Larson AM, et al. Complications and use of intracranial pressure monitoring in patients with acute liver failure and severe encephalopathy. Liver Transpl. 2005;**11**(12):1581–9.

15. Lee WM, Stravitz RT, Larson AM. Introduction to the revised American Association for the Study of Liver Diseases Position Paper on acute liver failure 2011. Hepatology 2012;**55**(3):965–7.

16. Agarwal B, Wright G, Gatt A, et al . Evaluation of coagulation abnormalities in acute liver failure. J. Hepatol. 2012;**57**(4):780–6.

17. O'Grady JG, Alexander GJ, Hayllar KM, Williams R. Early indicators of prognosis in fulminant hepatic failure. Gastroenterology 1989;**97**(2):439–45.

18. O'Grady J. Liver transplantation for acute liver failure. Best Pract. Res. Clin. Gastroenterol. 2012;**26**(1):27–33.

19. Yamashiki N, Sugawara Y, Tamura S, et al. Outcomes after living donor liver transplantation for acute liver failure in Japan: results of a nationwide survey. Liver Transpl. 2012;**18**(9):1069–77.

20. Montalti R, Busani S, Masetti M, et al. Two-stage liver transplantation: an effective procedure in urgent conditions. Clin Transplant. 2010;**24**(1):122–6.

21. Cash WJ, McConville P, McDermott E, McCormick PA, Callender ME, McDougall NI. Current concepts in the assessment and treatment of hepatic encephalopathy. Q. J. Med. 2010;**103**(1):9–16.

CHAPTER 27

Ascites and spontaneous bacterial peritonitis

Andrés Cárdenas,[1] Isabel Graupera,[2] and Pere Ginès[3]

[1] GI Unit, Institute of Digestive Diseases, Hospital Clinic, IDIBAPS, University of Barcelona, Barcelona, Spain
[2] Institut de Malalties Digestives i Metabolisme, Hospital Clinic, IDIBAPS, University of Barcelona, Barcelona, Spain
[3] Liver Unit, Institute of Digestive Diseases Hospital Clinic, IDIBAPS, Professor of Medicine, University of Barcelona, Spain

Introduction

Ascites is a common presenting sign in patients with various gastroenterological disorders. The most common cause of ascites is portal hypertension secondary to cirrhosis, which accounts for over 80% of patients with ascites [1]. Malignancy, congestive heart failure, tuberculosis, peritoneal diseases, and other causes are the etiology of ascites in approximately 20% of cases. The development of ascites is a major complication of cirrhosis associated with an impaired quality of life and decreased survival. Nearly 60% of patients with compensated cirrhosis develop ascites within a period of 10 years after diagnosis of the disease [2]. The development of ascites in cirrhosis is associated with a probability of survival of 85% at 1 year and 56% at 5 years [3]. Patients with cirrhosis and ascites are at a risk of developing complications associated with a poor prognosis such as dilutional hyponatremia, refractory ascites, spontaneous bacterial peritonitis (SBP), and/or hepatorenal syndrome (HRS) and as a result should always be considered for liver transplantation [4]. This chapter will discuss the management of ascites and in the setting of cirrhosis.

Pathophysiology of ascites in cirrhosis

Patients with advanced cirrhosis and portal hypertension develop an inability to maintain extracellular fluid volume within normal limits, which leads to the accumulation of fluid in the peritoneal and/or pleural cavities and interstitial tissue [5, 6]. The main cause of fluid accumulation is an abnormal increase in kidney sodium reabsorption. Patients with cirrhosis and portal hypertension develop splanchnic vasodilation likely secondary to local production and release of vasodilator factors such as nitric oxide, endocannabinoids, carbon monoxide, and glucagon among others [6]. With disease progression, vasodilatation of the splanchnic tree becomes so pronounced the total effective arterial blood volume decreases and systemic arterial pressure falls. The resulting compensatory response to this phenomenon is a homeostatic activation of vasoconstrictor and antinatriuretic factors (norepinephrine, renin–angiotensin, and vasopressin) triggered to compensate the relative arterial under filling described above, which leads to avid sodium and fluid retention. The pathogenesis of SBP involves passage of bacteria from the intestinal lumen to the systemic circulation through translocation of bacteria to mesenteric lymph nodes, bacteremia secondary to the impairment of the reticuloendothelial system phagocytic activity, and infection due to poor opsonization and defective bactericidal activity of ascitic fluid. A detailed review of the pathogenesis of ascites and SBP in cirrhosis is beyond the scope of this chapter and can be found elsewhere [7].

Clinical presentation of ascites and diagnosis

Clinical features

The main clinical symptom of patients with ascites is abdominal distension often accompanied by lower extremity edema. Some patients presenting with tense

---

Gastrointestinal Emergencies, Third Edition. Edited by Tony C. K. Tham, John S. A. Collins, and Roy Soetikno.

ascites have difficulty breathing and limited physical activity. Ascites usually develops slowly over the course of several weeks or months and in the initial stages, patients are asymptomatic. However, worsening liver disease, portal vein thrombosis, kidney failure due to parenchymal renal diseases, and development of hepatocellular carcinoma with tumor invasion of the portal vein may also precipitate the development of ascites. In severe alcoholic hepatitis, ascites may appear rapidly but in most cases there is resolution following therapy and abstinence. Dyspnea may also occur as a consequence of accompanying pleural effusions. Patients with SBP can present with fever, chills, abdominal pain, hepatic encephalopathy, and rebound abdominal tenderness. However, SBP may be asymptomatic in early stages or present with very few symptoms.

Other common manifestations of patients with ascites include fatigue, weakness, malnutrition, and jaundice. Abdominal hernias due to increased intra-abdominal pressure may occur in patients with cirrhosis and long-standing ascites [8]. Umbilical hernias may increase in size in untreated ascites and sometimes cause significant complications such as rupture and infection due to previous ulcer formation on the surface and delayed wound healing. Inguinal hernias can also be problematic in patients with ascites. Painful gynecomastia may occur in patients with cirrhosis and ascites either due to estrogen excess or the estrogenic effects of spironolactone, a diuretic commonly used in these patients.

It is considered that patients must have approximately 1.5 L of fluid for ascites to be detected reliably by physical examination [9]. The current classification of ascites defined by the International Ascites Club divides patients in three groups [10]. Patients with grade 1 ascites are those in whom ascites is detected only by ultrasonography. Patients with grade 2 ascites are those in which ascites causes moderate distension of the abdomen associated with mild/moderate discomfort. Patients with grade 3 ascites have large amounts of ascitic fluid causing marked abdominal distension and associated with significant discomfort. Patients with refractory ascites are those that do not respond to high doses of diuretics or develop side effects that preclude their use.

Evaluation

The evaluation of a cirrhotic patient either in the emergency room or in the hospital ward must include a detailed clinical history paying special attention to the use of drugs such as non-steroidal anti-inflammatory agents (NSAIDs) that could increment the risk of further sodium retention and development of ascites or impairment of kidney function, physical exam and standard hematology, electrolyte, kidney (serum creatinine and blood urea nitrogen), coagulation (prothombin time or International Normalized Ratio, INR), and liver tests (aminotransferases, bilirubin, albumin, total protein, alkaline phosphatase) [11]. An abdominal ultrasonography to rule out hepatocellular carcinoma and evaluate the patency of the portal venous system should always be performed [11, 12]. In addition, an upper gastrointestinal endoscopy to assess the presence and characteristics of esophageal and/or gastric varices is recommended [11]. In patients with kidney failure (serum creatinine greater than 1.5 mg/dL), urine sediment and 24-hour urine protein should be assessed and the kidneys examined by ultrasonography. Evaluation of circulatory function should include measurement of arterial pressure and heart rate. A checklist of tests that need to be performed in patients with cirrhosis and ascites is described in Table 27.1.

Table 27.1 Initial evaluation of patients with cirrhosis and ascites.

Checklist

1. Admission to the hospital: patients presenting with the first episode of ascites, those with known ascites and fever, abdominal pain, gastrointestinal bleeding, hepatic encephalopathy, hypotension or kidney failure
2. Anamnesis: check out for drugs that facilitate sodium retention (NSAIDs).
3. Monitor arterial pressure, pulse, intake and outtake, urine volume and daily weight.
4. Standard hematology, coagulation, liver tests and alpha-fetoprotein.
5. *Evaluation of ascitic fluid*
   a. Total protein and albumin measurement
   b. Cell count
   c. Culture in blood culture bottles
6. *Evaluation of kidney function**
   a. 24-h urine sodium
   b. Serum electrolytes, serum blood urea nitrogen and serum creatinine
   c. Urine sediment and protein excretion
7. Abdominal ultrasonography and Doppler flow (including the kidneys).
8. Upper gastrointestinal endoscopy to assess the presence of esophageal or gastric varices.

NSAID, non-steroidal anti-inflammatory drug.
*Kidney function should initially be assessed with the patient maintained on a low-sodium diet without diuretic therapy.

Ascitic fluid analysis

The technique for performing paracentesis has been described elsewhere [13, 14]. The risk of bleeding in cirrhotic patients when performing a paracentesis is extremely low; the frequency of severe hemorrhage after a tap is approximately 0.20% and a lethal outcome occurs is less than 0.01% of cases [15]. Most clinical trials assessing large volume paracentesis in patients with cirrhosis and ascites have excluded patients with an elevated prothrombin time >21 seconds or INR >1.6 or platelet count <50 000/μL. Therefore the risk of bleeding complications in patients with more severe coagulopathy is unknown and deserves investigation. Nonetheless consensus meetings, guidelines and expert opinion consider that the abnormal coagulation profile of the cirrhotic patient (mild prolonged prothrombin time and low platelets with a value <50 000/μL) is not an absolute contraindication for paracentesis and the routine administration of platelets or fresh frozen plasma as prophylaxis for bleeding is not recommended [12–14, 16, 17]. In a survey of the use of coagulation products in performing a paracentesis in patients with cirrhosis among practitioners, 50% indicated that they either never used prophylaxis or only used it if the INR of the patient was >2.5 [17]. In patients with severe thrombocytopenia with a platelet count < 40,000 per μL some authors recommend the administration of platelets, although the risk of bleeding in this situation has not been specifically assessed [16]. Patients with suspected disseminated intravascular coagulopathy should not undergo a paracentesis [12].

A diagnostic paracentesis (30 mL of fluid) is required in all patients presenting with their first episode of ascites and in those requiring hospitalization with any evidence of clinical deterioration such as fever, abdominal pain, gastrointestinal bleeding, hepatic encephalopathy, hypotension, or kidney failure. The ascitic fluid in cirrhotics is mostly transparent and yellow/amber in color. Necessary tests in the ascitic fluid include cell count, albumin, total protein, and cultures in blood culture bottles (10 mL of fluid injected at the bedside) [10–12, 16]. Glucose, lactate dehydrogenase (LDH), amylase, bilirubin, triglyceride, tuberculosis smear, and cytological analysis of the fluid are optional and may provide important information in the differential diagnosis of ascites in selected cases.

Patients with cirrhosis and ascites for the most part have a low total ascitic fluid protein; the vast majority have a protein concentration in ascitic fluid <15 g/L. A low protein concentration in ascitic fluid (<15 g/L) is associated with an increased risk of SBP [18, 19]. Selected patients with low ascitic fluid protein should be given prophylaxis with oral quinolones to reduce the risk of SBP and HRS (see later sections). The difference between serum albumin concentration and ascites albumin concentration (serum–ascites albumin gradient) in patients with cirrhosis and ascites is usually >11 g/L; values <11 g/L suggest a cause of ascites other than cirrhosis [12].

The cell count is the most helpful test in determining SBP. In most cases the ascitic fluid white blood cell count is <500/mm³ with a predominance of mononuclear cells (>75%) and a low number of neutrophils. An increased number of white blood cells with predominance of neutrophils indicates peritoneal infection. The diagnosis of SBP is made when the fluid sample has >250/mm³ neutrophils [20]. Reagent strips (that identify leukocytes by detecting esterase activity via colorimetric reaction) have been proposed as a useful technique for the rapid diagnosis of peritoneal fluid infection in the emergency department [21]. However, a recent review [22] has shown up that reagent strips have low sensitivity and a high risk of false negative results and thus cannot be recommended for the rapid diagnosis of SBP. Bloody ascites (>50 000 red blood cells/mm³), which may occur due to a traumatic tap or underlying hepatocellular carcinoma, may lead to a higher neutrophil count in the absence of infection; in this case a correction factor of 1 neutrophil per 250 red blood cells is recommended [20]. Although patients with SBP may develop a systemic inflammatory response syndrome, the classic criteria of this syndrome and serum C-reactive protein and procalcitonin levels have a suboptimal diagnostic accuracy in patients with cirrhosis. The cutoff values proposed for the diagnosis of infection in patients with advanced cirrhosis are 2 mg/dL for C-reactive protein (lower than that recommended in the general population) and 0.5 ng/mL for procalcitonin.

The distinction of secondary bacterial peritonitis (peritoneal infection arising from gut perforation or inflammation of intra-abdominal organs) from SBP is critical as mortality in the former is extremely high without surgical intervention. On the other hand, mortality is near 80% if a patient with advanced liver disease and SBP is subjected to an unnecessary exploratory laparotomy [23]. Patients with secondary bacterial peritonitis usually have a clinical picture of severe abdominal pain, fever, and a rigid abdomen and therefore an abdominal computerized tomography (CT) scan or ultrasonography should be performed. A multimicrobial positive ascitic fluid culture or a reduction in ascitic fluid neutrophil count of less than 25% of the pretreatment value after 2 days of antibiotic treatment suggests failure to respond to therapy and should raise the suspicion of secondary peritonitis. Patients with secondary bacterial peritonitis from gastrointestinal perforation can also have an elevation of the ascitic fluid total protein to levels >10 g/L, glucose <50 mg/dL, and LDH >225 mU/mL [24]. Also an ascitic fluid carcinoembryonic antigen >5 ng/mL or an ascitic fluid alkaline phosphatase >240 units/L have been proposed as accurate markers in detecting gut perforation into the ascitic fluid [25].

Treatment of ascites

Evaluation for liver transplantation

Figure 27.1 outlines the different treatment modalities applicable to patients with cirrhosis and ascites. After the initial evaluation described above, the most important aspect of the management of all patients with cirrhosis and ascites is an evaluation for possible liver transplantation. Most patients with cirrhosis and ascites have advanced liver disease with high Child–Pugh scores (>10 points). Patients with an elevated serum bilirubin level, an elevated prothrombin time, and a low serum albumin level have an impaired liver function that is associated with a poor prognosis without liver transplantation. Other important factors indicating a poor prognosis in cirrhosis with ascites are those related with kidney and circulatory function. These include dilutional hyponatremia (serum sodium <130 mEq/L), low arterial blood pressure, serum creatinine >1.2 mg/dL, and intense sodium retention (urine sodium less than 10 mEq/day) [26]. Patients with any of these abnormalities should be evaluated as potential candidates for liver transplantation as they have a poor outcome. Allocation for liver transplantation in some countries is based on the Model for End-Stage Liver disease (MELD) score that includes serum bilirubin, serum creatinine, and the INR as variables [27]. This scoring system is objective, includes a parameter of kidney function, and predicts survival in cirrhotics. In patients with cirrhosis and ascites the MELD score is

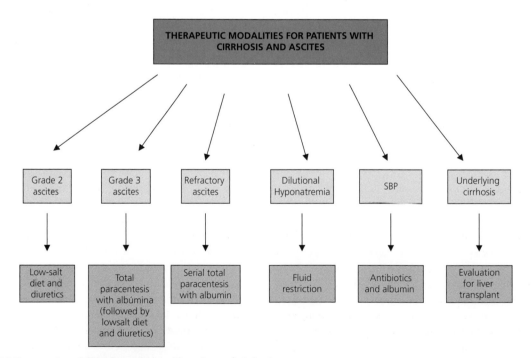

Fig. 27.1 Treatment modalities for patients with ascites and cirrhosis.

also predictive of survival and might be a reliable parameter that helps calculate risk in these patients.

Sodium restriction and nutritional recommendations

A reduction in sodium intake alone achieves a negative sodium balance in approximately 10% of patients. A low sodium diet with 80–90 mmol/day is recommended because a more severe restriction is usually unpalatable [10–12]. Patients with dilutional hyponatremia (serum sodium level <130 mEq/L) need fluid restriction of 1.5 L per day; however, this measure usually is ineffective but may prevent serum sodium levels dropping further. An evaluation by a nutritionist is recommended for appropriate education regarding an appropriate caloric and salt intake. Improvement of the nutritional status is extremely important because patients with advanced liver disease have decreased intake and absorption of nutrients, increased energy expenditure and altered fuel metabolism with an accelerated starvation metabolism [28, 29]. Nutritional therapy in cirrhotic patients can improve nutritional status, reduce infection rates, and decrease morbidity [28, 29]. It is also recommended that nutritional therapy be instituted for long periods of time or until patients reach liver transplantation. The goal is for nutritional supplementation to correct the underlying protein energy malnutrition. In extreme cases of malnutrition, enteral nutrition in cirrhotic patients with ascites may improve liver function and hepatic encephalopathy [28–31]. There is limited data that suggests that enteral feeding in decompensated cirrhosis is more effective than a conventional diet in improving liver function and survival [31].

Uncomplicated ascites

Patients with *Grade 1* ascites do not require any specific treatment, but should be advised of avoiding foods with high sodium content. Patients with *Grade 2* ascites should be treated with a low-sodium diet and diuretics [11]. The best initial regimen for reducing ascites is spironolactone (initial doses 50 to 100 mg/day), a drug that inhibits sodium reabsorption by binding to the mineralocorticoid receptor in the renal collecting tubules, thus blocking the effects of aldosterone. Furosemide (initial doses 20 to 40 mg/day) is useful in patients with concomitant peripheral edema or anasarca. Spironolactone alone may be used up to a dose of 400 mg/day in patients not responding to lower doses and furosemide

subsequently added up to 160 mg/day in progressively increasing doses [16, 32]. In patients that do not respond, compliance with the low sodium diet and the diuretics should be confirmed, afterwards the dose may be increased every 5–7 days. Spironolactone may cause painful gynecomastia in some patients and tamoxifen (20 mg p.o. bid) has been used in the management of this complication with some success [33]. Muscle cramps due to diuretic therapy may require a reduction in diuretic dosage. Quinidine (quinidine sulfate, 400 mg/day) [34] and intravenous albumin administration (25 g/week) [35] have been reported to reduce the frequency and intensity of muscle cramps in cirrhotic patients with ascites treated with diuretics but data on this approach is limited. The goal of treatment with diuretics in patients with ascites is to produce an average weight loss of 0.5 kg/day in patients without edema and 1 kg/day in those with peripheral edema.

Large volume paracentesis is the treatment of choice in the management of Grade 3 ascites [10–13, 16, 36]. Complete removal of ascites in one tap with intravenous albumin (8 g/L tapped) has been shown to be a fast and effective measure in controlling tense ascites and associated with a lower number of complications than conventional diuretic therapy [36]. A post-paracentesis circulatory dysfunction may develop after a large tap; this is a circulatory derangement that is accompanied by activation of the renin-angiotensin system that occurs few days after the procedure [36, 37]. This disorder although silent, may be associated with hyponatremia, kidney impairment, and decreased survival. It may be effectively prevented with the administration of plasma expanders particularly albumin [38, 39, 42]. When less than 5 L of ascites are removed, artificial plasma expanders, saline and albumin are equally effective [39–41]. However, if more than 5 L are removed, albumin is recommended [39–41]. Since in virtually all patients ascites will recur after a paracentesis ascites, they need to be started or continued on spironolactone in order to prevent a positive sodium balance and recurrence of ascites (43, 42). Recommendations for the management of ascites are summarized in Table 27.2.

Refractory ascites

The definition and diagnostic criteria of refractory ascites are listed in Table 27.3 [44]. The vast majority of patients with refractory ascites have very intense sodium retention and a severely impaired capacity to

Table 27.2 Management practice points in patients with ascites and cirrhosis (all patients must be evaluated for liver transplantation).

A. Treatment strategy for patients with cirrhosis and grade 2 ascites

Start with a low-sodium diet (90 mmol/day) and spironolactone (50–100 mg/day) to reach goal of weight loss: 500 g/day or 1000 g/day if edema is present. If needed, doses to be increased every 7 days up to 400 mg/day of spironolactone. Furosemide can be added at a starting dose of 40 mg/day and subsequently increased to 160 mg/day in patients not responding to lower doses with peripheral edema and anasarca.

B. Treatment strategy for patients with cirrhosis and grade 3 ascites

Large-volume paracentesis plus intravenous albumin (8 g/L of ascites removed) followed by a low-sodium diet (90 mmol/day) and diuretics if patient tolerated them beforehand.

C. Treatment strategy for patients with cirrhosis and refractory ascites

Large-volume paracentesis plus intravenous albumin can be performed as needed.

Consider use of TIPSS in patients with very frequent recurrent ascites and preserved hepatic function, loculated ascites, aged <70 years, and no hepatic encephalopathy.

Table 27.3 Definition and diagnostic criteria of refractory ascites in cirrhosis.

Diuretic-resistant ascites: Ascites that cannot be mobilized or the early recurrence of which cannot be prevented because of a lack of response to sodium restriction and diuretic treatment.

Diuretic-intractable ascites: Ascites that cannot be mobilized or the early recurrence of which cannot be prevented because of the development of diuretic-induced complications that preclude the use of an effective diuretic dosage

Requisites:

1. Treatment duration: Patients must be on intensive diuretic therapy (spironolactone 400 mg/day and furosemide 160 mg/day) for at least 1 week and on a salt-restricted diet of less than 90 mmol /day
2. Lack of response: Mean weight loss of <0.8 kg over 4 days and urinary sodium output less than the sodium intake.
3. Early ascites recurrence: Reappearance of grade 2 or 3 ascites within 4 weeks of initial mobilization.
4. Diuretic-induced complications: Diuretic-induced hepatic encephalopathy is the development of encephalopathy in the absence of any other precipitating factor. Diuretic-induced kidney impairment is an increase of serum creatinine by >100% to a value >2 mg/dL in patients with ascites responding to treatment. Diuretic-induced hyponatremia is defined as a decrease of serum sodium by >10 mmol/L to a serum sodium of <125 mmol/L. Diuretic induced hypo- or hyperkalemia is defined as a change in serum potassium to <3 mmol/L or > 6 mmol/L despite appropriate measures.

Source: Adapted from Moore KP, Wong F, Ginès P, et al. The management of ascites in cirrhosis: report on the consensus conference of the International Ascites Club. Hepatology. 2003;38:258–66. Reproduced with permission of John Wiley & Sons Ltd.

excrete solute-free water, the latter resulting in dilutional hyponatremia [44]. Moreover, most patients have a reduction in renal plasma flow and glomerular filtration rate. The main difference with non-refractory ascites is that sodium excretion may be increased with the use of diuretics, whereas in refractory ascites, sodium retention cannot be treated with diuretics either because patients do not respond to high doses or they develop side effects that preclude their use.

Current treatment strategies include repeated large volume paracentesis plus intravenous albumin or the use of a transjugular intrahepatic portosystemic shunt (TIPSS). TIPSS is a non-surgical method of portal decompression that consists of the insertion of an intrahepatic stent between one hepatic vein and the portal vein using a transjugular approach [45]. Reduction in portal pressure is accompanied by a resolution of ascites in most patients. This method is very effective for reducing ascites but might be associated with several side effects such as the development of hepatic encephalopathy and obstruction of the prosthesis.

Large volume paracentesis with albumin is the recommended therapy for refractory ascites [46]. Patients generally require a tap every 2 to 4 weeks which can be performed in an outpatient setting. This approach is therefore easy to perform and relatively inexpensive. Uncovered TIPSS are very effective in relieving ascites, but frequently complicated by obstruction of the prosthesis (70% in 1 year) [45]. Polytetrafluoroethylene-covered prostheses seem to improve TIPSS patency and decrease the number of clinical relapses and reinterventions without increasing the risk of encephalopathy [47]. Randomized clinical trials comparing TIPSS vs. repeated large volume paracentesis with albumin demonstrate that TIPSS controls ascites effectively and is associated with a lower rate of ascites recurrence [46, 48–51]. In addition patients with ascites that undergo TIPSS improve their nutritional status as measured by resting energy expenditure, total body nitrogen, body fat and food intake [52]. Hepatic encephalopathy occurs in approximately 30–50% of patients [46, 49, 50]. Two studies showed a survival benefit with TIPS [49, 51], but two other studies demonstrated no difference in survival [46, 50]. Meta-analyses of these randomized controlled studies conclude that TIPSS is better at controlling ascites but survival is not significantly different [53-55]. For the above reasons large-volume paracentesis is recommended as the initial treatment of choice in patients with refractory ascites [46, 56]. TIPSS placement may be considered for patients with very rapid recurrence of ascites and preserved liver function (usually Child-Pugh score <13, MELD score <18), loculated ascites, age <70, without hepatic encephalopathy or cardiopulmonary disease [55, 56]. Recommendations for the management of refractory ascites are summarized in Table 27.2.

Treatment and prophylaxis of SBP

SBP and urinary infections are the most frequent infections in patients with cirrhosis and ascites; other infections include by pneumonia, cellulitis, and bacteremia [57]. Approximately 30% of bacterial infections are community-acquired, 30% are health care-associated (HCA), and 35% to 40% are nosocomial [57]. Clinical risk factors include poor liver function, variceal bleeding, low protein ascites, and prior episodes of SBP. SBP is characterized by a monomicrobial infection of ascitic fluid in the absence of any intra-abdominal source of infection [20, 58]. The prevalence of SBP in hospitalized cirrhotic patients ranges between 10–30% [58]. Historically, Gram-negative bacteria were responsible for nearly 80% of cases with *Escherichia coli* accounting for most of them, but the epidemiologic pattern of SBP has experimented drastic changes over past two decades. The increasing presence of Gram-positive bacteria (mostly *Streptococcus viridans*, *Staphylococcus aureus*, and *Enterococcus faecalis*), in part as a consequence of invasive procedures during hospitalization, is one of them [59]. The second and most important is the alarming increase of infections caused by multi-resistant bacteria in cirrhosis [60]. The most common are extended-spectrum β-lactamase–producing Enterobacteriaceae, non-fermentable Gram-negative bacilli (i.e. *Pseudomonas aeruginosa*), methicillin-resistant *Staphylococcus aureus* (MRSA), vancomycin-susceptible *Enterococcus* (VSE), and vancomycin-resistant *Enterococcus* (VRE). Although resistance varies among different geographical areas, these multi-resistant bacteria are more frequently

isolated in nosocomial infections (35%–39%) compared with health care-associated (HCA) (14–20%) or community-acquired episodes (0–4%). Main risk factors for multiresistant bacterial infections are nosocomial acquisition of infection, long-term norfloxacin prophylaxis, treatment with β-lactams within the last 3 months and infection by multiresistant bacteria in the last 6 months [60]. Infections by multi-resistant bacteria not only diminish the efficacy of current first-line empiric regimens but also increases treatment failures of second line therapies [60–64].

The clinical spectrum of SBP is variable and ranges from an asymptomatic presentation to a full-blown picture of peritonitis; therefore the diagnosis relies on a high index of suspicion and prompt examination of the ascitic fluid. Additionally, patients with cirrhosis and sepsis-related infections including SBP may develop adrenal insufficiency in 50–70% of cases [65, 66]. The development of adrenal insufficiency is associated with hemodynamic instability and increased mortality (80% in those with adrenal insufficiency vs. 37% without adrenal insufficiency) [65]. Furthermore in cirrhotic patients with adrenal insufficiency (diagnosed by the short corticotropin test within the first 24 hours of admission) and septic shock, administration of intravenous hydrocortisone (50 mg every 6 hours) helps with the resolution of shock and improves survival in those with advanced Child C cirrhosis [66]. An important clinical feature of SBP is the development of hepatorenal syndrome during the infection as it develops in 30% of patients with SBP, and is a major cause of death [67, 68]. The risk may be decreased with infusion of intravenous albumin [68].

Therapy and prognosis
Antibiotic therapy should be initiated in patients with a neutrophil count in ascitic fluid greater than 250/mm³ before microbiologic results are obtained [20] and then modified according to the results of the culture. Although current guidelines recommend empiric antibiotic therapy with an intravenous third-generation cephalosporin (cefotaxime 2 g every 8–12 hours or ceftriaxone 1 g/24 hours) for 5 days [20, 46], this recommendation does not take into account the risk of multiresistant bacterial infections. The etiology and pattern of SBP mainly depends on the site of acquisition of the infection. In community acquired infection, Gram negative bacteria still are the main cause and the empiric

regimens with third-generation cephalosporins achieve the resolution of infection in the vast majority of cases [60]. In nosocomial infections multi-resistant bacteria are responsible for 30–40% of cases [60]. Although current empiric regimens are a good option for community acquired SBP, in nosocomial SBP empiric treatment should be adapted according to local patterns of resistance. In areas with a high prevalence of Enterobacteriaceae-producing Enterobacteriaceae, carbapenems are recommended in combination with antibiotics active against VSE/VRE and MRSA (i.e. glycopeptide, linezolid, or daptomycin) [69].

Assessment of response to therapy includes not only daily clinical evaluation but a repeat diagnostic paracentesis 2–3 days after beginning antibiotics. In case of treatment failure (worsening infection or no decrease in polymorphonuclear cell count), antibiotic therapy should be revised and appropriately changed. Despite achieving resolution of the infection with antibiotic treatment, hospital mortality remains between 10–30%, because most of these patients have advanced liver failure and complications like gastrointestinal bleeding, kidney failure, and hepatic encephalopathy.

The most important predictor of survival in patients with SBP, aside from the resolution of the infection, is the development of hepatorenal syndrome during the infection [67]. Hepatorenal syndrome is triggered by an impairment of circulatory function with activation of vasoconstrictor systems. The administration of albumin at a dose of 1.5 g/kg at the diagnosis of the infection and 1 g/kg 48 hours later prevents hepatorenal syndrome and improves survival in patients with SBP [68]. Recommendations for the management of SBP are summarized in Table 27.4.

Prophylaxis

Unfortunately, life expectancy after an episode of SBP is short, with a 1-year probability of survival of 30–50% if antibiotic prophylaxis is not given [58, 70]. Conditions associated with an increased risk of SBP include: gastrointestinal bleeding, low-protein concentration in ascitic fluid, advanced liver failure (high serum bilirubin and/or markedly prolonged prothrombin time), and past history of SBP. Because most episodes of SBP are caused by Gram-negative bacteria present in the normal intestinal flora, oral quinolones such as norfloxacin or ciprofloxacin have been used as prophylactic agents. The efficacy

Table 27.4 Recommendations for the management and prevention of spontaneous bacterial peritonitis.

Therapy

After diagnosis of peritonitis has been made (>250 neutrophils/mm^3 in ascitic fluid), start with third-generation cephalosporins (i.e. cefotaxime 2 g/8–12 h IV or ceftriaxone 1 g/24 h IV) unless risk factors for multirresistant bacteria are present*.

Infuse albumin (1.5 g/kg at diagnosis of the infection and 1 g/kg 48 hours later).

Maintain antibiotic therapy for at least 5 days or until disappearance of signs of infection. Patients should be evaluated daily to assess signs of infection. A follow-up paracentesis helps evaluate response to therapy.

After resolution of infection, start long-term oral norfloxacin 400 mg/day.

Prevention

1. Patients with gastrointestinal hemorrhage:
   a. Norfloxacin 400 mg/12 h orally or per gastric tube for 7 days in patients with preserved liver function and not actively bleeding.
   b. Intravenous ceftriaxone 1 g/day for 7 days in patients with advanced liver failure and/or actively bleeding.
2. Patients with ascites with a previous episode of SBP
   a. Norfloxacin 400 mg/day indefinitely
   b. Evaluation for liver transplantation
3. Patients with ascites and advanced liver disease** without a previous episode of SBP and low ascitic fluid protein concentration (<15 g/L):
   a. Norfloxacin 400 mg/day indefinitely

---

*Nosocomial acquisition of infection, long-term norfloxacin prophylaxis, B-lactams within the last 3 months.
**Serum bilirubin >3 mg/dL, Child–Pugh score >10, dilutional hyponatremia (serum sodium <130 mEq/L) and/or renal impairment.

of this approach has been demonstrated in patients with gastrointestinal hemorrhage [71–73] and patients who have recovered from the first SBP episode [74] and has been recommended by a panel of experts in an International Consensus Conference on SBP [20].

In patients with gastrointestinal hemorrhage, the short-term administration of norfloxacin or intravenous ceftriaxone reduces the incidence of SBP or bacteremia as compared with patients not receiving prophylactic antibiotics [71–73, 75, 76]. In patients with advanced liver disease who are actively bleeding intravenous ceftriaxone is preferred [75]. Previous meta-analyses indicate that antibiotic prophylaxis in patients with gastrointestinal bleeding not only prevents infection but also improve survival [71, 73]. Long-term norfloxacin administration is effective in the prevention of SBP recurrence (secondary prophylaxis) [74]. Antibiotic prophylaxis also appears to be effective in the prevention of SBP (primary prophylaxis) in patients with low ascitic fluid protein (<15 g/L), who are at high risk of developing the first episode of SBP. Primary prophylaxis with norfloxacin reduces the incidence of SBP, delays the development of HRS and improves survival in patients with advanced cirrhosis [77].

References

1. Cárdenas A, Ginés P, Arroyo V. Ascites. In *Clinical Gastroenterology and Hepatology*, Weinstein W, Hawkey CJ, Bosch J (eds). Elsevier Science: Oxford, 2005: 101–4.

2. Ginès P, Quintero E, Arroyo V, et al. Compensated cirrhosis: natural history and prognostic factors. *Hepatology* 1987;**7**: 122–8.

3. Planas R, Montoliu S, Ballesté B, et al. Natural history of patients hospitalized for management of cirrhotic ascites. *Clin. Gastroenterol. Hepatol.* 2006; **4**:1385–94.

4. Murray KL, Carithers RL. AASLD practice guidelines: Evaluation of the patient for liver transplantation. *Hepatology* 2005;**41**:1407–32.

5. Schrier RW, Arroyo V, Bernardi M, et al. Peripheral arterial vasodilation hypothesis: a proposal for the initiation of renal sodium and water retention in cirrhosis. *Hepatology* 1988;**8**:1151–7.

6. Cárdenas A, Arroyo V. Mechanisms of water and sodium retention in cirrhosis and the pathogenesis of ascites. *Best Pract. Res. Clin. Endocrinol. Metab.* 2003;**17**:607–22.

7. Weist R, Krag A, Gerbes A. Spontaneous bacterial peritonitis: recent guidelines and beyond. *Gut* 2012;**61**: 297–310.

8. Belghiti J, Durand F. Abdominal wall hernias in the setting of cirrhosis. *Semin. Liver Dis.* 1997;**17**:219–26.

9. Cattau EL Jr, Benjamin SB, Knuff TE, Castell DO. The accuracy of the physical exam in the diagnosis of suspected ascites. *JAMA* 1982;**247**:1164–6.

10. Moore KP, Wong F, Ginès P, et al. The management of ascites in cirrhosis: report on the consensus conference of the International Ascites Club. *Hepatology.* 2003;**38**: 258–266.

11. Ginès P, Cárdenas, A, Arroyo V, Rodés J. Management of cirrhosis and ascites. *N. Engl. J. Med.* 2004;**350**:1646–54.

12. Runyon B. Management of adult patients with ascites due to cirrhosis. *Hepatology* 2004;**39**:841–56.

13. Cárdenas A, Guevara M, Ginés P. Paracentesis. In *Clinical Gastroenterology and Hepatology*, Weinstein W, Hawkey CJ, Bosch J (eds). Elsevier Science: Oxford, 2005: 1097–100.

14. Thomsen TW, Shaffer RW, White B, Setnik GS. Videos in clinical medicine. *Paracentesis. N. Engl. J. Med.* 2006;**355**:e21.

15. Pache I, Bilodeau M. Severe haemorrhage following abdominal paracentesis for ascites in patients with liver disease. *Aliment. Pharmacol. Ther.* 2005;**21**:525–9.

16. Moore KP. Aithal GP. Guidelines on the management of ascites in cirrhosis. *Gut* 2006;**55**(Suppl 6):vi1–vi12

17. Caldwell S, Hoffmann M, Lisman B, et al. Coagulation disorders and hemostasis in liver disease: Pathophysiology and critical assessment of current management. *Hepatology* 2006;**44**:1039–46.

18. Runyon BA. Low-protein-concentration ascitic fluid is predisposed to spontaneous bacterial peritonitis. *Gastroenterology* 1986;**91**:1343–6.

19. Llach J, Rimola A, Navasa M, et al: Incidence and predictive factors of first episode of spontaneous bacterial peritonitis in cirrhosis with ascites. Relevance of ascitic fluid protein concentration. *Hepatology* 1992;**16**:742–7.

20. Rimola A, Garcia-Tsao G, Navasa M, et al. Diagnosis, treatment and prophylaxis of spontaneous bacterial peritonitis: a consensus document. *International Ascites Club. J. Hepatol.* 2000;**32**:142–53.

21. Castellote J, López C, Gornals J, et al. Rapid diagnosis of spontaneous bacterial peritonitis by use of reagent strips. *Hepatology* 2003;**37**:893–96.

22. Nguyen Khac E, Caldranel JF Thévenot T, et al. Review article: utility of reagent strips in diagnosis of infected ascites of cirrhotic patients. *Aliment. Pharmacol. Ther.* 2008;**28**:282–8.

23. Garrison RN, Cryer HM, Howard DA, Polk HC Jr. Clarification of risk factors for abdominal operations in patients with hepatic cirrhosis. *Ann. Surg.* 1984;**199**:648–55.

24. Runyon BA, Hoefs JC. Ascitic fluid analysis in the differentiation of spontaneous bacterial peritonitis from gastrointestinal tract perforation into ascitic fluid. *Hepatology* 1984;**4**:447–50.

25. Wu SS, Lin OS, Chen Y-Y, et al. Ascitic fluid carcinoembryonic antigen and alkaline phosphatase levels for the differentiation of primary from secondary bacterial peritonitis with intestinal perforation. *J. Hepatol.* 2001;**34**:215–21.

26. Llach J, Ginès P, Arroyo V, et al: Prognostic value of arterial pressure, endogenous vasoactive systems, and renal function in cirrhotic patients admitted to the hospital for the treatment of ascites. *Gastroenterology* 1988;**94**:482–7.

27. Kamath P, Wiesner R, Malinchoc M, et al. A model to predict survival in patients with end-stage liver disease. *Hepatology.* 2001;**33**:464–70.

28. Henkel AS, Buchman AL. Nutritional support in patients with chronic liver disease. *Nat. Clin. Pract. Gastroenterol. Hepatol.* 2006;**3**:202–9.

29. McCullough AJ. Nutrition and malnutrition in liver disease. In *Therapy of Digestive Disorders*, 2nd edn, Wolfe MM, Davis GL, Farraye F, Giannella RA, Malagelada JR, Steer ML (eds). Saunders: Philadelphia, 2006: 67–83.

30. Kearns PJ, Young H, Garcia G, et al. Accelerated improvement of alcoholic liver disease with enteral nutrition. *Gastroenterology* 1992;**102**:200–5.

31. Cabrè E, Gonzalez-Hux F, Abad-Lacruz A, et al. Effect of total enteral nutrition on the short-term outcome of severely malnourished cirrhotics. A randomized controlled trial. *Gastroenterology* 1990;**98**:715–20.

32. Santos J, Planas R, Pardo A et al: Spironolactone alone or in combination with furosemide in the treatment of moderate ascites in nonazotemic cirrhosis. A randomized comparative study of efficacy and safety. J. *Hepatol.* 2003;**39**: 187–92.

33. Li CP, Lee FY, Hwang SJ, et al. Treatment of mastalgia with tamoxifen in male patients with liver cirrhosis: a randomized crossover study. *Am. J. Gastroenterol.* 2000;**95**:1051–5.

34. Lee FY, Lee SD, Tsai YT, et al: A randomized controlled trial of quinidine in the treatment of cirrhotic patients with muscle cramps. *J. Hepatol.* 1991;**12**:236–40.

35. Angeli P, Albino G, Carraro P, et al. Cirrhosis and muscle cramps: evidence of a causal relationship. *Hepatology* 1996;**23**:264–73.

36. Ginès P, Arroyo V, Quintero E, et al: Comparison of paracentesis and diuretics in the treatment of cirrhotics with tense ascites. Results of a randomized study. *Gastroenterology* 1987;**93**:234–41.

37. Ruiz-del-Arbol L, Monescillo A, Jiménez W, et al. Paracentesis-induced circulatory dysfunction: mechanism and effect on hepatic hemodynamics in cirrhosis. *Gastroenterology* 1997;**113**:579–86.

38. Ginès P, Tito L, Arroyo V, et al. Randomized comparative study of therapeutic paracentesis with and without intravenous albumin in cirrhosis. *Gastroenterology* 1988;**94**: 1493–502.

39. Ginès A, Fernández-Esparrach G, Monescillo A, et al. Randomized trial comparing albumin, dextran 70, and polygeline in cirrhotic patients with ascites treated by paracentesis. *Gastroenterology* 1996;**111**:1002–10.

40. Moreau R, Valla DC, Durand-Zaleski I, et al: Comparison of outcome in patients with cirrhosis and ascites following treatment with albumin or a synthetic colloid: a randomised controlled pilot trail. *Liver Int.* 2006;**26**:46–54.

41. Sola-Vera J, Minana J, Ricart E, et al. Randomized trial comparing albumin and saline in the prevention of paracentesis-induced circulatory dysfunction in cirrhotic patients with ascites. *Hepatology* 2003;**37**:1147–53.

42. Bernardi, M., et al., Albumin infusion in patients undergoing large-volume paracentesis: a meta-analysis of randomized trials. *Hepatology*.2013; **55**(4):1172–81.

43. Fernández-Esparrach G, Guevara M, Sort P, et al: Diuretic requirements after therapeutic paracentesis in non-azotemic patients with cirrhosis. A randomized double-blind trial of spironolactone versus placebo. *J. Hepatol.* 1997;**26**:614–20.

44. Arroyo V, Ginès P, Gerbes A, et al: Definition and diagnostic criteria of refractory ascites and hepatorenal syndrome in cirrhosis. *Hepatology* 1996;**23**:164–76.

45. Boyer TD, Haskal Z. The role of transjugular intrahepatic portosystemic shunt in the management of portal hypertension. *Hepatology* 2005;**41**:386–400.

46. Ginès P,Angeli P, Lenz K, et al. EASL Clinical Practice Guidelines on the management of ascites, spontaneous bacterial peritonitis and hepatorenal syndrome in cirrhosis. *J. Hepatol.* 2010;**53**(3):397–417.

47. Bureau C, García-Pagan JC, Otal P, et al. Improved clinical outcome using polytetrafluoroethylene-coated stents for TIPS: results of a randomized study. *Gastroenterology* 2004;**126**:469–75.

48. Ginès P, Uriz J, Calahorra B, et al. Transjugular intrahepatic portosystemic shunting versus: paracentesis plus albumin for refractory ascites in cirrhosis. *Gastroenterology* 2002;**123**: 1839–47.

49. Rossle M, Ochs A, Gulberg V, et al. A comparison of paracentesis and transjugular intrahepatic portosystemic shunting in patients with ascites. *N. Engl. J. Med.* 2000; **342**:1701–7.

50. Sanyal A, Genning C, Reddy RK, et al. The North American Study for Treatment of Refractory Ascites. *Gastroenterology* 2003;**124**:634–41.

51. Salerno F, Merli M, Riggio O, et al. Randomized controlled study of TIPS versus paracentesis plus albumin in cirrhosis with severe ascites. *Hepatology* 2004;**40**:629–35.

52. Allard JP, Chau J, Sandokji K, Blendis LM, Wong F. Effects of ascites resolution after successful TIPS on nutrition in cirrhotic patients with refractory ascites. *Am. J. Gastroenterol.* 2001;**96**:2442–7.

53. Delterne P, Mathurin P, Dharancy S, et al. Transjugular intrahepatic portosystemic shunt in refractory ascites: a meta-analysis. *Liver Int.* 2005;**25**:349–56

54. Albillos A, Banares R, Gonzales M, et al: A meta-analysis of transjugular intrahepatic portosystemic shunt versus paracentesis for refractory ascites. *J. Hepatol.* 2005;**43**:990–6.

55. Garcia-Tsao, G., The transjugular intrahepatic portosystemic shunt for the management of cirrhotic refractory ascites. *Nat. Clin. Pract. Gastroenterol. Hepatol.* 2006;**3**:380–9.

56. Cárdenas A, Ginès P. Management of refractory ascites. *Clin. Gastroenterol. Hepatol.* 2005;**3**:1187–91.

57. Fernandez J, Acevedo A, Castro M, et al., Prevalence and risk factors of infections by multiresistant bacteria in cirrhosis: a prospective study. *Hepatology.* **55**: 1551–61.

58. Garcia-Tsao G. Bacterial infections in cirrhosis: treatment and prophylaxis. *J. Hepatol.* 2005;**42**(Suppl1):S85–92.

59. Fernándcz J, Navasa M, Gómez J, et al. Bacterial infections in cirrhosis: epidemiological changes with invasive procedures and norfloxacin prophylaxis. *Hepatology* 2002; **35**:140–8.

60. Fernandez J, Acevedo J, Castro M, et al. Prevalence and risk factors of infections by multiresistant bacteria in cirrhosis: a prospective study. *Hepatology* 2012;**55**:1551–61.

61. Depuydt PO, Vandijck DM, Beckaert MA, et al. Determinants and impact of multidrug antibiotic resistance in pathogens causing ventilator-associated-pneumonia. *Crit. Care* 2008;**12**:R142.

62. Angeloni S, Leboffe C, Parente A, et al. Efficacy of current guidelines for the treatment of spontaneous bacterial

peritonitis in the clinical practice. *World J. Gastroenterol.* 2008;**14**(17)1757.

63. Umgelter A, Reindl W, Miedaner M, et al. Failure of current antibiotic first-line regimens and mortality in hospitalized patients with spontaneous bacterial peritonitis. *Infection* 2009;**37**:2–8.

64. Song K, Jeon J, Park W, Oark S, et al. Clinical outcomes of spontaneous bacterial peritonitis due to extended-spectrum beta-lactamase-producing *Escherichia coli* and *Klebsiella* species: A retrospective matched case-control study. *BMC Infect. Dis.* 2009;**9**:41.

65. Tsai MH, Peng YS, Chen YC, et al. Adrenal insufficiency in patients with cirrhosis, severe sepsis and septic shock. *Hepatology* 2006;**43**:673–81.

66. Fernández J, Escorsell A, Zabalza M, et al. Adrenal insufficiency in patients with cirrhosis and septic shock: Effect of treatment with hydrocortisone on survival. *Hepatology* 2006;**4**:1288–95.

67. Follo A, Llovet JM, Navasa M, et al: Renal impairment after spontaneous bacterial peritonitis in cirrhosis: Incidence, clinical course, predictive factors and prognosis. *Hepatology* 1994;**20**:495–501.

68. Sort P, Navasa M, Arroyo V, et al. Effect of intravenous albumin on renal impairment and mortality in patients with cirrhosis and spontaneous bacterial peritonitis. *N. Engl. J. Med.* 1999;**341**:403–09.

69. Fernandez J, Arroyo V. Bacterial infections in cirrhosis: a growing problem with significant implications. *Clin. Liver Dis.* 2013;**2**(3):102–5.

70. Tito L, Rimola A, Ginès P, et al. Recurrence of spontaneous bacterial peritonitis in cirrhosis: frequency and predictive factors. *Hepatology* 1988;**8**:27–31.

71. Bernard B, Grangé JD, Nguyen K, et al. Antibiotics prophylaxis in cirrhotic patients with gastrointestinal bleeding: a meta-analysis. *Hepatology* 1999;**29**:1655–61.

72. Soriano G, Guarner C, Tomás A, et al: Norfloxacin prevents bacterial infection in cirrhotics with gastrointestinal hemorrhage. *Gastroenterology* 1992;**103**:1267–72.

73. Soares-Weiser K, Brezis M, Tur-Kaspa R, Leibovici L. Antibiotic prophylaxis for cirrhotic patients with gastrointestinal bleeding. *Cochrane Database Syst. Rev.* 2002; (**2**):CD002907.

74. Ginès P, Rimola A, Planas R, et al: Norfloxacin prevents spontaneous bacterial peritonitis recurrence in cirrhosis: Results of a double blind, placebo-controlled trial. *Hepatology* 1990;**12**:716–24.

75. Rimola A, Bory F, Terés J, et al. Oral, nonabsorbable antibiotics prevent infection in cirrhotics with gastrointestinal hemorrhage. *Hepatology* 1995;**5**:463–67.

76. Fernández J, Ruiz del Arbol L, Gomez C, et al. Norfloxacin versus ceftriaxone in the prophylaxis of infections in patients with advanced cirrhosis and hemorrhage. *Gastroenterology* 2006;**131**:1049–56.

77. Navasa M, Fernández J, Montoliu S, et al. Randomized, double-blind, placebo, controlled trial evaluating norfloxacin in the primary prophylaxis of spontaneous bacterial peritonitis in cirrhotics with renal impairment, hyponatremia or severe liver failure. *J. Hepatol.* 2006;**44**(suppl 2):114A.

CHAPTER 28

Alcoholic hepatitis

Brian J. Hogan and David W. M. Patch

Royal Free London NHS Foundation Trust, Royal Free Hospital, London, UK

Introduction

While many patients presenting with alcoholic liver disease will have cirrhosis, as many as 60% will have evidence of an alcohol-related hepatitis [1]. For the clinician, the critical point is that alcoholic hepatitis is potentially reversible both clinically and histologically, and those patients who survive the inpatient period, and remain abstinent, may have a dramatic recovery in liver function. However, the short-term mortality of alcoholic hepatitis is particularly high among those with indicators of severe disease: patients with a Maddrey score of ≥32 have a 28-day mortality of 30–40% [2, 3], and the 28-day mortality of patients with a Glasgow alcoholic hepatitis score ≥ 9 is 54% [4] (see later sections). Partly as a consequence, trials have tended to focus on this early period of the patient's care, as it has been assumed this is where there would be greatest impact. However, any such discussion has to be put in the overall context of the patient: the acute management of alcoholic hepatitis cannot be divorced from the prevention of further harmful drinking, and the latter will have an equal if not greater impact on the longer-term mortality and morbidity.

Pathogenesis

Ethanol is metabolized in the liver via two pathways: alcohol dehydrogenase and cytochrome P450 2E1. Both result in acetaldehyde formation, which is highly reactive, and may modify microtubular function as well as

form, putting the hepatocyte under significant oxidant stress. Alcohol also alters gut permeability, which is associated with an increased passage of lipopolysaccharide-endotoxin into portal blood, a combination of these insults is proposed to initiate an inflammatory response. This response involves an endotoxin-like cytokine cascade, characterized by neutrophil infiltration, high levels of nuclear factor κb (NFκb), tumor necrosis factor-α (TNFα), and interleukin-8 (IL8), and is modified between individuals by genetic polymorphisms identified in both CYP450 2E1 and acetaldehyde dehydrogenase, the hepatic enzyme responsible for the metabolism of acetaldehyde. While much of these proposed mechanisms are derived from animal models and evidence for these mechanisms in humans is either absent or, at best, indirect, they have largely provided the rationale for the treatment modalities evaluated thus far. In particular, the four therapies, corticosteroids, pentoxifylline, enteral nutrition and anti-TNFα antibodies, are all directed at various components of the endotoxin–cytokine cascade.

Clinical features

Patients typically present with a history of long-term harmful alcohol use (40–80 units per week), and *often* a preceding period of binging. Because the symptom onset may be relatively acute, the patient will often stop drinking just prior to admission, and indeed blame the continued deterioration in their clinical state on abstinence as opposed to the preceding alcohol use. Symptoms include anorexia, fever, malaise, malnutrition, and the

---

Gastrointestinal Emergencies, Third Edition. Edited by Tony C. K. Tham, John S. A. Collins, and Roy Soetikno.

onset of jaundice/ascites. On examination, the patients are usually jaundiced with stigmata of chronic liver disease, and fever may be present which is rarely >38.5°C. The liver may be enlarged and tender and a bruit may be present. Ascites is common, and the presence of encephalopathy is associated with a poor prognosis.

Biochemical features

Typical features of severe acute alcoholic hepatitis include polymorph leukocytosis and prolonged prothrombin time. Mean corpuscular volume is often increased and marked thrombocytopenia attributable to a direct effect of alcohol on the bone marrow is also recognized. The aspartate transaminase (AST) and alanine transaminase (ALT) are usually only mildly elevated (levels typically remain below 400 U/L (higher levels would suggest additional or other pathology such as viral hepatitis or drug toxicity), and the AST is usually greater than ALT. The serum bilirubin is elevated and can exceed 750 μmol/L (44 mg/dL). Gamma glutamyltransferase and serum immunoglobulin A concentrations are also often increased. Serum ferritin may be very high (above 1000 μg/L), even in the absence of hemochromatosis. The patient's condition, both clinical and biochemical may deteriorate following admission and alcohol withdrawal, suggesting continued inflammatory hepatic insult.

Investigations and diagnosis

All patients with suspected alcoholic hepatitis should have a full blood count, clotting studies, renal and liver function tests, and serum magnesium and phosphate. Other causes of liver disease should be excluded, such as autoimmune liver disease, hepatitis C virus (HCV), HBV, genetic hemochromatosis (ferritin and % iron saturation may be misleading in patients ingesting large quantities of alcohol or with acute illness), Wilson disease and alpha1-antitrypsin disease. Structural disease should be excluded with ultrasound or computerized tomography (CT) scan. Fatty infiltration of the liver is common, and may be focal, mimicking space-occupying lesions.

A definitive diagnosis requires histology; indeed clinical trials where this has not been routinely obtained have been criticized. The key pathological features are ballooned hepatocytes, with or without Mallory hyaline, neutrophil infiltration and pericellular fibrosis. Of these patients over 50% will have cirrhosis [6]. A biopsy adds both therapeutic and prognostic information and the histological diagnosis of steatohepatitis has been shown to correlate poorly with components of the systemic inflammatory response score (SIRS), suggesting that a clinical diagnosis may be inaccurate in up to 50% of cases [7, 8].

However, by the very nature of the disease, prothrombin time is prolonged, ascites is frequently present and the platelet count is low. Hence a percutaneous approach is contraindicated and a liver biopsy can usually only be safely obtained via the transjugular route, and while this is a straightforward procedure it is not commonly available. It is reasonable therefore to diagnose and treat patients on clinical grounds but to seek histological confirmation where possible, and in particular in patients where there are inconsistencies in clinical course.

Prognostic factors

Death usually results from hepatorenal failure, uncontrollable sepsis, or variceal hemorrhage. These events can occur throughout the inpatient stay and in the author's opinion are often consequences of a poor response to predictable changes.

There are a number of validated scoring systems that may be applied to patients presenting with acute alcoholic hepatitis. The most recognized is the mDF (modified Maddrey's discriminate function) [2]:

$$mDF = \left(bilirubin(\mu mol/L)/17 \, or \, bilirubin \, in \, mg/dl + 4.6 \right) \times [PT \, prolongation]$$

A score of >32 predicts a 28-day mortality of around 35%.

Serum bilirubin, the prolongation of prothrombin time (PT) and the presence of hepatic encephalopathy and renal impairment have been shown to be independent predictors of short-term survival and a value of 32 or greater has been shown in several prospective studies to predict a 28-day mortality of around 35% [9]. As a consequence most treatment trials have focused on patients with a mDF more than 32 and/or encephalopathy and have examined short-term (usually 1 month) mortality only. Patients with less severe disease appear to have a good short-term prognosis even when jaundiced [9].

Table 28.1 The Glasgow alcoholic hepatitis score.

	Score given		
	1	2	3
Age	<50	≥50	—
WCC (10⁹/L)	<15	≥15	—
Urea (mmol/L)	<5	≥5	—
PT ratio	<1.5	1.5–2.0	>2.0
Bilirubin (μmol/L)	<125	125–250	>250
Urea (mg/dL)	<7.4	7.4–15	>15

A score of ≥ 9 at day 1 was associated with a 28-day mortality of 46% and at day 7 with a 28-day survival of 47%.
PT, prothrombin time; WCC, white cell count.

Accordingly, in these patients, and in severe patients surviving their initial presentation, treatment is focused on achieving abstinence, which has been convincingly shown to improve long-term outcome [10]. Long-term mortality remains poor with rates of 61% at 10 years in patents who maintain abstinence and 91% in those unable to reduce alcohol intake with 71% of deaths due to liver related causes [11].

Other prognostic indices include MELD (Model for End-stage Liver Disease), GAHS (Glasgow Alcoholic Hepatitis Score), and the ABIC (Age, serum Bilirubin, INR, and serum Creatinine) score. Both MELD and the ABIC score have been shown to predict 90 day mortality [12, 13].

The Glasgow scoring system GAHS (see Table 28.1) is a simpler and more accurate means of predicting mortality compared to the MELD [9]. The *GAHS* is based on the following intuitively logical factors: age, markers of renal and liver function, as well as sepsis/inflammation. The GAHS has also been shown to predict patients who may improve without corticosteroids [14].

Both the US and European guidelines for the management of alcoholic hepatitis suggest the use of the mDF to identify patient with the most severe disease [15, 16].

Management

General

Patients with severe alcoholic hepatitis should be considered as being nutritionally deficient, immunosuppressed, and with critical renal impairment. Thus baseline interventions should include aggressive fluid resuscitation, intravenous B vitamin supplementation and gastric acid suppression (with H_2 antagonists), early use of antibiotics following a full septic screen (including diagnostic ascitic tap) when there is clinical suspicion of sepsis and *early* use of vasoactive agents such as Terlipressin if hepatorenal syndrome is developing. The focus should be on the prevention and early treatment of acute kidney injury and *not* on the management of ascites, when present, since this can be tapped for comfort.

It is the authors' opinion that successful management of this fragile group of patients is labor intensive and requires an awareness of the events that can occur combined with regular clinical assessment (2–3 times each day) and regular review of fluid and pharmacological therapy in response to altering physiological parameters. Diuretics should only be used when the renal function is stable and normal.

A recent national confidential enquiry into patient outcome and death in the UK reviewed the care received by patients admitted to hospitals with alcohol related liver disease. This audit revealed significant deficiencies and areas where there was cause for concern. One quarter of all patients were not reviewed by a gastroenterologist or a hepatologist during their admission, timely investigation and management was lacking and some patients were inappropriately denied escalation to intensive care. Importantly, 71% of the patients who died had been admitted to hospital at least once in the previous 2 years, suggesting missed opportunities for intervention.

Alcohol withdrawal should be managed with oral benzodiazepines, and these should be titrated according to the severity of withdrawal, and the possible presence of encephalopathy. While there are no guidelines on who to refer to specialist liver units, it is the author's opinion that those in whom it is the first presentation, and the young, should be considered for maximal support, and hence should be discussed with the regional liver unit.

This chapter does not deal with the (perhaps more difficult) topic of maintaining abstinence. It does however seem obvious that having struggled to get a patient through a severe attack of alcoholic hepatitis, to then discharge them without any provision for outpatient care is both illogical and poor medicine.

Specific

Steroids

Steroid therapy has been the most intensively studied therapy in alcoholic hepatitis and there have been over 20 published studies of steroid therapy for alcoholic hepatitis since 1971. The majority has found no overall benefit from steroid treatment and a recent systematic review employing the Cochrane methodology did not support their use [17]. Despite this corticosteroids are the most widely applied treatment and are likely to be offered to all patients with severe disease (mDF > 32).

There has been only one randomized clinical trial in which all patients had a histologically proven diagnosis of alcoholic hepatitis using transjugular biopsy where necessary. This trial has been the subject of two reports [18, 19], the second including an open treatment prednisolone group ($n = 61$), in addition to the placebo ($n = 29$) and randomized prednisolone ($n = 32$) groups. The overall survival at 6 months in the two treated groups was 73% and 84%, compared with 41% in the placebo group ($p = 0.02$). However by 2 years the mortality in all three groups was identical. Thus, in this study, prednisolone was associated with a short-term improvement in mortality in patients with histologically proven alcoholic hepatitis.

Rather than performing a further conventional meta-analysis, the authors of three large randomized controlled trials pooled individual patient data, only including patients with encephalopathy and/or a mDF greater than 32 [20]. This study showed that steroids improved survival versus placebo (85% versus 65%), with placebo treatment, increasing age and creatinine independent predictors of mortality on multivariate analysis. A weakness of this study is that two of the three original trials included gastrointestinal bleeding as a contraindication, while one did not, and only one trial required a liver biopsy for diagnosis. The same authors recently updated these results including 387 patients with severe alcoholic hepatitis from five trials. They reported 28-day survival of $74.2 \pm 2.9\%$ in the 202 who received corticosteroids and $64.1 \pm 3.5\%$ in the 185 who did not ($p = 0.0005$) [21].

Further analysis of steroid trial data has identified a group who appear to show a good response to steroids, identified by an early change in bilirubin levels (ECBL) at 7 days [22]. It has been suggested from this data that patients who do not have an ECBL should therefore stop steroids, and the Lille model was developed to better identify this group [23]. It is the authors' opinion that this is an over-interpretation of the trial data. Not having an ECBL only identifies a poor prognosis – it does not indicate that steroids should be ceased because of lack of efficacy.

Pentoxifylline

Following the identification of high levels of TNF in patients with acute alcoholic hepatitis, pentoxifylline (PTX; an inhibitor of TNF synthesis) was compared with placebo in a randomized placebo-controlled trial [24]. One hundred patients were enrolled, all with severe disease as evidenced by a mDF of >32. PTX was administered for 3 weeks, at a dose of 400 mg three times a day. In the PTX group 12/49 (24.5%) died compared to 24/52 (46.1%) in the placebo group during the index hospitalization ($p = 0.037$). The principal benefit for the agent appeared to be a reduction in the development of hepatorenal syndrome. Unlike steroids, PTX could be administered following recent gastrointestinal bleeding and during evidence of sepsis. The trial was criticized however for the absence of a steroid arm. A Cochrane review could not confirm any mortality benefit of pentoxifylline and a more recent meta-analysis of 10 trials including 884 patients suggested pentoxifylline reduced the risk of fatal HRS (RR 0.47), but was not associated with increased short-term survival [25, 26].

STOPAH trial

In an attempt to clarify the roles of both corticosteroids and pentoxifilline in alcoholic hepatitis a large, multicenter, double-blind, randomized, controlled trial of 1200 participants is currently nearing the end of recruitment in the UK. The Steroids Or Pentoxyphilline in Alcoholic Hepatitis (STOPAH) trial randomizes participants to one of four groups: prednisolone and placebo; pentoxyphilline and placebo; prednisolone and pentoxyphilline; or placebo alone.

Antioxidants

Although initial trials of antioxidants did not show any benefit [27], a recent multicenter French study of corticosteroids with N-acetylcystine or corticosteroids alone suggested a 1 month mortality rate of 24% in the prednisolone alone group versus 8% in the prednisolone–N-acetylcysteine group (hazard ratio, 0.58; 95% CI, 0.14 to 0.76; $p = 0.006$). The primary outcome, however, was mortality at 6 months which was 38% in the prednisolone-only group (34 of 89) and 27% in the prednisolone–N-acetylcysteine group (23 of 85) (HR 0.62; 95% CI, 0.37 to 1.06; $p = 0.07$) [28].

Nutritional therapy

Because of the evidence of malnutrition in many patients with alcoholic hepatitis, as well as the association between mortality and nutritional status, this is a significant opportunity for intervention. While there have been a number of small trials, the two main studies were both done by the same group. In the first, enteral tube feeding of an energy-dense formula supplying 2000 kcal/day was compared with a standard oral diet [29]. In-hospital mortality was 12% in the tube-fed patients, compared to 47% in the oral diet group. Although only 37 (admittedly malnourished and sick) patients were randomized, this prompted a further study comparing enteral feeding to steroids. A total of 71 patients were randomized, and while there was no difference in mortality during the 28 days duration of the trial, deaths occurred earlier in the steroid-treated patients and the mortality rate was lower in the enterally fed group in the year following treatment [30]. The overall mortality rate at one year was 61% in the steroid-treated group and 38% in the enteral group ($p = 0.26$). Although a metanalysis of seven randomized controlled studies failed to show a mortality benefit associated with nutritional supplementation the authors advocate enteral feeding in all patient with severe alcoholic hepatitis [31].

One of the benefits of nasogastric tube feeding is a reliable source of hydration, and its ease of use should make this a more popular therapy. The presence of varices is not a contraindication to nasogastric tube placement (though softer, fine-bore tubes are recommended) and the use of bridles usually will stop even the most determined of individuals from removing the tube.

Anti-TNF antibodies

Early enthusiasm for the potential of these (expensive) drugs was fueled by initial reports of improved liver function tests in patients with alcoholic hepatitis, either when used alone or in combination with steroids [32, 33]. However, this was rapidly tempered by the early cessation of a randomized trial of infliximab in conjunction with steroids, principally because of sepsis [34]. This is perhaps not surprising, since sepsis is such a common event in patients with advanced liver disease, and has been a well-described complication of anti-TNF therapy. While the trial has been criticized on the grounds of excessive dosing, and the choice of antibody, it should

also be borne in mind that TNFα is required for hepato-cellular regeneration [35], and as in many of the sepsis studies, blocking one part of the various cascades runs the risk of 'shooting the messenger'.

Molecular absorbent recirculating system

The molecular absorbent recirculating system (MARS) involves hemofiltration against an albumin gradient, aiming to remove metabolites. Despite initial enthusiasm [36], the recent RELIEF study including 189 patients with decompensated chronic liver disease (over 80% due to alcohol) did not show any benefit and its use is not recommended [37].

Liver transplantation

The utility of donated organs in patients with alcoholic hepatitis requires careful consideration, and has been the subject of much debate. A recent French study selected 26 patients with histologically proven severe alcoholic hepatitis and a high Lille score (indicating a poor response to corticosteroids). Patients had a perceived low risk of return to alcohol misuse (supportive family members, no severe coexisting conditions, and a commitment to alcohol abstinence). The 6-month survival rate was 77 ± 8% and infection (particularly from invasive aspergillus) was a significant cause of early mortality.

The low availability of donor organs UK mean it is ethically questionable to consider liver transplantation in this high-risk group of patients. In addition, we have analyzed our own patient subgroup who would have fulfilled the French transplant listing criteria, and have found high survival rates. Clearly, patient selection is critical, and requires further fine-tuning.

Other therapies

Other therapies that have been studied and shown to be ineffective include propylthiouracil [38, 39], milk thistle [40], and anabolic steroids [41].

Conclusion

Acute alcoholic hepatitis is an increasing burden for the attending clinician. There can at times be a sense of therapeutic nihilism with a difficult group of patients. However, it is also true that with attentive medical care, excellent results can be achieved. While the data is unsatisfactory, steroids, pentoxifylline, and nutritional support have been shown to improve survival. One could use all three modalities, but this also needs to be combined with close attention to prevention of sepsis, withdrawal, and fluid/electrolyte balance, as well as provision of long-term alcohol services once the patient has been discharged.

References

1. Maddrey WC, Boitnott JK, Bedine MS, Weber FL, Jr., Mezey E, White RI, Jr. Corticosteroid therapy of alcoholic hepatitis. *Gastroenterology* 1978;**75**(2):193–9.

2. Carithers RL, Jr., Herlong HF, Diehl AM, et al. Methylprednisolone therapy in patients with severe alcoholic hepatitis. A randomized multicenter trial. Ann. Intern. Med. 1989;**110**(9):685–90.

3. Mathurin P, O'Grady J, Carithers RL, et al. Corticosteroids improve short-term survival in patients with severe alcoholic hepatitis: meta-analysis of individual patient data. *Gut*. 2011;**60**(2):255–60.

4. Forrest EH, Evans CDJ, Stewart S, et al. Analysis of factors predictive of mortality in alcoholic hepatitis and derivation and validation of the Glasgow alcoholic hepatitis score. *Gut* 2005;**54**(8):1174–9.

5. Roberts SE, Goldacre MJ, Yeates D. Trends in mortality after hospital admission for liver cirrhosis in an English population from 1968 to 1999. *Gut* 2005;**54**(11):1615–21.

6. Spahr L, Rubbia-Brandt L, Genevay M, Hadengue A, Giostra E. Early liver biopsy, intraparenchymal cholestasis, and prognosis in patients with alcoholic steatohepatitis. *BMC Gastroenterol* 2011;**11**:115.

7. Mookerjee RP, Lackner C, Stauber R, et al. The role of liver biopsy in the diagnosis and prognosis of patients with acute deterioration of alcoholic cirrhosis. *J. Hepatol.* 2011;**55**(5): 1103–11.

8. Hardy T, Wells C, Kendrick S, et al. White cell count and platelet count associate with histological alcoholic hepatitis in jaundiced harmful drinkers. *BMC Gastroenterol.* 2013;**13**(1):55.

9. Goldberg S, Mendenhall C, Anderson S, et al. VA Cooperative Study on Alcoholic Hepatitis. IV. The significance of clinically mild alcoholic hepatitis – describing the population with minimal hyperbilirubinemia. Am. J. Gastroenterol. 1986;**81**(11):1029–34.

10. Alexander JF, Lischner MW, Galambos JT. Natural history of alcoholic hepatitis. II. The long-term prognosis. Am. J. Gastroenterol. 1971;**56**(6):515–25.

11. Aljoudeh A, E. M, M. K, Gleeson D. Decompensated alcoholic liver disease (ALD): high long-term mortality despite initial survival. In The International Liver Congress, April 2013. D.S. (ed।)., Amsterdam: Elsevier, **2013**: S211.

12. Dunn W, Jamil LH, Brown LS, et al. MELD accurately predicts mortality in patients with alcoholic hepatitis. *Hepatology* 2005;**41**(2):353–8.

13. Dominguez MMD, Rincon DMD, Abraldes JGMD, et al. A new scoring system for prognostic stratification of patients with alcoholic hepatitis. Am. J. Gastroenterol. 2008; **103**(11):2747–56.

14. Forrest EH, Morris AJ, Stewart S, et al. The Glasgow alcoholic hepatitis score identifies patients who may benefit from corticosteroids. *Gut* 2007;**56**(12):1743–6.

15. O'Shea RS, Dasarathy S, McCullough AJ. Alcoholic liver disease. *Hepatology* 2010 Jan;**51**(1):307–28.

16. EASL clinical practical guidelines: management of alcoholic liver disease. *J. Hepatol.* 2012;**57**(2):399–420.

17. Rambaldi A, Saconato HH, Christensen E, Thorlund K, Wetterslev J, Gluud C. Systematic review: glucocorticosteroids for alcoholic hepatitis – a Cochrane Hepato-Biliary Group systematic review with meta-analyses and trial sequential analyses of randomized clinical trials. *Aliment. Pharmacol. Ther* 2008;**27**(12):1167–78.

18. Ramond M-JMD, Poynard TMD, Rueff BMD, et al. A Randomized Trial of Prednisolone in patients with severe alcoholic hepatitis. N. Engl. J. Med. 1992;**326**(8):507–12.

19. Mathurin P, Duchatelle V, Ramond MJ, et al. Survival and prognostic factors in patients with severe alcoholic hepatitis treated with prednisolone. *Gastroenterology* 1996;**110**(6): 1847–53.

20. Mathurin P, Mendenhall CL, Carithers RL, Jr., et al. Corticosteroids improve short-term survival in patients with severe alcoholic hepatitis (AH): individual data analysis of the last three randomized placebo controlled double blind trials of corticosteroids in severe AH. *J. Hepatol.* 2002;**36**(4):480–7.

21. Mathurin P OGJ, Carithers RL, Martin P, et al. AASLD Abstract 738. *Hepatology*. 2008;**48**(S1):609A–706A.

22. Mathurin P, Abdelnour M, Ramond MJ, et al. Early change in bilirubin levels is an important prognostic factor in severe alcoholic hepatitis treated with prednisolone. *Hepatology* 2003 Dec;**38**(6):1363–9.

23. Louvet A, Naveau S, Abdelnour M, et al. The Lille model: A new tool for therapeutic strategy in patients with severe alcoholic hepatitis treated with steroids. *Hepatology* 2007; **45**(6):1348–54.

24. Akriviadis E, Botla R, Briggs W, Han S, Reynolds T, Shakil O. Pentoxifylline improves short-term survival in severe acute alcoholic hepatitis: a double-blind, placebo-controlled trial. *Gastroenterology* 2000 Dec;**119**(6):1637–48.

25. Parker R, Armstrong MJ, Corbett C, Rowe IA, Houlihan DD. Systematic review: pentoxifylline for the treatment of severe alcoholic hepatitis. *Aliment. Pharmacol. Ther.* 2013; **37**(9):845–54.

26. Whitfield K, Rambaldi A, Wetterslev J, Gluud C. Pentoxifylline for alcoholic hepatitis. *Cochrane Database Syst. Rev* 2009(**4**):CD007339.

27. Phillips M, Curtis H, Portmann B, Donaldson N, Bomford A, O'Grady J. Antioxidants versus corticosteroids in the treatment of severe alcoholic hepatitis–a randomised clinical trial. *J. Hepatol.* 2006;**44**(4):784–90.

28. Nguyen-Khac E, Thevenot T, Piquet M-A, et al. Glucocorticoids plus N-acetylcysteine in severe alcoholic hepatitis. *N. Engl. J. Med.* 2011;**365**(19):1781–9.

29. Cabre E, Gonzalez-Huix F, Abad-Lacruz A, et al. Effect of total enteral nutrition on the short-term outcome of severely malnourished cirrhotics. A randomized controlled trial. *Gastroenterology* 1990 Mar;**98**(3):715–20.

30. Cabre E, Rodriguez-Iglesias P, Caballeria J, et al. Short- and long-term outcome of severe alcohol-induced hepatitis treated with steroids or enteral nutrition: a multicenter randomized trial. *Hepatology* 2000;**32**(1):36–42.

31. Antar R, Wong P, Ghali P. A meta-analysis of nutritional supplementation for management of hospitalized alcoholic hepatitis. *Can. J. Gastroenterol.* 2012;**26**(7):463–7.

32. Spahr L, Rubbia-Brandt L, Frossard JL, et al. Combination of steroids with infliximab or placebo in severe alcoholic hepatitis: a randomized controlled pilot study. *J. Hepatol.* 2002 Oct;**37**(4):448–55.

33. Menon KVNMD, Stadheim LRN, Kamath PSMD, et al. A Pilot Study of the Safety and Tolerability of Etanercept in patients with alcoholic hepatitis. *Am. J. Gastroenterol.* 2004;**99**(2):255–60.

34. Naveau S, Chollet-Martin S, Dharancy S, et al. A double-blind randomized controlled trial of infliximab associated with prednisolone in acute alcoholic hepatitis. *Hepatology* 2004;**39**(5):1390–7.

35. Akerman P, Cote P, Yang SQ, et al. Antibodies to tumor necrosis factor-alpha inhibit liver regeneration after partial hepatectomy. *Am. J. Physiol.* 1992;**263**(4 Pt 1):G579–85.

36. Jalan R, Sen S, Steiner C, Kapoor D, Alisa A, Williams R. Extracorporeal liver support with molecular adsorbents recirculating system in patients with severe acute alcoholic hepatitis. *J. Hepatol.* 2003;**38**(1):24–31.

37. Bañares R, Nevens F, Larsen FS, et al. Extracorporeal albumin dialysis with the molecular adsorbent recirculating system in acute-on-chronic liver failure: The RELIEF trial. *Hepatology* 2013;**57**(3):1153–62.

38. Halle P, Pare P, Kaptein E, Kanel G, Redeker AG, Reynolds TB. Double-blind, controlled trial of propylthiouracil in patients with severe acute alcoholic hepatitis. *Gastroenterology* 1982;**82**(5 Pt 1):925–31.

39. Rambaldi A, Gluud C. Propylthiouracil for alcoholic liver disease. *Cochrane Database Syst. Rev.* 2002;(**2**):CD002800. PubMed PMID: 12076451.

40. Rambaldi A, Jacobs BP, Iaquinto G, Gluud C. Milk thistle for alcoholic and//or hepatitis B or C liver diseases – a Systematic Cochrane Hepato-Biliary Group Review with Meta-Analyses of Randomized Clinical Trials. *Am. J. Gastroenterol.* 2005;**100**(11):2583–91.

41. Rambaldi A, Iaquinto G, Gluud C. Anabolic-androgenic steroids for alcoholic liver disease: a Cochrane review. *Am. J. Gastroenterol.* 2002;**97**(7):1674–81.

CHAPTER 29

Perforation of the gastrointestinal tract

Ian McAllister

Ulster Hospital, Dundonald, Belfast, UK

Introduction

The incidence of hospital admissions for peptic ulcer disease has been in decline in recent decades, falling by 30% between 1993 and 2006 in the United States [1]. This has largely been attributed to the introduction of proton pump inhibitors and eradication of *Helicobacter pylori*. However, complicated peptic ulcer disease, particularly perforation, remains associated with mortality rates approaching 30%, and higher in elderly patients [2]. The incidence of peptic perforation has been reported at rates between 3.8 and 14 per 100 000 [3].

Infection with *H. pylori* has been shown to be important in the development of peptic ulceration [4]. In cases of peptic perforation, 60–70% of patients are infected with this rate rising to 80–90% if users of non-steroidal anti-inflammatory drugs (NSAIDs) are excluded [5,6].

NSAID use is associated with an increased risk of peptic ulcer perforation irrespective of *Helicobacter* infection [4,6,7] It would appear that peptic ulcer disease and therefore perforation is rare in patients who are *Helicobacter* negative and non-NSAID users [4].

Other etiological factors include ingestion of low-dose aspirin, corticosteroids, and smoking [8]. In younger patients, smoking increases the risk of peptic ulcer perforation by tenfold with a significant dose response correlation, but there is no additional risk for those who have managed to stop smoking [9].

Clinical presentation

History

Peptic ulcer perforation typically presents as severe, sudden upper abdominal pain, which then becomes generalized. Over one-third of patients will have a prior history of peptic ulcer disease and many will have been prescribed various antacid medications. In excess of 40% of patients will be using NSAIDs or corticosteroids and a high proportion will be smokers [10]. A majority of patients will have other significant comorbidity, and up to 15% of patients are hospitalized for another complaint at the time of perforation [10].

Examination

The patient may exhibit signs of systemic inflammatory response syndrome with tachycardia, pyrexia, and tachypnea. Abdominal peritonism is a consistent finding, described in 60% of patients. Loss of liver dullness on percussion suggests free intraperitoneal air.

Elderly and critically ill patients with peptic perforation may present atypically and physical signs may be subtle or even absent. Care must be taken in the elderly patient who may present with vague symptoms such as mild abdominal pain, nausea, dyspepsia, or anorexia. Clinical examination in the elderly may also be misleading with a significant proportion not exhibiting abdominal tenderness.

Investigations

Laboratory investigations often demonstrate a leukocytosis and elevated inflammatory markers in a case of peptic ulcer perforation.

Sub-diaphragmatic free gas may be evident on an erect chest radiograph in 50–70% of cases [11,12]. A combination of classical clinical findings and radiological pneumoperitoneum will often be sufficient to warrant proceeding straight to laparotomy. If diagnostic doubt persists, other imaging may be utilized.

The addition of water-soluble oral contrast will confirm the presence of an intraperitoneal leak. However, this modality does not exclude a sealed perforation [13]. Abdominal ultrasound may demonstrate evidence of intraperitoneal free fluid and reduced intestinal peristalsis, but these findings are not specific for gastroduodenal perforation.

Multidetector computerized tomography (CT) scanning may assist in differentiating between a sealed-off duodenal perforation and other causes of an acute abdomen. Water soluble oral contrast is used and CT allows detection of even small amounts of free air and free fluid in the abdomen [14,15].

Prognosis

Most deaths related to peptic ulcer disease are due to perforation. Gastroduodenal perforation produces a severe chemical peritonitis, resulting in a systemic inflammatory response and eventual multiorgan dysfunction. Several studies have examined scoring systems for outcomes following peptic ulcer perforation. These include the Boey and, more recently, PULP scores [16,17]. The most important factors identified as increasing morbidity and mortality rates are patient comorbidity, age >65 years and preoperative shock. Limiting the perforation to operation interval has been reported as a critical determinant of survival [18,19].

Management

Following patient resuscitation and optimization with nasogastric aspiration, intravenous proton pump inhibitor and broad-spectrum antibiotics, the mainstay of treatment remains prompt surgical intervention. In the next section we shall consider conventional surgical treatment, examine the role of minimally invasive surgery and discuss the non-operative approach.

Conventional surgical treatment

Historically, perforated peptic ulcers were managed operatively by closing the perforation and surgically reducing acid secretion. Closure was performed either primarily or with a pedicled (Cellan–Jones) or free (Graham) omental patch [20,21]. In the 1940s the acid suppression approach would have been via a truncal vagotomy and a drainage procedure to overcome delayed gastric emptying. By the 1960s the process was refined to a highly selective vagotomy, which eliminated the requirement for a drainage procedure. The long-term ulcer recurrence rates following these operations were in the region of 5–15%.

In 1999, Chu et al. reported that recurrent ulcer disease in patients with a history of perforated duodenal ulcer and simple patch repair was related to *Helicobacter* infection [22]. Subsequent studies concluded that eradication of *Helicobacter*, with acid suppression and antibiotics, following the simple surgical closure of a perforated peptic ulcer reduces the recurrence rate to less than 5% [23,24].

We therefore conclude that simple omental patch closure and peritoneal lavage alongside *Helicobacter* eradication reduces ulcer recurrence rates following perforation, thus consigning definitive ulcer surgery to the history books.

Minimally invasive surgery

Since 1990 laparoscopic techniques have been used to repair perforated peptic ulcers. However, there is still significant debate with regard to the merits of the minimally invasive approach. Laparoscopically, the perforation may be patched by suturing omentum as at open repair or equally well plugged with gelatine sponge and fibrin glue [25].

Siu et al. reported that laparoscopic patients had shorter operating times, reduced respiratory complications, shorter postoperative stay, earlier return to normal activity, required significantly less parenteral analgesia, and had lower pain scores in the initial postoperative period. There was no difference in nasogastric aspirate and time to tolerating oral intake between the two approaches and there were more reoperations and intra-abdominal collections within the laparoscopic group in this study [26]. The Dutch LAMA trial concluded that laparoscopic repair is safe, feasible for the experienced laparoscopic surgeon, and causes less post-operative pain. However, operating times were longer and there was no difference in length of hospital stay or incidence of postoperative complications [27].

A meta-analysis of 13 studies comprising 658 patients also reported a reduction in postoperative pain and less analgesic requirements. However, the success rate was only 87%, and a significantly higher reoperation rate was noted with the laparoscopic approach [28]. A systematic review of the literature published in 2005, based on 1113 patients represented by 15 studies, concluded that laparoscopic repair seemed better than open repair for low-risk patients, and that for high-risk patients with significant comorbidity the open approach may be more appropriate [29]. This was echoed in a further review in 2010, which reported less pain, lower morbidity and mortality, and shorter hospital stay with laparoscopic repair. However, laparoscopy was associated with an overall conversion rate of 12.4%, significantly longer operating times, and higher incidence of recurrent leakage [30].

A recently published Cochrane review suggested that the laparoscopic approach probably reduces septic abdominal complications but concluded that the laparoscopic results were not clinically different from those of open surgery [31]. Again, a recent meta-analysis reported that current evidence does not clearly demonstrate the advantages of laparoscopic versus open repair of perforated peptic ulcers [32].

On balance, it would seem that minimally invasive surgery for perforated peptic ulcers confers some short-term benefits. However, this is traded against an increase in reoperation rates and no earlier return of gut function. Further studies are required to identify subgroups of patients, probably those of low risk, who may gain most from the minimally invasive approach. High-risk patients should undergo open repair.

Non-operative approach

A randomized trial of non-operative treatment for peptic ulcer perforation compared to standard surgical intervention has been published [33]. A total of 83 patients were entered in the study; 40 patients were randomly assigned to conservative treatment consisting of intravenous fluid resuscitation, nasogastric suction, antibiotics, and acid suppression. After 12 hours almost 30% did not improve and proceeded to emergency surgery. The overall morbidity and mortality between the two groups was similar but the hospital stay was 35% longer for those treated conservatively. There was a higher incidence of sepsis and intra-abdominal abscess for the non-operative approach, and those patients over 70 years old were less likely to respond to conservative measures.

Donovan et al. reported the non-operative management of patients in whom a perforated but sealed peptic ulcer had been demonstrated via gastroduodenogram. This was found to be a safe approach, with just 3% abscess formation and <2% re-leak [34]. Although conservative treatment is possible, it may not be optimal for patients with perforated peptic ulceration, but should be reserved for those with a sealed perforation who are too frail for surgical intervention.

Special circumstances
Perforated gastric cancer

It has been estimated that less than 1% of gastric cancer cases will perforate and it has been reported that around 10–15% of all gastric perforations are caused by gastric carcinoma.

Patients will present with symptoms and signs similar to that of peptic ulcer perforation but may have additional symptoms such as anorexia, lethargy, and weight loss. During emergency laparotomy it is often very difficult to identify the etiology of the perforation due to the surrounding edema and inflammation. It is therefore prudent to obtain tissue biopsies from the edges of the perforation for histopathological examination.

Management of perforated gastric malignancy involves two often incompatible aims: dealing with the peritonitis and performing an oncologically sound procedure. Roviello et al. identified factors that can help decide the most appropriate management option. Decisions should be made based on the general condition of the patient and the curability of the malignancy. If the patient's general condition is acceptable and the tumor is resectable then a radical total or subtotal gastrectomy should be performed. When the tumor is at an advanced stage and cure is unlikely, but the patient is in a reasonable condition, then a palliative gastrectomy is recommended. A simple patch repair as used for perforated peptic ulcers is reserved for patients who are too frail for surgical resection [35].

Most of these patients present with advanced disease and therefore the outlook is bleak. A number of patients do have an early-stage tumor, when a curative operation can be performed. Survival rates after gastric perforation are similar to the rates observed for elective patients [36].

Colonic perforation

Introduction

Perforation of the colon is associated with significant morbidity and high mortality. This is partly due to the systemic insult of fecal peritonitis and in part the group of patients involved, who are often elderly with significant comorbidity. Prompt, appropriate intervention is vital in improving survival and reducing long-term morbidity for this group.

Diverticular disease remains the single commonest cause for large bowel perforation, accounting for 40–60% of cases with a reported increase in the prevalence of perforated sigmoid diverticulitis from 2.4 per 100 000 in 1986 to 3.8 per 100 000 in 2000 [37]. Perforation of colonic carcinoma accounts for around 10–20% [38], and perforation due to ischemia for approximately 10%. The remaining miscellaneous group comprise iatrogenic, trauma, foreign body, and stercoral perforation (see Table 29.1).

Perforation occurs in diverticular disease when a fecolith obstructs the neck of the diverticulum. The release of enteric organisms into the peritoneal cavity results in a polymicrobial-induced peritonitis. There is a predominance of Gram-negative organisms and common pathogens include *Escherichia coli*, *Enterobacter*, *Klebsiella*, and anaerobic species, including *Bacteroides* and *Clostridium*.

The release of bacteria into the normally sterile environment of the peritoneal cavity initiates the host defense to eliminate or indeed contain the infecting agent by compartmentalization. A reduction in fibrinolytic activity produces fibrinous exudates, into which large numbers of bacteria are sequestered, limiting the spread of peritoneal contamination. The residual effect of this process is the formation of an abscess cavity, which matures to protect the bacteria from the host's defense mechanisms. If a contained abscess cavity does not develop then generalized purulent or fecal peritonitis will be the outcome, precipitating a more aggressive immune response. This leads to a systemic inflammatory response syndrome (SIRS) and, if unchecked, ultimately to multiple organ failure.

Diagnosis

The presentation of patients with colonic perforation varies from localized left lower quadrant pain to extreme circulatory collapse. This is dependent on the degree of contamination, the site, and etiology of the perforation, together with the patient's comorbidity and duration of the symptoms.

History

A precise clinical history is important when considering the diagnosis and etiology of colonic perforation. Abdominal pain is evident in around 70% of patients diagnosed with colonic perforation with the time of onset, duration and localization of the pain all important [39]. A past history of left-sided abdominal pain over many years suggests possible diverticular disease, whereas a history of weight loss, altered bowel habit, and rectal bleeding may indicate a colonic carcinoma. Identifying immunocompromised patients, those with diabetes, peripheral vascular disease, or colitis may facilitate the decision-making process with regard to management and prognosis.

Examination

Physical examination will reveal signs of systemic sepsis with tachycardia, hypotension, tachypnea, and fever [39]. Abdominal palpation may elicit localized tenderness corresponding to the site of perforation. An immobile patient with a board-like abdomen, generalized percussion tenderness, and absent bowel sounds is suggestive of more widespread peritonitis.

Investigations

Laboratory tests often show evidence of leukocytosis and elevated inflammatory markers, such as C-reactive protein. Severe sepsis often results in renal dysfunction, acidosis,

Table 29.1 Etiology of colonic perforation.

Etiology	Number (%)
Diverticulitis	133 (63%)
Carcinoma	30 (14%)
Ischemia	20 (9.4%)
Iatrogenic	13 (6.1%)
Other	16 (7.5%)
Total	212

Source: Biondo 2002. Reproduced by permission of Lippincott, Williams & Wilkins.

and may also lead to a significant coagulopathy requiring correction before or during any surgical procedure.

Plain radiography demonstrates free air in only one-third of cases of colonic perforation and should not be relied upon for reassurance [40]. In suspected colonic perforation, multidetector CT scan with oral and intravenous contrast will identify free air in up to 100% of cases. Other CT findings include the presence of an inflammatory phlegmon, pericolic inflammatory stranding, extraluminal fluid collection, and bowel wall thickening around the perforation site [40]. A report by Lohrmann et al. demonstrated that CT identified the perforation site in 86% of patients with perforated sigmoid diverticulitis [41]. CT has the added advantage that it may help differentiate between a neoplastic or diverticular perforation and possibly identify liver metastases. Reports suggest that the presence of enlarged pericolic lymph nodes, with a short (<10 cm) length of colonic wall thickening and a luminal mass, were findings more suggestive of carcinoma [42].

Classification

In 1978, Hinchey et al. proposed a classification of peritoneal inflammation and contamination following colonic diverticular perforation and this remains the most widely used grading system (Table 29.2) [43]. Although designed for complicated diverticulitis the categories would also apply to non-diverticular perforations. Although the Hinchey classification describes the degree of contamination, it does not consider other factors which are important for prognostic evaluation.

The Mannheim peritonitis index (MPI) (Table 29.3) is a well-validated method of classification and risk assessment for patients with peritonitis of all causes, and has been shown to be as efficient as APACHE II in predicting the risk of death [44]. The reliability of the MPI was assessed in a multicenter study of 2003 patients in an effort to select high-risk patients for more aggressive intervention. The mortality rate for patients with an MPI score of <21 was 2.3%, 21–29 was 22.5%, and MPI >29 was 59.1%; overall the index had an accuracy of 83% in predicting death [45].

Management
General measures

The initial management of a patient with a colonic perforation involves fluid resuscitation, intravenous antibiotics to cover aerobic and anaerobic organisms, analgesia,

Table 29.2 Hinchey classification of peritoneal contamination in perforated diverticular disease.

Stage I	Pericolic or mesenteric abscess
Stage II	Walled-off pelvic abscess
Stage III	Generalized purulent peritonitis
Stage IV	Generalized fecal peritonitis

Source: Hinchey 1978.

Table 29.3 Mannheim peritonitis index.

Age >50	5
Female	5
Organ failure	7
Malignancy	4
Peritonitis <24hr preop	4
Origin of sepsis not colonic	4
Diffuse generalized peritonitis	6
Clear exudate	0
Purulent exudate	6
Fecal exudate	12

Source: Linder et al. 1987 [44]. Reproduced with permission of Springer.

a urinary catheter for monitoring output and, based on the clinical findings, a definitive treatment plan.

Conservative

If the patient is hemodynamically stable and the abdominal signs are localized, a non-operative approach may be indicated, with a CT assessment as described above [46]. Antibiotics are continued and any small localized abscess (<5 cm) should resolve, whereas a larger abscess should be drained percutaneously under radiological guidance [47]. Regular clinical assessment is required to identify any deterioration in the patient's condition. Failure of medical management in association with percutaneous drainage warrants surgical intervention.

Surgical

If there is evidence of severe sepsis, progression from localized to generalized peritonitis, or failure to resolve with conservative measures then surgery is necessary. CT is not required in the patient with signs of severe sepsis and generalized peritonitis. If the patient is relatively stable a CT may be useful to identify the exact site of perforation and the degree of intra-abdominal contamination [41].

Having decided to operate, the next surgical dilemma is the selection of the most appropriate procedure and more recently, whether to use a conventional or minimally invasive approach.

Three-stage procedure

Historically, at laparotomy, if the colonic perforation had precipitated purulent or fecal peritonitis, a three-stage approach was used. This involved initially draining the perforated colon and fashioning a diverting transverse loop colostomy. After an interval, the diseased segment was resected with primary anastomosis. Finally, the loop colostomy was reversed, thus restoring bowel continuity.

However, in 1984, a review by Krukowski identified a significant disadvantage in morbidity and a mortality rate approaching 25% when the diseased colon was retained, and this approach is no longer used [46].

Two-stage procedure

In the late 1970s, a number of units advocated the two-stage procedure, which involved primary resection of the diseased segment, the formation of an end colostomy and oversewing of the rectal stump (Hartmann procedure) [48,49] This was followed by stoma reversal, when the intra-abdominal sepsis had settled. The adoption of this two-stage approach more than halved the operative mortality and became the standard approach [46].

However, colostomy reversal can be a complex procedure. Several authors have shown a high incidence of post-reversal morbidity [50,51]. Often, many patients tolerate and manage their colostomy well and up to 50% are satisfied not to pursue reversal [52].

Several studies and two comprehensive literature reviews favor colonic resection with primary anastomosis over Hartmann's procedure [53,54]. In most of these studies, a diverting stoma was routinely performed and these were thus also two-stage procedures. Primary anastomosis with diverting ileostomy was associated with higher stoma reversal rate and reduced overall complication rate, hospital stay, operating time and cost when compared with Hartmann's procedure in a recent randomized trial [55].

One-stage procedure

Concerns remain about fashioning an anastomosis on an unprepared bowel in the presence of peritoneal contamination with edema in the colonic wall. Maneuvers such as on-table colonic lavage and formation of a defunctioning loop ileostomy have been utilized to reduce the likelihood and effects of an anastomotic leak. The evidence is weak, however, and some authors suggest that lavage and diversion may not be mandatory [56,57].

Other reports have shown favorable results with primary anastomosis, even without a diverting stoma, and particularly in patients with localized or generalized purulent peritonitis [58]. This approach has been mainly reserved for those patients without fecal peritonitis, but a prospective non-randomized study demonstrated no difference in mortality between a one-stage and two-stage procedure; for patients with Hinchey stage III/IV diverticulitis [59].

Constantinides et al. performed a meta-analysis of 15 studies, only 2 of which were prospective, and none was randomized. They demonstrated similar mortality rates for both one and two-stage procedures (14.1% vs 14.4%) for a colonic perforation with purulent or fecal peritonitis (Hinchey stage >II). If the peritonitis was classified as Hinchey I/II then there was a significant improvement in mortality and morbidity for patients undergoing a one-stage procedure. However, the authors highlighted a significant selection bias in all of the papers examined as patients with significant peritoneal contamination and poor physiological status were often subjected to a Hartmann procedure [54].

It is therefore difficult to draw strong conclusions until a randomized controlled trial is performed comparing one- and two-stage procedures, in patient groups matched for age, sex, degree of contamination, and physiological status.

Minimally invasive surgery

Laparoscopic resection has been increasingly performed in the treatment of both uncomplicated and complicated diverticulitis. Large series have reported similar outcomes to open resection in the management of complicated diverticulitis [60,61]. This has largely been in cases of localized perforation; however, comparable outcomes have also been reported in cases of Hinchey III/IV peritonitis [62].

Laparoscopic peritoneal lavage has emerged as a promising alternative to sigmoid resection in Hinchey III/IV peritonitis [63,64]. A systematic review has shown use of this method for purulent peritonitis to be associated with low morbidity and mortality rates, while

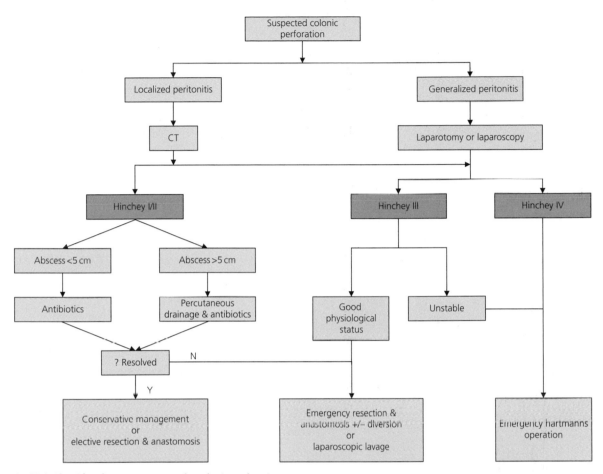

Fig. 29.1 Algorithm for management of a colonic perforation.

avoiding stoma formation [65]. Others have reported feculent peritonitis to be a contraindication to minimally invasive lavage, and even in purulent peritonitis, patients with significant comorbidity, a high C-reactive protein concentration and a high MPI are at risk of failure of lavage [66].

Laparoscopic lavage is the subject of several ongoing trials and it is hoped that these studies will help to define the role of minimally invasive surgery in patients with perforated diverticular disease [67–70].

Management algorithm

Based on the data available, a management algorithm has been constructed suggesting a management plan for the patient presenting with a suspected perforation of the colon (Fig. 29.1).

References

1. Wang YR, Richter JE, Dempsey DT. Trends and outcomes of hospitalizations for peptic ulcer disease in the United States, 1993 to 2006. *Ann. Surg.* 2010;**251**:51.

2. Thorsen K, Soreide JA, Kvaloy JT, et al. Epidemiology of perforated peptic ulcer: age- and gender-adjusted analysis of incidence and mortality. *World J. Gastroenterol.* 2013;**19**(3):347–54.

3. Lau JY, Sung J, Hill C et al. Systematic review of the epidemiology of complicated peptic ulcer disease: incidence, recurrence, risk factors and mortality. *Digestion* 2011;**84**: 102–13.

4. Huang JQ, Sridhar S, Hunt RH. Role of *Helicobacter pylori* infection and non-steroidal anti-inflammatory drugs in peptic-ulcer disease: a meta-analysis. *Lancet* 2002;**359** (9300):14–22.

5. Ng EK, Chung SC, Sung JJ, et al. High prevalence of Helicobacter pylori infection in duodenal ulcer perforations

not caused by non-steroidal anti-inflammatory drugs. *Br. J. Surg.* 1996;**83**:1779–81.

6. Gisbert JP, Legido J, Garcia-Sanz I, et al. *Helicobacter pylori* and perforated peptic ulcer: prevalence of the infection and role of non-steroidal anti-inflammatory drugs. *Dig. Liver Dis.* 2004;**36**(2):116–20.

7. Armstrong CP, Blower AL. Non-steroidal anti-inflammatory drugs and life threatening complications of peptic ulceration. *Gut* 1987;**28**(5):527–32.

8. Hermansson M, Ekedahl A, Ranstam J, et al. Decreasing incidence of peptic ulcer complications after the introduction of the proton pump inhibitors, a study of the Swedish population 1974–2002. *BMC Gastroenterol.* 2009;**9**:25.

9. Svanes C, Soreide JA, Skarstein A, et al. Smoking and ulcer perforation. *Gut* 1997;**41**(2):177–80.

10. Gunshefski L, Flancbaum L, Brolin RE, et al. Changing patterns in perforated peptic ulcer disease. *Am. Surg.* 1990;**56**(4):270–4.

11. Miller RE, Nelson SW. The roentgenologic demonstration of tiny amounts of free intraperitoneal gas: experimental and clinical studies. Am. J. Roentgeno*l. Radium Ther. Nucl. Med.* 1971;**112**(3):574–85.

12. Chen CH, Yang CC, Yeh YH. Role of upright chest radiography and ultrasonography in demonstrating free air of perforated peptic ulcers. *Hepatogastroenterology* 2001;**48**:1082–4.

13. Wellwood JM, Wilson AN, Hopkinson BR. Gastrografin as an aid to the diagnosis of perforated peptic ulcer. *Br. J. Surg.* 1971; **58**(4):245–9.

14. Pinto A, Scaglione M, Giovine S, et al. Comparison between the site of multislice CT signs of gastrointestinal perforation and the site of perforation detected at surgery in forty perforated patients. *Radiol. Med. (Torino)* 2004;**108**(3):208.–17.

15. Yeung KW, Chang MS, Hsiao CP, et al. CT evaluation of gastrointestinal tract perforation. *Clin. Imaging* 2004;**28**:329.

16. Boey J, Choi SK, Poon A, et al. Risk stratification in perforated duodenal ulcers. A prospective validation of predictive factors. Ann. Surg. 1987;**205**:22–6.

17. Moller MH, Engebjerg MC, Adamsen S, et al. The peptic ulcer perforation (PULP) score: a predictor of mortality following peptic ulcer perforation.A cohort study. Acta Anaesthesiol. *Scand.* 2012;**56**(5):655–62.

18. Surapaneni S, Reddy AVB. The perforation–operation time interval; an important indicator in peptic ulcer perforation. *J. Clin. Diagn. Res.* 2013;**7**(5):880–2.

19. Buck DL, Vester-Anderson M, Moller MH. Surgical delay is a critical determinant of survival in perforated peptic ulcer. *Br. J. Surg.* 2013;**100**(8):1045–9.

20. Cellan-Jones CJ. A rapid method of treatment in perforated duodenal ulcer. *BMJ* 1929;**1076–7**.

21. Graham RR. The treatment of perforated duodenal ulcers. *Surg. Gynecol. Obstet.* 1937:**235–8**.

22. Chu KM, Kwok KF, Law SY, et al. *Helicobacter pylori* status and endoscopy follow-up of patients having a history of perforated duodenal ulcer. *Gastrointest. Endosc.* 1999; **50**(1):58–62.

23. Ng EK, Lam YH, Sung JJ, et al. Eradication of *Helicobacter pylori* prevents recurrence of ulcer after simple closure of duodenal ulcer perforation: randomized controlled trial. *Ann. Surg.* 2000; **231**(2):153–8.

24. Tomtitchong P, Siribumrungwong B, Vilaichone RK, et al. Systematic review and meta-analysis: Helicobacter pylori eradication therapy after simple closure of perforated duodenal ulcer. *Helicobacter* 2012;**17**(2):148–52.

25. Lau WY, Leung KL, Kwong KH, et al. A randomized study comparing laparoscopic versus open repair of perforated peptic ulcer using suture or sutureless technique. *Ann. Surg.* 1996;**224**(2):131–8.

26. Siu WT, Leong HT, Law BK, et al. Laparoscopic repair for perforated peptic ulcer: a randomized controlled trial. *Ann. Surg.* 2002;**235**(3):313–19.

27. Bertleff MJOE, Halm JA, Bemelman WA, et al. Randomized clinical trial of laparoscopic versus open repair of the perforated peptic ulcer: the LAMA trial. *World J. Surg.* 2009;**33**:1368.–73.

28. Lau H. Laparoscopic repair of perforated peptic ulcer: a meta-analysis. *Surg. Endosc.* 2004;**16**:1013–21.

29. Lunevicius R, Morkevicius M. Systematic review comparing laparoscopic and open repair for perforated peptic ulcer. *Br. J. Surg.* 2005; **92**(10):1195–207.

30. Bertleff MJOE, Lange JF. Laparoscopic correction of perforated peptic ulcer: first choice? A review of literature. *Surg. Endosc.* 2010;**24**:1231–9.

31. Sanabria A, Villegas MI, Morales Uribe CH. Laparoscopic repair for perforated peptic ulcer disease. *Cochrane Database Syst. Rev.* 2013;**2**:CD004778.

32. Antoniou SA, Antoniou GA, Koch OO, et al. Meta-analysis of laparoscopic versus open repair of perforated peptic ulcer. *JSLS* 2013;**17**(1):15–22.

33. Crofts TJ, Park KG, Steele RJ. A randomized trial of nonoperative treatment for perforated peptic ulcer. *N. Engl. J. Med.* 1989;**320**:970–3.

34. Donovan AJ, Berne TV, Donovan JA. Perforated duodenal ulcer: an alternative therapeutic plan. *Arch. Surg.* 1998;**133**:1166.–71.

35. Roviello F, Rossi S, Marrelli D, et al. Perforated gastric carcinoma: a report of 10 cases and review of the literature. *World J. Surg. Oncol.* 2006;**4**:19.

36. Cuschieri A, Weeden S, Fielding J, et al. Patient survival after d1 and d2 resections for gastric cancer: long-term results of the MRC randomized surgical trial. *Surgical Cooperative Group. Br. J. Cancer* 1999;**79**(9–10):1522–30.

37. Makela J, Kiviniemi H, Laitinen S. Prevalence of perforated sigmoid diverticulitis is increasing. *Dis Colon Rectum* 2002;**45**(7):955–61.

38. Biondo S, Pares D, Marti Rague J, et al. Emergency operations for nondiverticular perforation of the left colon. *Am. J. Surg.* 2002; **183**(3):256–60.

39. Gedebou TM, Wong RA, Rappaport WD, et al. Clinical presentation and management of iatrogenic colon perforations. *Am. J. Surg.* 1996; **172**(5):454–7.

40. Miki T, Ogata S, Uto M, et al. Multidetector-row CT findings of colonic perforation: direct visualization of ruptured colonic wall. *Abdom. Imaging* 2004;**29**(6):658–62.

41. Lohrmann C, Ghanem N, Pache G, et al. CT in acute perforated sigmoid diverticulitis. *Eur. J. Radiol.* 2005;**56**(1):78.–83.

42. Chintapalli KN, Chopra S, Ghiatas AA, et al. Diverticulitis versus colon cancer: differentiation with helical CT findings. *Radiology* 1999;**210**(2):429–35.

43. Hinchey EJ, Schaal PG, Richards GK. Treatment of perforated diverticular disease of the colon. *Adv. Surg.* 1978; **12**:85–109.

44. Linder MM, Wacha H, Feldmann U, et al. The Mannheim peritonitis index: an instrument for the intraoperative prognosis of peritonitis. *Chirurg* 1987; **58**(2):84–92.

45. Billing A, Frohlich D, Schildberg FW. Prediction of outcome using the Mannheim peritonitis index in 2003 patients. *Peritonitis Study Group. Br. J. Surg.* 1994; **81**(2):209–13.

46. Krukowski ZH, Matheson NA. Emergency surgery for diverticular disease complicated by generalized and faecal peritonitis: a review. *Br. J. Surg.* 1984; **71**(12):921–7.

47. Stabile BE, Puccio E, van Sonnenberg E, et al. Preoperative percutaneous drainage of diverticular abscesses. *Am. J. Surg.* 1990; **159**(1):99–104.

48. Eng K, Ranson JH, Localio SA. Resection of the perforated segment: a significant advance in treatment of diverticulitis with free perforation or abscess. *Am. J. Surg.* 1977; **133**(1):67–72.

49. Rugtiv GM. Diverticulitis: selective surgical management. *Am. J. Surg.* 1975; **130**(2):219–25.

50. Bell C, Asolati M, Hamilton E, et al. A comparison of complications associated with colostomy reversal versus ileostomy reversal. *Am. J. Surg.* 2005; **190**(5):717–20.

51. Aydin HN, Remzi FH, Tekkis PP, et al. Hartmann's reversal is associated with high postoperative adverse events. *Dis. Colon Rectum* 2005;**48**(11):2117–26.

52. Keck JO, Collopy BT, Ryan PJ, et al. Reversal of Hartmann's procedure: effect of timing and technique on ease and safety. *Dis. Colon Rectum* 1994;**37**(3):243–8.

53. Abbas S. Resection and primary anastomosis in acute complicated diverticulitis, a systematic review of the literature. *Int. J. Colorectal Dis.* 2007;**22**:351–7.

54. Constantinides VA, Tekkis PP, Athanasiou T, et al. Primary resection with anastomosis vs. Hartmann's procedure in nonelective surgery for acute colonic diverticulitis: a systematic review. Dis. *Colon Rectum* 2006;**49**(7):966–81.

55. Oberkofler CE, Rickenbacher A, Raptis DA, et al. A multi center randomized clinical trial of primary anastomosis or Hartmann's procedure for perforated left colonic diverticulitis with purulent or fecal peritonitis. *Ann. Surg.* 2012;**256**(5):819–26.

56. Patriti A, Contine A, Carbone E, et al. One-stage resection without colonic lavage in emergency surgery of the left colon. *Colorectal Dis.* 2005; **7**(4):332–8.

57. Ambrosetti P, Michel JM, Megevand JM, et al. Left colectomy with immediate anastomosis in emergency surgery. *Ann. Chir.* 1999;**53**(10):1023–8.

58. Biondo S, Perea M, Rague J, et al. One-stage procedure in non-elective surgery for diverticular disease complications. *Colorectal Dis.* 2001;**3**:42–5.

59. Regenet N, Pessaux P, Hennekinne S, et al. Primary anastomosis after intraoperative colonic lavage vs. Hartmann's procedure in generalized peritonitis complicating diverticular disease of the colon. Int. J. *Colorectal Dis.* 2003;**18**(6):503.–7.

60. Jones OM, Stevenson AR, Clark D, et al. Laparoscopic resection for diverticular disease: follow-up of 500 consecutive patients. *Ann. Surg.* 2008;**248**(6):1092–7.

61. Pendlimari R, Touzios JG, Azodo IA, et al. Short-term outcomes after elective mimally invasive colectomy for diverticulitis. *Br. J. Surg.* 2011;**98**(3):431–5.

62. Royds J, O'Riordan JM, Eguare E, et al. Laparoscopic surgery for complicated diverticular disease: a single-centre experience. *Colorectal Dis.* 2012;**14**(10):1248–54.

63. Taylor CJ, Layani L, Ghusn MA, et al. Perforated diverticulitis managed by laparoscopic lavage. *ANZ J. Surg.* 2006;**76**(11):962–5.

64. Myers E, Hurley M, O'Sullivan GC, et al. Laparoscopic peri toneal lavage for generalized peritonitis due to perforated diverticulitis. *Br. J. Surg.* 2008;**95**(1):97–101.

65. Toorenvliet BR, Swank H, Schoones JW, et al. Laparoscopic peritoneal lavage for perforated colonic diverticulitis: a systematic review. *Colorectal Dis* 2010;**12**(9):862–7.

66. Swank HA, Mulder IM, Hoofwijk AG, et al. Early experience with laparoscopic lavage for perforated diverticulitis. *Br. J. Surg.* 2013;**100**(5):704–10.

67. Swank HA, Vermeulen J, Lange JF, et al. The ladies trial: laparoscopic peritoneal lavage or resection for purulent peritonitis and Hartmann's procedure or resection with primary anastomosis for purulent or faecal peritonitis in perforated diverticulitis (NTR2037). *BMC Surg.* 2010;**10**:29.

68. Thornell A, Angenete E, Gonzales E, et al. Treatment of acute diverticulitis laparoscopic lavage vs. resection (DILALA): study protocol for a randomised controlled trial. *Trials* 2011;**12**:186.

69. Schultz JK, Oresland T. Scandanavian Diverticulitis Trial (SCANDIV). [Online] Available at http://www.clinicaltrials.gov/show/NCT01047462 (accessed 2 July 2015).

70. Hogan A, Winter DC. The LapLAND Trial: Laparoscopic Lavage for Acute Non-Faeculent Diverticulitis. [Online] Available at http://www.clinicaltrials.gov/show/NCT01019239 (accessed 2 July 2015).

CHAPTER 30

Intestinal obstruction

Kevin McCallion

Ulster Hospital, Dundonald, Belfast, UK

Introduction

Intestinal obstruction is defined as the impedance or restriction to the normal passage of intestinal contents through the gastrointestinal tract. It is a common surgical emergency and is broadly classified into two categories: mechanical (dynamic) and paralytic ileus (adynamic). Mechanical obstruction occurs when intestinal peristalsis is actively working against a physical blockage. Ileus occurs where there is a loss of normal peristalsis, without a physical blockage present.

Further subdivision and clinical presentation is based on:
- level of obstruction: proximal or distal
- speed of onset: acute or chronic
- etiology: intraluminal, mural, extrinsic
- nature/pathophysiology: simple mechanical, strangulated (ischemic), perforated, closed loop, volvulus, intussusception.

Clinical presentation varies depending on the site, speed of onset, and etiology of the obstruction but broadly, the classical symptoms are: colicky abdominal pain, abdominal distension, constipation (especially with distal obstruction), and vomiting (especially with proximal obstruction).

Etiology

Mechanical (dynamic) obstruction

Causes of mechanical obstruction can be divided into three subgroups: intraluminal, mural (intrinsic), and extrinsic.

Intraluminal

Ingested foreign bodies can cause obstruction especially in children and people with learning difficulties. Fecal impaction can cause severe constipation with overflow diarrhea. In rare cases, usually in frail or elderly people, this can result in obstruction and perforation at the site of impaction (stercoral perforation). Gallstone ileus results when a large gallstone erodes through the gallbladder into the intestine via a cholecyst–duodenal fistula, causing mechanical obstruction (making the term ileus a misnomer) when it impacts at the ileocecal valve. Occasionally, the gallstone impacts in the duodenum causing gastric outlet obstruction (Bouveret syndrome).

Mural (intrinsic)

Lesions intrinsic to the bowel wall form strictures, which obstruct the passage of intestinal contents. Malignant strictures are the most common cause of intrinsic obstruction in adults but benign strictures from inflammatory bowel disease (most commonly Crohn's disease), diverticular disease and iatrogenic strictures following drugs (e.g. non-steroidal anti-inflammatory drugs), radiation, or surgery are also found. In infants, congenital atresia or stenosis are the most common causes of intrinsic obstruction.

Extrinsic

The most common cause of intestinal obstruction is extrinsic compression from adhesions. The incidence of adhesions causing obstruction is decreasing due to the use of powder-free gloves and improved operative techniques (including laparoscopic surgery). Hernias cause

Gastrointestinal Emergencies, Third Edition. Edited by Tony C. K. Tham, John S. A. Collins, and Roy Soetikno.
© 2016 John Wiley & Sons, Ltd. Published 2016 by John Wiley & Sons, Ltd.

extrinsic obstruction by constricting the intestine as it passes through the neck of the hernia sac. This results in an obstructed, irreducible hernia. If the blood supply to the herniated bowel becomes compromised then the bowel will become ischemic (strangulated hernia). Inguinal hernias (due to the fact that they are the most common type of hernia) are responsible for most cases of hernial obstruction. However, a greater percentage of femoral hernias present with obstruction, due to the femoral canal being narrow and rigid. Femoral hernias often present after significant weight loss with loss of fat from the femoral canal.

A volvulus occurs when a portion of the intestine twists around itself resulting in a closed-loop obstruction. A closed-loop obstruction refers to an obstruction where the intestine is obstructed both proximally and distally (i.e. there is no point of decompression). Volvulus can affect any part of the intestine, including a gastric volvulus, sigmoid volvulus, cecal volvulus, or small bowel volvulus. The kink or twist that obstructs the lumen can also involve the blood supply resulting in ischemia, necrosis and perforation if untreated. This swirling of the mesenteric blood vessels can be identified on a computerized tomography (CT) scan. In the case of malrotation, a mid-gut volvulus can occur around the super mesenteric artery, resulting in necrosis of the entire small bowel.

In a strangulated obstruction the viability of the bowel is threatened due to inadequate perfusion. Initially venous return is compromised, resulting in congestion and edema of the affected segment of bowel. As the congestion and edema progresses, the pressure exceeds that of arterial pressure, resulting in ischemia. As the viability of the bowel mucosa is affected, there is a great loss of electrolytes and fluid, and spread of bacteria into the bloodstream with associated toxins, resulting in sepsis and endotoxemia. Strangulation occurs, most commonly, secondary to hernias but is also found secondary to adhesive bands, internal hernias, or volvulus. Differentiation between simple and strangulated hernias is clinically difficult. However, the absence of pyrexia, tachycardia, abdominal or hernia tenderness, and leukocytosis make strangulation less likely.

Paralytic ileus (adynamic obstruction)

Lack of transmission of normal peristalsis via the myenteric plexus causes an adynamic obstruction or paralytic ileus. When affecting the colon this is usually termed a pseudo-obstruction (Ogilvie syndrome). Failure of contraction leads to stasis, with accumulation of gas and fluid. It is most commonly seen as a result of abdominal surgery and usually lasts no longer than 48–72 hours. Prolonged postoperative ileus should give rise to suspicion of another cause of obstruction such as intra-abdominal sepsis, hemorrhage, metabolic upset, or port-site hernia following a laparoscopic procedure. Other causes of ileus include pneumonia, electrolyte abnormalities, spinal injury, retroperitoneal trauma or hemorrhage, drugs such as tricyclic antidepressants, mesenteric ischemia, and acute pancreatitis.

History

The level of the obstruction is important in determining the symptoms with which the patient will present. High small bowel obstruction tends to be of sudden onset, with vomiting, while low small bowel obstruction has a more gradual onset. Large bowel obstruction usually has an insidious onset, starting with constipation. The classic symptoms of mechanical obstruction are abdominal pain, vomiting, distension, and constipation. In contrast, adynamic obstruction is usually painless.

The pain of obstruction is experienced as a colicky visceral pain. Patients tend to be restless with the pain and unable to find a position of relief. Pain that is relieved by lying still raises the possibility of obstruction complicated with peritonitis. The area where the pain is felt is dependent on the embryological origin of the intestine that is affected. Embryological mid-gut obstruction (second part of the duodenum to two-thirds along the transverse colon) presents with periumbilical discomfort. Hindgut obstruction (distal to two-thirds along transverse colon) is felt as lower abdominal colic. Very high small bowel obstruction may be associated with a more continuous epigastric pain, relieved by vomiting.

The degree of abdominal distension is also dependent on the level of obstruction. In all patients, there is overgrowth of both aerobic and anaerobic organisms, which results in increased gas production. Absorption of fluids and electrolytes by the intestine is inhibited, while production continues unabated. Intestine proximal to the level of obstruction therefore becomes dilated as a result of accumulation of fluid and gas. In distal obstruction (colonic or distal small bowel), distension can therefore be marked. In contrast, high small bowel or any closed-loop obstruction can present with minimal distension.

Absolute constipation is failure to pass either flatus or feces and is an early sign of large bowel obstruction. Patients with small bowel obstruction may still pass flatus or feces due to residual colonic matter, and therefore the absence of constipation does not exclude intestinal obstruction. If the obstruction is partial it may be associated with overflow diarrhea rather than constipation, for example fecal impaction, gallstone ileus, and colonic cancer.

Vomiting is an early feature of high small bowel obstruction and may result in relief from the associated pain. In general, the more distal the level of obstruction the later is the onset of vomiting as a feature. In some cases with distal colonic obstruction vomiting may even be absent. The longer the history of the obstruction the more feculent is the nature of the vomitus.

In taking the medical history of a patient with suspected intestinal obstruction, direct questioning concerning previous abdominal surgery and any lumps or hernias in the groin is essential. Care should also be exercised to inquire of weight loss, symptoms of anaemia, altered bowel habit, respiratory symptoms, recent surgery, trauma, and medications. It is important to inquire about any change in the nature of the pain as a shift from colicky pain to a more constant pain may indicate strangulation and ischemia with impending perforation. Depending on the underlying cause, perforation may occur at the point of obstruction or in the proximally dilated bowel. A detailed medical history is important, as this may point towards a likely cause of obstruction and will be important when considering treatment options.

Examination

In the early stages of intestinal obstruction the patient may look well and vital signs appear normal. Often by the time the patient presents for help, the intestinal obstruction, however, is advanced and he or she is severely ill. Persistent vomiting and diminished luminal absorption of fluid and electrolytes can lead to potentially fatal imbalances. Patients may exhibit signs of dehydration, with reduced skin turgor, dry mucous membranes, tachycardia, and hypotension. If the temperature is raised, complications such as intestinal ischemia or perforation should be considered. Alternatively the temperature could be raised because the obstructing pathology involves inflammation,

for example acute diverticulitis, pericolic abscess, or inflammatory bowel disease.

Abdominal inspection focuses on the presence of scars from previous surgery, indicating a possible etiology from adhesions, and the presence of abdominal wall or groin hernias. Together, they are the two commonest causes of obstruction. Abdominal distension is usual, and the more distal the obstruction the more obvious it is. In some thin patients it may be possible to see visible peristalsis. Patients with gastric outlet obstruction may have an audible succussion splash.

Mild tenderness is commonly present. Marked tenderness indicates the progression to a complication such as ischemia or perforation. Palpation may reveal a mass, such as in acute diverticulitis or an obstructing cancer. The need to carefully examine the hernial orifices cannot be overstated. Redness of the overlying skin or tenderness of the hernia may indicate strangulation.

On auscultation, the presence of high-pitched, tinkling, hyperactive bowel sounds indicate dynamic obstruction, whereas absent bowel sou nds are indicative of adynamic obstruction.

Rectal examination is usually normal but may demonstrate an obstructing rectal cancer, fecal impaction or a ballooned, empty rectum in adynamic pseudo-obstruction.

Investigations

In the early phase all laboratory investigations may be normal. A raised white blood cell count or C-reactive protein (CRP) may indicate an inflammatory cause for the obstruction or the development of complications, such as ischemia or perforation. Dehydration is common in small bowel obstruction and prerenal failure may be seen with a raised serum urea and creatinine. High small bowel obstruction with profuse vomiting may be associated with hypochloremic, hypokalemic alkalosis. A marked acidosis or raised serum amylase may indicate intestinal ischemia as a complication, though these are not universally reliable.

Plain, supine abdominal radiography is the initial imaging modality of choice. This can be used to demonstrate the presence of obstruction and reveal the distinctive features of large and small bowel dilatation. Small bowel loops tend to be central in position and have striations that pass across the full width of the bowel. The large bowel, in contrast, tends to be peripherally located and its haustra (caused by the taenia coli) do not cover the whole width of the bowel. With a sigmoid volvulus there is grossly dilated bowel, which is seen to arise from the pelvis and extend into the upper abdomen. An erect chest radiograph, looking for subdiaphragmatic gas, is useful to help exclude perforation. An erect abdominal radiograph may demonstrate the presence of fluid levels, though these may also be caused by other non-obstructing conditions such as pancreatitis and abscess. In obstruction due to gallstone ileus, pneumobilia due to the enterobiliary fistula may be seen on abdominal radiography in association with distal small bowel obstruction and (in approximately 10% of cases) a radio-opaque gallstone in the right iliac fossa (Rigler's triad). Plain abdominal radiographs will not differentiate between mechanical obstruction and paralytic ileus.

Previously a water-soluble enema was used to confirm and demonstrate the level of suspected colonic obstruction and a contrast follow-through to assess suspected small bowel obstruction.

The current investigation of choice for suspected intestinal obstruction is CT scanning, which will differentiate between mechanical obstruction and ileus. The etiology of mechanical obstruction can be characterized and potential complications identified (e.g. imminent or actual perforation). In neoplastic conditions, a scan can provide cancer staging information that may influence treatment, such as the presence of metastases. A CT scan may also provide information regarding the urgency of surgical intervention. For example, evidence of a perforation or volvulus will require urgent intervention whereas incomplete obstruction secondary to adhesions may settle with conservative management. An abrupt transition point between dilated proximal and collapsed distal bowel is unlikely to resolve with conservative management. A CT scan is particularly useful in differentiating between obstruction and other causes of the acute abdomen.

Management

The primary aim of initial management is aggressive resuscitation. Patients should be treated with oxygen, intravenous fluids, nasogastric tube decompression, and a urinary catheter. Usually, successful resuscitation improves the patient's symptoms and signs and one should be careful not to be falsely reassured that surgery is not required.

Adynamic or paralytic ileus is usually treated by conservative, non-operative measures that rely on nasogastric decompression and resuscitation of fluid and electrolyte abnormalities. The aim should be to diagnose and treat the underlying medical or surgical cause of the problem. Surgery may be required if the cause is an acute abdominal problem such as peritonitis. Intra-abdominal abscess as a cause of ileus is usually best managed by CT- or ultrasound-guided drainage.

While surgery is often required early in the management of mechanical obstruction there are some exceptions when it may be wiser to observe the patient expectantly. These include: multiple previous operations for obstruction, postoperative ileus, abdominal carcinomatosis, prior abdominal or pelvic radiation, and inflammatory bowel disease. The timing of any surgical intervention is dependent on the level of the obstruction, the assessment of whether the obstruction is simple or involves strangulated intestine, the degree or severity of electrolyte imbalance and the likelihood of the patient's condition and organ function being improved by delaying surgery.

High small bowel obstruction is rarely complicated by strangulation and the priority of management is correction of the fluid and electrolyte imbalances that are frequently severe due to profuse vomiting. Often it is possible to defer surgery until after full investigation. Mid to lower small bowel obstruction is at a higher risk of strangulation and surgery is more often required soon after the initial resuscitation. In the absence of any features of strangulation it is safe to defer surgery and investigate with CT scanning – occasionally the water-soluble oral contrast (an osmotic laxative) may prove therapeutic. Surgery for uncomplicated large bowel obstruction can usually be deferred until after investigations which may include a flexible sigmoidoscopy. Caution should be exercised when a closed-loop obstruction is suspected. Right iliac fossa tenderness associated with colonic obstruction should prompt intervention.

Specific management is dependent on the etiology of the obstruction and the likelihood of strangulation. Incomplete adhesive obstruction may be treated successfully using the above conservative measures. Obstruction due to other mechanical causes should be treated surgically following appropriate preoperative resuscitation, and is tailored to the cause. For example, an obstruction due to a hernia requires reduction of the hernia, resection of non-viable intestine, and hernia repair.

An exploratory laparotomy is required for cases due to conditions other than a hernia. Adequate exposure is by a midline incision appropriate for the suspected pathology. A previous incision is used if present and it is safest to enter the abdomen via an extension of the old wound where adhesions are least likely. The main considerations during the laparotomy are to determine the site and nature of the obstruction as well as the viability of the gut. The site of obstruction will usually have been determined on the CT scan. Decompression of small bowel loops by milking contents back to stomach and aspiration via nasogastric tube is preferable to decompression via an enterotomy. Decompression of a massively distended colon can usually be accomplished using a large-bore needle connected to suction and inserted through one of the taenia coli. Particularly when the obstruction is due to adhesions, inflammatory bowel disease or diffuse cancer, it is important to examine the entire length of the small bowel as more than one level of obstruction may be present.

An obstructing colonic cancer can be treated with an appropriate resection dependent on the site of the tumor. The decision to perform a primary anastomosis or fashion a stoma following resection will depend upon many factors including patient comorbidity, hemodynamic status, presence of ischemia, degree of peritoneal cavity contamination (by feces or pus), site of obstruction, as well as surgeon experience. An uncomplicated cecal obstruction is likely to be treated by right hemicolectomy and primary anastomosis. A sigmoid stercoral obstruction with perforation and fecal contamination in a frail patient is likely to be treated with a Hartmann's procedure (segmental resection and end colostomy). Due to the high chance of an often permanent stoma following emergency surgery for left-sided colonic obstructing tumors, self-expanding metal colonic stents can be used as a bridge to surgery or as definitive treatment in a palliative setting, such as the presence of diffuse metastatic disease. When used as a bridge to surgery, colonic stenting allows decompression of the bowel, resuscitation of the patient, and converts an emergency operation into a (semi-)elective one. The intent is to reduce the risks associated with emergency surgery as well as enable a primary anastomois to be performed. There were early concerns regarding tumor perforation by emergency colonic stenting and ongoing trials are taking place to clarify which approach is optimal (emergency surgery or delayed surgery following emergency stenting).

In cases of obstruction due to irresectable disease a defunctioning stoma or bypass may be performed. For example, an obstructing cecal tumour can be palliatively bypassed with an ileotransverse anastomosis. Obstruction associated with diffuse intra-abdominal malignancy can be treated with a combination of antiemetics, antisecretory drugs (octreotide or hyoscine), analgesics and corticosteroids.

Acknowledgment

We are grateful to the previous writers of this chapter, Andrew B.C. Crumley and Robert C. Stuart.

CHAPTER 31
Acute appendicitis

Ian McAllister

Ulster Hospital, Dundonald, Belfast, UK

Introduction

Acute appendicitis is the most common indication for emergency abdominal surgery. It may occur at any age, but most commonly during young adulthood, with a further peak during the seventh decade of life. Its incidence has risen in the United States during the last two decades [1]. Male and female lifetime risks for appendicitis are 8.6% and 5.7%, respectively [2]. Mortality rates are under 1% and most deaths are due to perforated appendicitis and peritonitis at the extremes of age [3].

An accurate clinical assessment is required to achieve a timely diagnosis. Patients may present atypically, and therefore a thorough history and physical examination remain essential in discriminating patients with acute appendicitis from the large differential diagnosis (Table 31.1). An early diagnosis of acute appendicitis is paramount to avoiding the increased morbidity and mortality associated with the sequelae of perforation, namely abscess and peritonitis.

Etiology

Acute appendicitis is probably caused by obstruction of the appendiceal lumen. Obstruction may be triggered by fecoliths, lymphoid hyperplasia, parasitic worms, or neoplasms of the cecum or appendix itself. Low-fiber diets and various infective agents, including *Yersinia*, have also been associated with an increased risk of appendicitis [4, 5].

Approximately 1% of cases of acute appendicitis are caused by an appendiceal carcinoid tumor. The appendix is the most common site for carcinoid tumors of the intestinal tract. Most are less than 1 cm in size, located at the tip, rarely metastasize, and approximately half will present as appendicitis.

Obstruction causes increasing intraluminal and intramural pressures, leading to vascular and lymphatic compromise. This results in ischemia, bacterial overgrowth, and eventually full-thickness inflammation, which may involve adjacent structures such as small bowel, omentum, and parietal peritoneum. Transmural necrosis may precipitate perforation, leading to a localized abscess or more diffuse peritonitis.

History

The presentation of acute appendicitis is variable. Approximately half of patients will describe the classical symptom of periumbilical pain migrating to the right iliac fossa over a 12–24 hour period. Other common symptoms include anorexia, nausea, and vomiting. Thorough systemic, urological, and gynecological histories should also be obtained.

Examination

On general examination patients may exhibit a tachycardia and pyrexia. The typical abdominal finding is peritonism in the right iliac fossa, and classically, over McBurney's

---

Gastrointestinal Emergencies, Third Edition. Edited by Tony C. K. Tham, John S. A. Collins, and Roy Soetikno.
© 2016 John Wiley & Sons, Ltd. Published 2016 by John Wiley & Sons, Ltd.

Table 31.1 Differential diagnosis of acute appendicitis.

Site of pathology	Diagnosis
Gynecological	Pelvic inflammatory disease
	Ectopic pregnancy
	Ovarian cyst (rupture/torsion)
	Tubo-ovarian abscess
	Endometriosis
Gastrointestinal	Crohn's disease
	Ileal perforation
	Meckel's diverticulum
	Cecal/small bowel neoplasm
	Gastroenteritis
	Intestinal obstruction
	Omental torsion
	Pancreatitis
	Cholecystitis
	Peptic ulcer
	Diverticulitis
Genitourinary	Urinary tract infection
	Renal calculus
	Pyelonephritis
	Testicular torsion
Other	Infective (tuberculosis/*Yersinia*)
	Pulmonary
	Systemic (diabetes, porphyria)
	Mesenteric adenitis
	Non-specific abdominal pain

point. This may be demonstrated by percussion tenderness. Positive Rosving's (right iliac fossa pain elicited by left iliac fossa palpation) and Dunphy's (increased pain on coughing) signs also indicate localized peritonism, and are suggestive of appendicitis. A positive psoas stretch (right iliac fossa pain on passive right hip extension) may signal retrocecal appendicitis. Unless the appendix lies within the pelvis, a digital rectal examination does not provide additional diagnostic information, particularly when the abdominal findings are suggestive [6].

Unusual presentations

Variations in the position of the appendix may produce atypical presentations and signs. Retrocecal appendicitis may cause a dull abdominal ache and minimal, or even absent, abdominal signs. Left-sided pain, urinary urgency, frequency, dysuria, or diarrhea may signal a pelvic

appendicitis. Again, there may be minimal abdominal findings, but rectal tenderness will often be present and a pelvic mass palpable if an associated abscess has developed.

Appendicitis is most difficult to diagnose at the extremes of age. The very young may present late and without a history. Elderly patients may have subtle signs and symptoms and are subject to a wider differential diagnosis. These factors, compounded by a lower level of suspicion in assessing these age-groups, may result in a delayed diagnosis and increased morbidity in these vulnerable patients.

Chronic or grumbling appendicitis remains a controversial diagnosis, but it is accepted that recurrent episodes of luminal obstruction may result in a chronically inflamed or fibrotic appendix. Rarely, an episode of acute appendicitis will spontaneously resolve, resulting in a chronically inflamed and symptomatic appendix. These patients are often cured by appendicectomy. Chronic appendicitis should be a diagnosis of exclusion, having considered chronic non-specific abdominal pain amongst other causes, before undertaking operative management.

Appendicitis during pregnancy may produce right upper quadrant rather than right iliac fossa tenderness, as the appendix migrates cephalad with the enlarging uterus. The gravid uterus may also displace the parietal peritoneum anteriorly, resulting in less peritonism.

Investigation

Although clinical assessment is the mainstay of diagnosis, this may be complemented by laboratory and imaging findings. Most patients exhibit a leukocytosis (with neutrophilia) and/or elevated C-reactive protein. If levels of both these inflammatory markers are normal then appendicitis is unlikely [7]. Urinalysis may help to exclude significant urinary tract disease.

The Alvorado score is the most widely recognized of several scoring systems devised to aid the diagnosis of appendicitis. Eight criteria are used to predict the likelihood of appendicitis and direct management. These variables include: migratory right iliac fossa pain, anorexia, nausea/vomiting, right iliac fossa tenderness, rebound tenderness, fever, and leukocytosis with left shift [8]. Used as adjuncts to clinical judgment, these scoring systems may improve specificity and reduce negative appendicectomy rates. However, they are not definitively diagnostic, are seldom used, and remain inferior to senior clinical assessment.

Imaging should be performed if appendicitis is suspected but the diagnosis is unclear. Transabdominal ultrasound has an unclear role in the diagnosis of appendicitis. Sensitivity and specificity rates are 86% and 81% respectively [9]. It may help to confirm the clinical diagnosis of appendicitis but cannot be relied upon to exclude appendicitis. Ultrasonography may also be of benefit in the identification of other causes of right iliac fossa pain such as ovarian, urinary, or biliary pathology without exposure to ionizing radiation.

Computerized tomography (CT) is probably more accurate in diagnosing appendicitis with 94% sensitivity and 95% specificity [9]. It also has the advantage of visualization of the entire abdomen. It is of particular benefit in patients with a palpable right iliac fossa mass who may have an associated neoplasm or have developed an appendiceal abscess or phlegmon.

However, despite the increased use of imaging modalities, rates of negative appendicectomy and perforated appendicitis remain unchanged [10, 11]. Diagnostic imaging is unnecessary if the clinical diagnosis of appendicitis has been made and should be reserved for cases when the diagnosis of appendicitis is clinically suspected but unclear. Women of child-bearing age have the highest incidence of negative appendicectomy (up to 20%), and this sub-group of patients may benefit most from imaging as the diagnosis is often gynecological. The role of laparoscopy will be discussed below.

Management

If acute appendicitis is suspected, the patient should be fluid resuscitated and adequate analgesia administered (see Fig 31.1). Narcotic analgesia does not compromise diagnostic accuracy and should not be withheld [12].

Prompt appendicectomy remains the management of choice and may be performed either by an open or laparoscopic approach. A single preoperative antibiotic dose covering both aerobic and anaerobic organisms should be administered within 1 hour of surgery as this

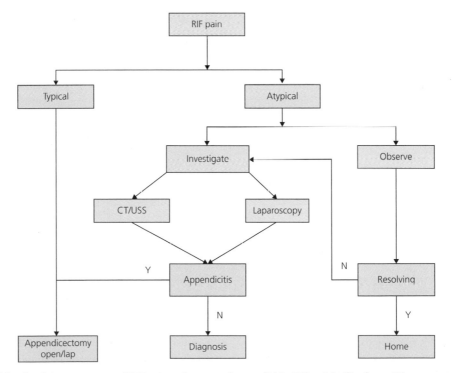

Fig. 31.1 Algorithm for the management of RIF pain and suspected appendicitis. RIF = right iliac fossa, CT = computerized tomography scan, USS = ultrasound scan.

reduces the incidence of post-appendicectomy wound infection and intra-abdominal abscess [13]. Thromboprophylaxis should also be routinely prescribed.

Open appendicectomy

A conventional appendicectomy is performed via either a gridiron or Lanz incision in the right iliac fossa. A muscle-splitting technique is used to enter the peritoneal cavity. The appendix stump should be short and simply ligated. Stump burial is unnecessary [14]. Should the appendix be perforated at its base then a cuff of cecal pole can be excised en bloc with a linear stapling device. All free fluid should be aspirated but formal lavage is unnecessary unless the appendix has perforated resulting in peritoneal contamination. Postoperative antibiotics are also reserved for cases of perforated appendicitis, and most surgeons would advocate a 5-day broad-spectrum regimen. Early return to regular diet and mobilization are encouraged postoperatively and most patients achieve discharge within 48 hours.

Laparoscopic appendicectomy

A pneumoperitoneum is created after bladder and gastric decompression. A 3-port approach via paraumbilical, left iliac fossa, and suprapubic port-sites is most commonly used. The appendiceal base is divided following loop ligation or with a laparoscopic stapler. The appendix is retrieved in a specimen bag and lavage performed if necessary. Postoperative management mirrors the open approach.

Meta-analyses have shown laparoscopic appendicectomy to be associated with lower wound infection rates, less postoperative pain, and shorter hospital stay. However, longer operative times, higher rates of intra-abdominal abscess, and higher costs compared with the open approach were also evident, particularly in cases of complicated appendicitis [15].

Laparoscopic appendicectomy has gained widespread acceptance and rates are rising. This trend has been associated with decreasing rates of open conversion and complications. Provided the surgical expertise and equipment are available, laparoscopic appendicectomy has definite advantages over the open approach. In particular, it is the preferred approach in women of child-bearing age as it may reveal other pelvic pathology and is associated with reduced morbidity and mortality in obese and elderly patients [16, 17].

If a normal appendix is found, laparoscopy provides comprehensive abdomino-pelvic visualization which may reveal an alternative diagnosis. Removal of a normal appendix at laparoscopy is controversial. However, in the absence of alternative pathology, the normal appendix should be excised. Microscopic appendicitis is evident in approximately a third of grossly normal appendices and, furthermore, appendicitis can be excluded from the differential diagnosis of further right iliac fossa pain.

Non-operative management

Whilst the majority of patients undergo appendicectomy, there is evidence that some patients can be managed non-operatively with antibiotic therapy alone. However, there is a significant risk of recurrent appendicitis within 1 year and approximately 30% of conservatively managed patients will ultimately require surgery [18, 19]. Unless the operative risks are prohibitive, appendicectomy remains the gold standard [20, 21].

Management of complicated appendicitis

Appendix mass

Patients presenting with a history of abdominal pain in excess of 5–7 days may be found to have a palpable, tender, right iliac fossa mass. This may represent a phlegmon centered upon an inflamed appendix and involving adherent omentum and small bowel. The diagnosis is best confirmed with CT. Alternative diagnoses, such as Crohn's disease in younger patients or cecal carcinoma in older patients, should also be considered and further imaging or colonoscopy may be required.

An appendix mass should be treated non-operatively with intravenous antibiotics. Surgery is occasionally required for non-responders but is associated with significant rates of ileocecectomy and morbidity including enteric injury and fistulation [22]. Delaying surgery for a further 6–12 weeks was traditionally advocated in such cases. However, recent evidence suggests that, provided other significant pathology has been excluded, interval appendicectomy is no longer justified due to low rates of recurrent symptoms [23].

Appendix abscess

A localized perforation of the appendix can result in a periappendiceal abscess. This may provoke significant sepsis and often requires radiological or, less commonly, surgical drainage. Once resolved, the decision whether to continue a conservative approach or perform an interval appendicectomy is again based on the risks of further symptoms versus operative morbidity.

Postoperative complications

Around 15% of patients will develop a post-appendicectomy wound infection and those with a perforated appendix are at particular risk. Superficial infections mostly respond to antibiotics but a wound abscess usually requires formal drainage.

Appendiceal perforation also increases the risk of postoperative abdominal and pelvic collections. A pelvic abscess may cause systemic sepsis, pain, or diarrhea. Most cases respond to antibiotic therapy but some will require either image-guided or open drainage.

Although historically thought to be associated with risk of infertility, a recent study reported increased pregnancy rates following appendicectomy [24].

References

1. Anderson JE, Bickler SW, Chang DC, Talamini MA. Examining a common disease with unknown etiology: trends in epidemiology and surgical management of appendicitis in California, 1995–2009. *World J. Surg.* 2012;**36**(12):2787–94.
2. Addiss DG, Shaffer N, Fowler BS, Tauxe RV. The epidemiology of appendicitis and appendectomy in the United States. *Am. J. Epidemiol.* 1990;**132**(5):910–25.
3. Baigrie RJ, Dehn TC, Fowler SM, Dunn DC. Analysis of 8651 appendicectomies in England and Wales during 1992. *Br. J. Surg.* 1995;**82**(7):933.
4. Black J. Acute appendicitis in Japanese soldiers in Burma: support for the "fibre" theory. *Gut* 2002;**51**(2):297.
5. Lamps LW. Infectious causes of appendicitis. *Infect. Dis. Clin. N. Am.* 2010;**24**(4):995–1018.
6. Dixon JM, Elton RA, Rainey JB, Macleod DA. Rectal examination in patients with pain in the right lower quadrant of the abdomen. *BMJ* 1991;**302**(6773):386–8.
7. Anderson REB. Meta-analysis of the clinical and laboratory diagnosis of appendicitis. *Br. J. Surg.* 2004;**91**:28–37.
8. Ohle R, O'Reilly F, O'Brien KK, Fahey T, Dimitrov BD. The Alvarado score for predicting acute appendicitis: a systematic review. *BMC Med.* 2011;**9**:139.
9. Teresawa T, Blackmore CC, Bent S, Kohlwes RJ. Systematic review: computed tomography and ultrasonography to detect acute appendicitis in adults and adolescents. *Ann. Intern. Med.* 2004;**141**(7):537–46.
10. Wagner PL, Eachempati SR, Soe K, Pieracci FM, Shou J, Barie PS. Defining the current negative appendectomy rate: for whom is preoperative computed tomography making an impact? *Surgery* 2008;**144**(2):276–82.
11. Flum DR, McClure TD, Morris A, Koepsell T. Misdiagnosis of appendicitis and the use of diagnostic imaging. *J. Am. Coll. Surg.* 2005;**201**(6):933–9.
12. Amoli HA, Golozar A, Keshavarzi S, Tavakoli H, Yaghoobi A. Morphine analgesia in patients with acute appendicitis: a randomised double-blind clinical trial. *Emerg. Med. J.* 2008;**25**(9):586–9.
13. Andersen BR, Kallehave FL, Andersen HK. Antibiotics versus placebo for prevention of postoperative infection after appendicectomy. *Cochrane Database Syst. Rev.* 2005;(**3**):CD001439.
14. Engström L, Fenyö G. Appendicectomy: assessment of stump invagination versus simple ligation: a prospective, randomized trial. *Br. J. Surg.* 1985;**72**(12):971–2.
15. Sauerland S, Jaschinski T, Neugebauer EA. Laparoscopic versus open surgery for suspected appendicitis. *Cochrane Database Syst. Rev.* 2010;(**10**):CD001546.
16. Masoomi H, Nguyen NT, Dolich MO, et al. Comparison of laparoscopic versus open appendectomy for acute nonperforated and perforated appendicitis in the obese population. *Am. J. Surg.* 2011;**202**(6):733–8.
17. Harrell AG, Lincourt AE, Novitsky YW, et al. Advantages of laparoscopic appendectomy in the elderly. *Am. Surg.* 2006;**72**(6):474–80.
18. Varadhan KK, Neal KR, Lobo DN. Safety and efficacy of antibiotics compared with appendicectomy for treatment of uncomplicated acute appendicitis: meta-analysis of randomised controlled trials. *BMJ* 2012;**344**:e2156.
19. Vons C, Barry C, Maitre S, et al. Amoxicillin plus clavulanic acid versus appendicectomy for treatment of acute uncomplicated appendicitis: an open-label, non-inferiority, randomised controlled trial. *Lancet* 2011;**377**(9777):1573–9.
20. Wilms IM, de Hoog DE, de Visser DC, Janzing HM. Appendectomy versus antibiotic treatment for acute appendicitis. *Cochrane Database Syst. Rev.* 2011;(**11**): CD008359.
21. Fitzmaurice GJ, McWilliams B, Hurreiz H, Epanomeritakis E. Antibiotics versus appendectomy in the management of acute appendicitis: a review of the current evidence. *Can. J. Surg.* 2011;**54**(5):307–14.
22. Andersson RE, Petzold MG. Nonsurgical treatment of appendiceal abscess or phlegmon: a systematic review and meta-analysis. *Ann. Surg.* 2007;**246**(5):741–8.
23. Deakin DE, Ahmed I. Interval appendicectomy after resolution of adult inflammatory appendix mass – is it necessary? *Surgeon* 2007;**5**(1):45–50.
24. Wei L, Macdonald TM, Shimi SM. Appendicectomy is associated with increased pregnancy rate: a cohort study. *Ann. Surg.* 2012;**256**(6):1039–44.

CHAPTER 32

Middle gastrointestinal bleeding

Andres Sanchez-Yague

Vithas Xanit International Hospital, Benalmadena, Spain
Hospital Costa del Sol, Marbella, Spain

Introduction

Middle gastrointestinal bleeding (MGIB) represents approximately 5% of all gastrointestinal bleeds. With the advent of capsule endoscopy and balloon-assisted enteroscopy (BAE), a new classification of MGIB with easier to identify landmarks has been proposed [1] – MGIB is considered when the source is located between the ampulla of Vater and the ileocecal valve. Prior classification considered MGIB to be when the source of bleeding was located distal to the ligament of Treitz or proximal to the terminal ileum. MGIB is often an exclusion diagnosis made in the context of obscure gastrointestinal bleeding (OGIB), but although synonymous to some, both terms are not the same. Obscure bleeding is bleeding from the gastrointestinal tract that persists or recurs without obvious etiology despite endoscopic or radiologic evaluation. OGIB can be occult, this is without a visible proof of bleeding or overt with bleeding present in the form of hematemesis, melena, hematochezia, or rectorragia. Occult bleeding is considered an emergency when presenting with profound anemia. Overt bleeding is typically an emergency.

Evaluation

When should we think of MGIB?

MGIB should be considered in patients with occult obscure bleeding and profound anemia or in patients with overt obscure bleeding who have a negative upper endoscopy and colonoscopy However, MGIB should not be pursued in all the patients presenting with suspected blood loss from an unknown origin. For example, further testing is not recommended in patients with obscure bleeding and negative standard workup, but without anemia [2], or in patients with iron deficiency without anemia.

History and examination

A thorough clinical history and physical examination are crucial to reach a diagnosis. Although some information may point towards MGIB, the diagnosis of MGIB is typically considered after causes of upper and lower gastrointestinal bleeding have been excluded.

Patients may present for evaluation of anemia or iron deficiency anemia (considered occult OGIB) or overt gastrointestinal bleeding that can suggest an upper (hematemesis, melena) or lower (hematochezia – bleeding with passage of stool, rectorragia – i.e. bleeding without defecation, or melena) source of bleeding.

Clinical information is very important to determine the next diagnostic step. Hematemesis suggests a bleeding located proximal to the ligament of Treitz while rectorragia suggests a distal bleeding unless rapid passage is suspected. Melena, on the other hand, has little value to predict the bleeding location. The past medical history and use of non-steroidal anti-inflammatory drugs (NSAIDs), anticoagulation, and antiplatelet agents should be reviewed for diseases related to MGIB. Diseases and conditions related to middle gastrointestinal bleed are as follows:

• NSAID intake
• Antiplatelet medication

Gastrointestinal Emergencies, Third Edition. Edited by Tony C. K. Tham, John S. A. Collins, and Roy Soetikno.
© 2016 John Wiley & Sons, Ltd. Published 2016 by John Wiley & Sons, Ltd.

- Anticoagulation
- Chronic renal failure
- Prior abdominal radiotherapy
- Aortic stenosis (Heyde's syndrome)
- Aortic aneurysm repair
- Inflammatory bowel disease
- Celiac disease
- Acquired immune deficiency syndrome
- Hemorrhagic hereditary telangiectasias
- Blue rubber nevus syndrome
- Plummer–Vinson syndrome
- Tylosis
- Pseudoxanthoma elasticum
- Ehlers–Danlos syndrome
- Schönlein–Henoch syndrome
- Neurofibromatosis
- Malignant atrophic papulosis
- Klippel–Trenaunay syndrome
- Behçet's disease.

Patients younger than 40 years old are more prone to have a Meckel's diverticulum, Crohn's disease or other forms of inflammatory bowel disease, Dieulafoy's lesions, or small bowel tumors while older patients present with vascular lesions or NSAID-related enteropathy. A detailed physical, including skin, examination should be performed as some of the abovementioned entities have a dermatological expression.

The causes of middle gastrointestinal bleeding are:
- Vascular
  - Angiodysplasias
  - Arteriovenous malformations
  - Dieulafoy's lesions
  - Ischemic enteritis
  - Varices
- Inflammatory
  - Anastomotic ulcers
  - Crohn's disease
  - Eosinophilic enteritis
  - NSAID enteropathy
  - Radiation enteritis
  - Ulcers
- Autoimmune
  - Amyloidosis
  - Behçet's disease
- Tumors
  - Adenocarcinoma
  - Gastrointestinal stromal tumor
  - Leiomyosarcoma
  - Lymphoma
  - Metastasis
- Malformation
  - Meckel's diverticulum
- Infection
  - Whipple's disease
  - Cytomegalovirus
  - Mycobacterium avium complex disease (MAC)
  - Tuberculosis.

What to do after a negative initial workup on OGIB?

Prior to making the diagnosis of MGIB, a repeat upper, lower or both endoscopies may be necessary to exclude a source in the upper or lower gastrointestinal tract. In cases of overt OGIB featuring hematemesis, repeat upper endoscopy with a forward view endoscope should be performed with special care to rule out ulcers in a hernia sac (Cameron's ulcers). In patients with prior abdominal aortic aneurysm repair the presence of aortoenteric fistulas typically in the distal duodenum. The posterior wall of the duodenal bulb and the duodenal C-loop must be thoroughly studied. A cap attached to the upper endoscope could be useful to exclude posterior duodenal wall ulcers while a duodenoscope would allow us to better study the papilla and rule out hemobilia and, hemosuccus pancreaticus. Colonoscopy should be repeated if there is a high suspicion of a lower gastrointestinal bleeding or the initial colonoscopy was performed under suboptimal conditions (e.g. poor preparation). In patients with occult OGIB duodenal biopsies should be taken to rule out celiac disease if not done before [2].

How do we study the small bowel?

Until the advent of capsule endoscopy (CE) and double balloon enteroscopy (DBE), imaging techniques were the mainstay for the study of OGIB (AGA 2000) [3]. At that time angiography was considered the technique to evaluate overt OGIB, while repeat endoscopy, and small bowel series and computerized tomography (CT) enterography were used to study occult OGIB. With the development of CE and DBE there has been a paradigm shift towards the use of endoscopic examinations to rule out lesions in the small bowel [2]. As we will see, the role of the different endoscopic techniques has also changed, displacing techniques like push enteroscopy and intraoperative enteroscopy to a historical role and enhancing the role of capsule endoscopy and deep enteroscopy techniques.

Endoscopic examinations
Push enteroscopy
Push enteroscopy is performed inserting an enteroscope or a pediatric colonoscope orally. Available enteroscopes range from 200 to 250 cm long and feature a 2.8 mm working channel. A pediatric colonoscope is not as long (around 170 cm) but features a larger diameter, and in some cases a variable stiffness system that provides more rigidity.

Using push enteroscopy the small bowel examination is limited due to looping and patient discomfort. Push enteroscopy allows only a study of 60–80cms distal to the ligament of Treitz. This can be extended by a small distance using an overtube that is designed to reduce looping in the stomach.

The diagnostic yield of push enteroscopy ranges from 24% to 56% when lesions reachable by a standard upper endoscope are excluded. This is important because push enteroscopy can reveal lesions within the reach of a standard upper endoscope in 6–37% [4,5] of cases thus emphasizing the need to perform a careful repeat upper endoscopy prior to push enteroscopy. The use of the aforementioned overtube has not improved the diagnostic yield of push enteroscopy [6,7].

Capsule endoscopy (see Fig. 32.1)
Several meta-analyses have reported a diagnostic yield of CE in OGIB ranging from 36 to 62% [14,15]. CE features a higher yield (55 to 76%) of OGIB detection as compared to push enteroscopy (21–32%) [16–18]. CE is a complimentary tool to DBE [14]. CE shows a similar diagnostic yield when compared to DBE (62% vs 56%), but the yield of DBE rose to 75% when performed after a positive CE while it was only 27.5% if the CE resulted negative. This study confirms other studies that recommended using CE to determine further steps on OGIB management [19].

A negative CE in a patient with overt OGIB or persistent anemia should be taken with caution and alternative methods to study the small bowel should be recommended. As noted above, there were a 27.5% of DBE findings in patients with negative CE [19]. The overall rebleeding rate in patients with a negative CE on overt OGIB has been as high as 28.4%. This rate was higher in patients with positive findings on CE and

especially on those that had to resume anticoagulation after the OGIB episode [20]. CE has also shown a tendency to miss small bowel tumors [21]. Capsule retention is always a concern. As a preventive measure, prior testing using the AGILE patency capsule is recommended in patients with suspected small bowel strictures [22]. Capsule endoscopy should not be used in patients with intestinal diversions such as Roux-en-Y surgery as it would be unable to explore the small bowel completely.

Deep enteroscopy (Fig. 32.2)
Deep enteroscopy can be performed using enteroscopes with modified overtubes. The most extensively studied is DBE followed by single-balloon enteroscopy. Because both feature balloon-tipped overtubes the term balloon-assisted enteroscopy has been proposed [23]. Another option is spiral enteroscopy that uses a spiral-shaped overtube. Deep enteroscopy can be perfomed per orum (antegrade) or per rectum (retrograde). CE can be useful to guide to determine route of insertion [2]. When CE is performed before DBE increases its diagnostic yield from 56% to 71% [14]. However, balloon assisted enteroscopy without prior CE may be considered in patients with significant bleeding [24]. All the enteroscopes designed for deep enteroscopy systems allow for therapeutic intervention and the depth of insertion, rate of therapeutic intervention and procedure times have been considered similar [25,26].

Deep enteroscopy techniques should also be used in cases of altered small bowel anatomy [27].

Double-balloon enteroscopy
DBE features an enteroscope and an overtube with latex-balloons attached to the tip. The insertion technique is also called push–pull·enteroscopy, as it is comprised of a series of steps:
- pushing of the enteroscope;
- inflation of the enteroscope-tip balloon;
- advancement of the overtube;
- inflation of the overtube-tip balloon;
- pull of both;
- deflation of the enteroscope-tip balloon;
- then begin the process again.

Total enteroscopy either with a single insertion or through a combined approach has been achieved in 16–86% of patients [1,28]. Although different studies have reported a diagnostic yield of DBE for OGIB

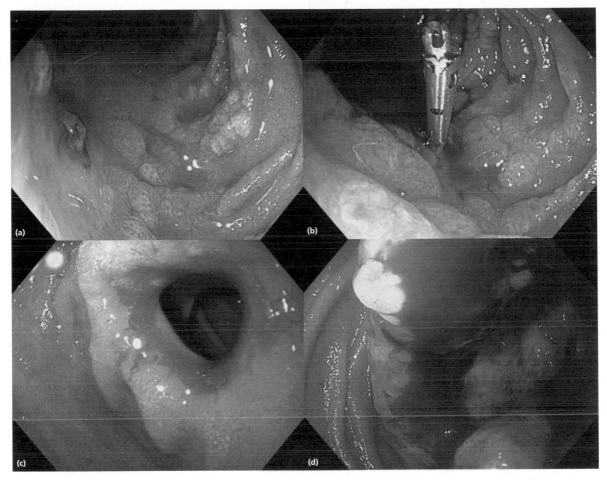

Fig. 32.1 Deep enteroscopy images. (a) Duodenal ulcer with a visible vessel. (b) Duodenal ulcer with visible vessel after endoscopic clipping. (c) Same under NBI. (d) Jejunal tumor. (*see insert for color representation of the figure.*)

ranging from 43 to 81%, an updated meta-analysis has reported a diagnostic yield of DBE of 56% but this percentage increased to 75% when DBE was performed directed by a positive CE examination [14].

Single balloon enteroscopy

Single-balloon enteroscopy (SBE) features a regular 200 cm enteroscope and an overtube with a balloon on the tip. SBE features also a push–pull·technique:

- the enteroscope is pushed forward;
- the overtube-balloon is deflated, the overtube is then advanced;
- the overtube-balloon is inflated;
- both are pulled back;
- the process begins again.

Some authors advocate SBE as easier to use due to the lack of one of the balloons.

The experience with SBE is significantly less than with DBE. The diagnostic yield for OGIB has ranged from 60% to 64.6% in two series [29,30]. Comparison studies have shown similar rates of total enteroscopy rate of SBE and DBE without significant differences (11% compared to 18%) [31].

Spiral enteroscopy

Spiral enteroscopy features an overtube with a spiral-shaped section. There is an overtube designed for anterograde exploration that can be used with any enteroscope under 9.4 mm of diameter and another for colonoscopy and retrograde examination that can be

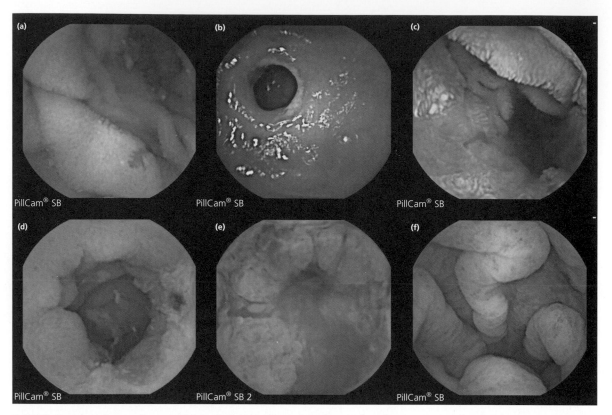

Fig. 32.2 Capsule endoscopy images. (a) Intestinal AVM. (b) Meckel's diverticulum opening. (c) Duodenal ulcer with bleeding visible vessel. (d) NSAID enteropathy with a visible clot. (e) Bleeding ileal tumor. (f) Active gastric bleeding in a patient with portal hypertensive gastropathy. (*see insert for color representation of the figure.*)

used with a pediatric colonoscope. The overtube has a rotatable handle that allows movement of the spiral section. The endoscope is inserted into the overtube that is positioned 25 cm from the tip of the endoscope. The anterograde enteroscopy is performed with advancement and withdrawal maneuvers achieved by rotatory clockwise and counterclockwise movements until the ligament of Treitz is reached. At this point the overtube is left in place and the enteroscope is advanced [32]. Likewise the retrograde examination uses the same movements to advance to the ileocecal valve.

The rate of complete examinations of SE was significantly lower compared to DBE (8% vs 92%) [33].

Intraoperative endoscopy

Intraoperative endoscopy is performed through an enterotomy site during surgery. After insertion the surgeon advances the enteroscope through the bowel.

The diagnostic yield has been shown as high as 84% [34]. On the other hand intraoperative endoscopy has been associated with a high mortality rate up to 17% [35].

At this point intraoperative endoscopy is reserved to patients in which deep enteroscopy cannot be performed for technical difficulties or anatomical conditions (e.g. adhesions, prior surgery, etc.).

Imaging techniques
Small bowel series and enteroclysis

Small bowel series is performed following ingestion of a dilute barium solution and serial abdominal X-rays. In the case of enteroclysis a catheter is advanced to the duodenum and infusion of barium dilute, methylcellulose, and air is performed.

The diagnostic yield of small bowel series is very low compared to capsule endoscopy in OGIB (8% vs 67%)

(15), especially due to the inability to detect small bowel angiodisplasias. Enteroclysis although presenting a diagnostic yield a little bit higher still remains under 20%. Small bowel series should be reserved for situations in which all the other tests are unavailable or when a small bowel stricture is suspected and the AGILE patency capsule is not available.

Cross-sectional imaging enterography and enteroclysis

Cross-sectional imaging enterography and enteroclysis result from the combination of CT and magnetic resonance imaging (MRI) techniques with luminal contrast, either by ingestion of a low density oral contrast (enterography), or infusion through a duodenal catheter (enteroclysis).

A recent meta-analysis has reported a diagnostic yield of CT enterography of 40% [36]. When compared to CE the yield of CT was significantly lower (53% vs 34%) than with DBE (38% vs 78%).

These techniques require a long and complex preparation that precludes their use in overt OGIB [37]. Cross-sectional imaging techniques should be reserved for patients with suspected strictures, intestinal masses, or extramural pathology.

Angiography

Angiography is performed by administering intravenous contrast and is capable of detecting a blood loss over 0.5 mL/min. Anigiography has the abililty to detect bleeding and also non-bleeding lesions like angioectasias.

Two studies comparing CE with angiography have revealed a higher diagnostic yield for CE (53–72% vs 20–56%) [38,39]. CE also provides comparable long-term outcomes compared to angiography [38]. Provocative angiography has been performed with modest results [40] although large studies have not been performed to date. At this point provocative angiography cannot be recommended.

The advantage of angiography is the possibility of therapy by means of embolization or coiling of the bleeding vessel.

CT angiography

CT angiography is performed by administering intravenous contrast and detecting the extravasation of such contrast into the small bowel. A study comparing CT angiography with CE found a lower diagnostic yield than the former (72% vs 24%) [39].

The main limitation is the inability to perform therapy so regular angiography is needed for therapeutic purposes.

Radionuclide scan with technetium 99m-labeled red blood cells

Also known as a bleeding scan, this allows the detection of active bleeding as low as 0.1 mL/min.

This is the most sensitive technique for detecting active gastrointestinal bleeding but lacks the ability to determine the exact cause or location of bleeding especially in the small bowel nor does it allow performing therapy [41].

Scintigraphy with technetium 99m pertechnetate

Also known as Meckel's scan, this allows for the detection of gastric mucosa, including ectopic gastric mucosa. This test does not detect bleeding, but a Meckel's diverticulum is considered a potential bleeding source especially in children and young adult. The sensitivity of a Meckel's scan ranges from 50% to 91% [42].

Management

Treatment of bleeding lesions in the middle gastrointestinal tract

Of all the causes of MGIB (see list previously) only vascular lesions are amenable to endoscopic treatment. Angiodysplasias are venous lesions that can be cauterized with argon plasma, while Dieulafoy's lesions and arteriovenous malformations can cause arterial bleeding, so clipping is necessary. If these lesions are not reached by endoscopic means directed angiographic therapy can be instituted or otherwise surgery might be necessary. Infectious diseases require medical treatment.

Inflammatory and autoimmune conditions require specific treatment, and in some cases surgery, if the treatment is not effective. Tumors are an indication for surgery if the stage is adequate. Meckel's diverticulum should be resected surgically.

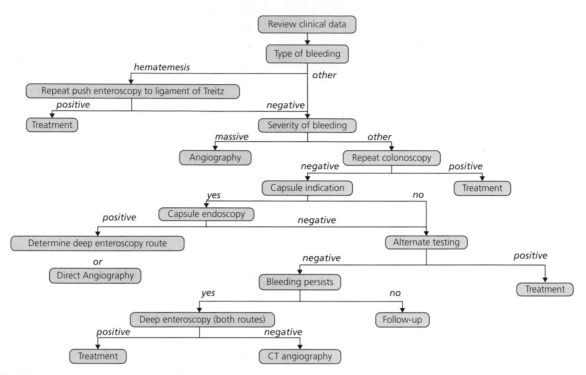

Fig. 32.3 Overt obscure gastrointestinal bleeding algorithm.

Management of OGIB (see Fig. 32.3).

In patients with overt OGIB the first step would be to review the clinical information. If the patient presented with hematemesis repeat upper endoscopy or push enteroscopy to reach the ligament of Treitz should be performed. If this is negative, or the patient presented with other type of bleeding, we should focus on the severity of bleeding; massive bleeding would indicate angiography to detect the bleeding area. Otherwise, repeat colonoscopy should be considered and, if negative, proceed immediately to capsule endoscopy. We favor this approach, as the colon preparation could improve detection of lesions in the small bowel. If available, or CE is unavailable or not indicated (like in altered anatomy patients), other testing options like a bleeding scan, cross-sectional imaging techniques, or deep enteroscopy could be considered. If the capsule is positive we should use it to determine the route of insertion for deep enteroscopy or direct angiographic treatment. If negative, we should continue testing for MGIB using other available techniques. If bleeding persists we would go for deep enteroscopy from both routes in the same session. If incomplete, CT angiography would be performed to detect vessel abnormalities.

The management of OGIB with significant anemia (Fig. 32.4)

In patients with occult OGIB presenting with significant anemia the first step would be to review clinical data. If there is data suggesting an upper or lower lesion repeat upper endoscopy or colonoscopy respectively should be undergone. If repeat testing is negative capsule endoscopy should be performed. If capsule endoscopy is unavailable or not indicated (like in altered anatomy patients) other testing options like cross-sectional imaging techniques or deep enteroscopy should be considered. If the capsule is positive we should use it to determine the route of insertion for deep enteroscopy or direct angiographic treatment. If negative, we should decide whether to continue testing for MGIB using other available techniques or institute medical treatment and follow the patient.

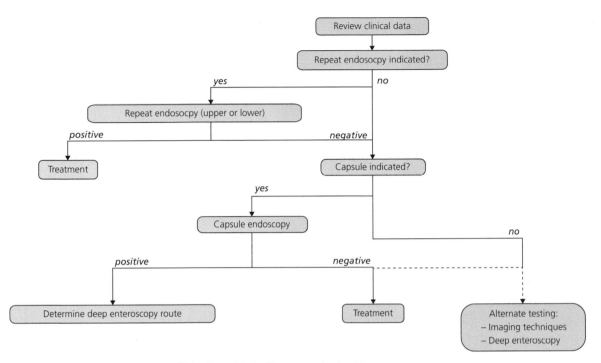

Fig. 32.4 Occult obscure gastrointestinal bleeding with significant anemia algorithm.

References

1. Ell C, May A. Mid-gastrointestinal bleeding: capsule endos-copy and push-and-pull enteroscopy give rise to a new med-ical term. *Endoscopy*. 2006; **38**(1):73–5.

2. Raju GS, Gerson L, Das A, Lewis B; American Gastroenterological Association. American Gastroenterological Association (AGA) Institute technical review on obscure gastrointestinal bleeding. *Gastroenterology*. 2007;**133**(5):1697–717.

3. Zuckerman GR, Prakash C, Askin MP, Lewis BS. AGA technical review on the evaluation and management of occult and obscure gastrointestinal bleeding. *Gastroenterology*. 2000;**118**(1):201–21.

4. Descamps C, Schmit A, Van Gossum A. "Missed" upper gas-trointestinal tract lesions may explain "occult" bleeding. *Endoscopy*. 1999;**31**(6):452–5.

5. Lara LF, Bloomfeld RS, Pineau BC. The rate of lesions found within reach of esophagogastroduodenoscopy during push enteroscopy depends on the type of obscure gastrointestinal bleeding. *Endoscopy*. 2005;**37**(8):745–50.

6. Benz C, Jakobs R, Riemann JF. Do we need the overtube for push-enteroscopy? *Endoscopy*. 2001;**33**(8):658–61.

7. Taylor AC, Chen RY, Desmond PV. Use of an overtube for enteroscopy – does it increase depth of insertion? A prospec-tive study of enteroscopy with and without an overtube. *Endoscopy*. 2001;**33**(3):227–30.

8. Koulaouzidis A, Rondonotti E, Karargyris A. Small-bowel capsule endoscopy: A ten-point contemporary review. *World J. Gastroenterol.* 2013;**19**(24):3726–46.

9. Matsumura T, Arai M, Sato T, et al. Efficacy of computed image modification of capsule endoscopy in patients with obscure gastrointestinal bleeding. *World J. Gastrointest. Endosc.* 2012;**4**(9):421–8.

10. Hartmann D, Eickhoff A, Damian U, Riemann JF. Diagnosis of small-bowel pathology using paired capsule endoscopy with two different devices: a randomized study. *Endoscopy*. 2007;**39**(12):1041–5.

11. Cave DR, Fleischer DE, Leighton JA, et al. A multicenter randomized comparison of the Endocapsule and the Pillcam SB. *Gastrointest. Endosc.* 2008;**68**(3):487–94.

12. Pioche M, Gaudin JL, Filoche B, Jet al.; French Society of Digestive Endoscopy. Prospective, randomized comparison of two small-bowel capsule endoscopy systems in patients with obscure GI bleeding. Gastrointest. *Endosc.* 2011;**73**(6):1181–8.

13. Choi EH, Mergener K, Semrad C, et al. A multicenter, pro-spective, randomized comparison of a novel signal trans-mission capsule endoscope to an existing capsule endoscope. *Gastrointest. Endosc.* 2013;**78**(2):325–32.

14. Teshima CW, Kuipers EJ, van Zanten SV, Mensink PB. Double balloon enteroscopy and capsule endoscopy for obscure gastrointestinal bleeding: an updated meta-analysis. *J. Gastroenterol. Hepatol.* 2011;**26**(5):796–801.

15. Triester SL, Leighton JA, Leontiadis GI, et al. A meta-analysis of the yield of capsule endoscopy compared to other diagnostic modalities in patients with obscure gastrointestinal bleeding. *Am. J. Gastroenterol.* 2005;**100**(11):2407–18.

16. Lewis BS, Swain P. Capsule endoscopy in the evaluation of patients with suspected small intestinal bleeding: Results of a pilot study. *Gastrointest. Endosc.* 2002;**56**(3):349–53.

17. Mylonaki M, Fritscher-Ravens A, Swain P. Wireless capsule endoscopy: a comparison with push enteroscopy in patients with gastroscopy and colonoscopy negative gastrointestinal bleeding. *Gut.* 2003;**52**(8):1122–6.

18. Hartmann D, Schilling D, Bolz G, et al. Capsule endoscopy versus push enteroscopy in patients with occult gastrointestinal bleeding. *Z. Gastroenterol.* 2003;**41**(5):377–82.

19. Gerson L, Kamal A. Cost-effectiveness analysis of management strategies for obscure GI bleeding. *Gastrointest. Endosc.* 2008;**68**(5):920–36.

20. Koh SJ, Im JP, Kim JW, et al. Long-term outcome in patients with obscure gastrointestinal bleeding after negative capsule endoscopy. *World J. Gastroenterol.* 2013;**19**(10):1632–8.

21. Postgate A, Despott E, Burling D, et al. Significant small-bowel lesions detected by alternative diagnostic modalities after negative capsule endoscopy. *Gastrointest. Endosc.* 2008;**68**(6):1209–14.

22. Herrerias JM, Leighton JA, Costamagna G, et al. Agile patency system eliminates risk of capsule retention in patients with known intestinal strictures who undergo capsule endoscopy. *Gastrointest Endosc.* 2008;**67**(6):902–9.

23. Mönkemüller K, Fry LC, Bellutti M, Malfertheiner P. Balloon-assisted enteroscopy: unifying double-balloon and single-balloon enteroscopy. *Endoscopy.* 2008;**40**(6):537.

24. Mönkemüller K, Neumann H, Fry LC. Middle gastrointestinal bleeding. In *Interventional and Therapeutic Gastrointestinal Endoscopy*, Monkemuller K, Wilcox M, Muñoz-Navas M (eds). Karger, Basel (Switzerland), 2010: 221–39.

25. Elena RM, Riccardo U, Rossella C, Bizzotto A, Domenico G, Guido C. Current status of device-assisted enteroscopy: Technical matters, indication, limits and complications. *World J. Gastrointest. Endosc.* 2012;**4**(10):453–61.

26. Efthymiou M, Desmond PV, Brown G, et al. SINGLE-01: a randomized, controlled trial comparing the efficacy and depth of insertion of single- and double-balloon enteroscopy by using a novel method to determine insertion depth. *Gastrointest. Endosc.* 2012;**76**(5):972–80.

27. Kim DH, Byeon JS, Lee SK, et al. Usefulness of double balloon endoscopy in patients with surgically distorted intestinal anatomy. *J. Clin. Gastroenterol.* 2009;**43**(8):737–42.

28. Yamamoto H, Sekine Y, Sato Y, et al. Total enteroscopy with a nonsurgical steerable double-balloon method. *Gastrointest. Endosc.* 2001;**53**(2):216–20.

29. Ramchandani M, Reddy DN, Gupta R, et al. Diagnostic yield and therapeutic impact of single-balloon enteroscopy: series of 106 cases. *J. Gastroenterol. Hepatol.* 2009;**24**(10):1631–8.

30. Kushnir VM, Tang M, Goodwin J, et al. Long-term outcomes after single-balloon enteroscopy in patients with obscure gastrointestinal bleeding. *Dig. Dis. Sci.* 2013;**58**(9):2572–9.

31. Domagk D, Mensink P, Aktas H, et al. Single- vs. double-balloon enteroscopy in small-bowel diagnostics: a randomized multicenter trial. *Endoscopy.* 2011;**43**(6):472–6.

32. Akerman PA, Agrawal D, Chen W, Cantero D, Avila J, Pangtay J. Spiral enteroscopy: a novel method of enteroscopy by using the Endo-Ease Discovery SB overtube and a pediatric colonoscope. *Gastrointest. Endosc.* 2009;**69**(2):327–32.

33. Messer I, May A, Manner H, Ell C. Prospective, randomized, single-center trial comparing double-balloon enteroscopy and spiral enteroscopy in patients with suspected small-bowel disorders. *Gastrointest. Endosc.* 2013;**77**(2):241–9.

34. Jakobs R, Hartmann D, Benz C, et al. Diagnosis of obscure gastrointestinal bleeding by intra-operative enteroscopy in 81 consecutive patients. *World J. Gastroenterol.* 200614;**12**(2):313–6.

35. Desa LA, Ohri SK, Hutton KA, Lee H, Spencer J. Role of intraoperative enteroscopy in obscure gastrointestinal bleeding of small bowel origin. *Br. J. Surg.* 1991;**78**(2):192–5.

36. Wang Z, Chen JQ, Liu JL, Qin XG, Huang Y. CT enterography in obscure gastrointestinal bleeding: a systematic review and meta-analysis. *J. Med. Imaging Radiat. Oncol.* 2013;**57**(3):263–73.

37. Huprich JE, Fletcher JG, Alexander JA, Fidler JL, Burton SS, McCullough CH. Obscure gastrointestinal bleeding: evaluation with 64-section multiphase CT enterography – initial experience. *Radiology.* 2008;**246**(2):562–71.

38. Leung WK, Ho SS, Suen BY, et al. Capsule endoscopy or angiography in patients with acute overt obscure gastrointestinal bleeding: a prospective randomized study with long-term follow-up. *Am. J. Gastroenterol.* 2012;**107**(9):1370–6.

39. Saperas E, Dot J, Videla S, et al. Capsule endoscopy versus computed tomographic or standard angiography for the diagnosis of obscure gastrointestinal bleeding. *Am. J. Gastroenterol.* 2007;**102**(4):731–7.

40. Bloomfeld RS, Smith TP, Schneider AM, Rockey DC. Provocative angiography in patients with gastrointestinal hemorrhage of obscure origin. *Am. J. Gastroenterol.* 2000;**95**(10):2807–12.

41. Howarth DM, Tang K, Lees W. The clinical utility of nuclear medicine imaging for the detection of occult gastrointestinal haemorrhage. *Nucl. Med. Commun.* 2002;**23**(6):591–4.

42. Kiratli PO, Aksoy T, Bozkurt MF, Orhan D. Detection of ectopic gastric mucosa using 99mTc pertechnetate: review of the literature. *Ann. Nucl. Med.* 2009;**23**(2):97–105.

CHAPTER 33

Ischemic bowel

Ryan B. Perumpail[1] and Shai Friedland[2]

[1] Stanford Hospital and Clinics, Stanford, CA, USA
[2] Stanford University School of Medicine and VA Palo Alto, Stanford, CA, USA

Introduction

Intestinal ischemia occurs when perfusion to the bowel is inadequate to meet metabolic demands. Ischemia can be classified as acute or chronic, and it can occur in response to arterial or venous insults. In acute mesenteric ischemia, all or part of the small bowel is affected. In addition, the right colon can be involved since its blood supply is also derived from the superior mesenteric artery (SMA). Acute mesenteric ischemia is a clinical emergency with a mortality rate of over 60% [1]. A high index of suspicion is required for early detection before bowel necrosis occurs. In contrast, the more common syndrome of ischemic colitis often has a milder clinical course characterized by transient bloody diarrhea and mild lower abdominal pain [2]. Chronic mesenteric ischemia, also called intestinal angina, is relatively rare and is characterized by abdominal pain following meals and weight loss. It can develop into an emergency if bowel viability is compromised by further deterioration in the blood supply [3].

Diagnosis of intestinal ischemia can be challenging; clinical suspicion and eliciting an adequate history from the patient play a more significant role than in many other gastrointestinal emergencies. Multidetector computerized tomography (CT) angiography is now commonly performed as the initial non-invasive test for acute and chronic mesenteric ischemia [4]. In patients who are diagnosed prior to bowel infarction, percutaneous treatment using angiography is often possible. Colonoscopy is often performed to diagnose ischemic colitis and in some cases to assess viability of the colon when there is doubt.

Acute mesenteric ischemia

Etiology

Superior mesenteric artery embolus is present in 50% of cases with sudden catastrophic abdominal pain out of proportion to physical findings. Atrial fibrillation is a common risk factor.

Non-occlusive mesenteric ischemia (25%) is a splanchnic vasoconstriction in response to a preceding cardiovascular event and may persist after the precipitating event has been corrected. SMA thrombosis (10%) is typically in an area of severe baseline atherosclerosis. Patients may have chronic mesenteric ischemia before thrombosis occurs. Mesenteric venous thrombosis (10%) may have a more subacute course. Patients often have risk factors such as hypercoagulable state or inflammation from other abdominal disorders.

Presentation

The patient may complain of severe, acute abdominal pain, sometimes accompanied by forceful bowel evacuation. The abdomen is initially often soft and nontender but increasing abdominal tenderness, rebound and guarding develop as bowel infarcts. Occult blood in the stool is common, but maroon stool is less common. Leukocytosis, elevated amylase, elevated lactate, and metabolic acidosis are increasingly common as bowel infarcts.

Investigations

Multi-detector CT angiography may detect embolic occlusion of the SMA just beyond the origin of the middle colic artery. Proximal SMA occlusion is typically

Gastrointestinal Emergencies, Third Edition. Edited by Tony C. K. Tham, John S. A. Collins, and Roy Soetikno.
© 2016 John Wiley & Sons, Ltd. Published 2016 by John Wiley & Sons, Ltd.

seen with thrombosis, and collaterals are visualized in patients with preceding chronic symptoms. Superior mesenteric vein and portal vein thrombosis may be detected on CT. Non-occlusive ischemia may be difficult to detect. Other findings on CT include bowel wall thickening, abnormal bowel wall enhancement and intramural or venous gas.

Magnetic resonance angiography is less commonly used than CT as it is typically less readily available and has lower spatial resolution in comparison. Advantages include absence of radiation (children) and no iodinated contrast. Angiography is now more commonly performed for treatment following a positive CT.

Management

The patient should be resuscitated and broad-spectrum antibiotics administered. In the absence of active bleeding, systemic anticoagulation should be administered to prevent thrombus formation or propagation. Angiography can permit papaverine infusion for treatment of vasoconstriction. Papaverine can be safely infused for up to 5 days. Thrombolytics, angioplasty, and stenting are used increasingly although there is some controversy as to their preferred role. Surgery provides the definitive assessment of viability and the decision can be made between resection of necrotic bowel, embolectomy or revascularization. Local infusion of thrombolytic therapy, a less well-established modality, can be considered if angiography occurs within 8 hours of the onset of abdominal pain in patients who do not have clinical evidence of bowel infarction or other contraindications to thrombolytic therapy [5].

Ischemic colitis

Etiology

This condition is usually due to non-occlusive ischemia. A precipitating event such as hypotension or arrhythmia may or may not be identified. Other causes include coagulopathy, emboli, vasculitis, abdominal aortic aneurysm surgery, cocaine or amphetamine abuse, and volvulus. Involvement of the ascending colon should raise suspicion of small bowel involvement (acute mesenteric ischemia). The splenic flexure and rectosigmoid are "watershed" areas that are commonly involved, but all other regions of colon and rectum can be involved.

Presentation

The patient will usually complain of sudden, mild, left lower quadrant abdominal pain. There may an urge for urgent defecation with bloody diarrhea. On examination there will be mild to moderate abdominal tenderness over the involved area. Many cases resolve spontaneously, however, and some patients do not seek medical attention. Increasing tenderness, guarding, fever, and ileus occur with infarction and colonic strictures may occur with healing.

Investigations

Colon blood flow has often normalized by the time that symptoms occur.

CT and plain radiography may show colon wall thickening or thumb-printing due to edema of the bowel wall. Colonoscopy may show submucosal hemorrhage, ulcers, or gangrenous bowel in severe cases.

Management

Resuscitation and broad-spectrum antibiotics are the initial emergency steps in management. Peritoneal signs suggest the need for emergency laparotomy and colon resection. Recurrent sepsis, bloody diarrhea and chronic diarrhea with protein loss occur with segmental ulcerating colitis. This is a chronic form of ischemic colitis and is sometimes mistaken for inflammatory bowel disease. Surgery is often required. Symptomatic strictures may occur following healing. While some may resolve spontaneously, surgical resection may be required.

Chronic mesenteric ischemia

Etiology

This condition is usually due to atherosclerosis of mesenteric arteries, and rarely, due to vasculitis. Abdominal pain typically occurs within 30 minutes of eating. This is likely due to reduced small intestine blood flow as blood preferentially flows to the stomach.

Traditionally, the diagnosis of chronic mesenteric ischemia requires a compatible history and significant angiographic lesions in at least two of the three major arteries supplying the gut: the celiac, superior mesenteric, and inferior mesenteric arteries. Some patients with occlusion of all three arteries are asymptomatic due to collaterals.

Presentation

The patient will complain of abdominal pain within 30 minutes of meals that resolves within 3 hours. Severity of pain is mild initially, but becomes severe within months. As pain worsens, patients develop a fear of eating, and weight loss occurs. Pain may become continuous as infarction occurs.

Investigations

CT angiography is useful to assess the splanchnic vessels for calcified plaques, stenosis, or occlusion. It has higher spatial and temporal resolution than magnetic resonance angiography. Duplex ultrasound is favored in some centers to demonstrate elevated peak systolic velocity in the celiac and superior mesenteric arteries as an indication of significant stenosis. Newer techniques include specialized magnetic resonance sequences for evaluating blood flow after meals and endoscopic oximetry. Gastrointestinal tonometry, which uses an intraluminal catheter to measure the post-prandial jejunal pH, utilizes the correlation between abdominal pain and intramural acidosis as a diagnostic tool for chronic mesenteric ischemia [6]. Endoscopic oximetry directly assesses the intestinal mucosa for ischemia and may be particularly valuable in patients with chronic vascular disease who have compensated for occlusion of major vessels with collaterals [7].

Management

Surgical revascularization may be attempted in suitable cases – generally younger patients with fewer comorbid conditions. Surgical options include bypass grafting, endarterectomy, and reimplantation. Percutaneous techniques, including stenting, are used increasingly and are now favored for most patients [8]. These techniques have been associated with high recurrence rates in the past, but improvements in initial treatment and successful percutaneous treatment of restenosis makes this approach increasingly attractive.

References

1. Chang RW, Chang JB, Longo WE. Update in management of mesenteric ischemia. *World J. Gastroenterol.* 2006;**12**: 3243–7.
2. Elder K, Lashner BA, Al Solaiman F. Clinical approach to colonic ischemia. *Cleve. Clin. J. Med.* 2009;**76**(7):401–9.
3. Pecoraro F, Rancic Z, Lachat M, et al. Chronic mesenteric ischemia: critical review and guidelines for management. *Ann. Vasc. Surg.* 2013;**27**:113–22.
4. Johnson JO. Diagnosis of acute gastrointestinal hemorrhage and acute mesenteric ischemia in the era of multi-detector row CT. *Radiol. Clin. N. Am.* 2012;**50**:173–82.
5. Schoots IG, Levi MM, Reekers JA, et al. Thrombolytic therapy for acute superior mesenteric artery occlusion. *J. Vasc. Interv. Radiol* 2005;**16**:317–29.
6. Mensink PB, Geelkarken RH, Huisman AB, et al. Twenty-four hour tonometry in patients suspected of chronic gastrointestinal ischemia. *Dig. Dis. Sci.* 2008;**1**:133–9.
7. Friedland S, Benaron D, Coogan S, Sze DY, Soetikno R. Diagnosis of chronic mesenteric ischemia by visible light spectroscopy during endoscopy. *Gastrointest. Endosc.* 2007;**65**: 294–300.
8. Gibbons CP, Roberts DE. Endovascular treatment of chronic arterial mesenteric ischemia: a changing perspective? *Semin. Vasc. Surg.* 2010;**23**:47–53.

CHAPTER 34

Acute severe ulcerative colitis

Subrata Ghosh and Marietta Iacucci

University of Calgary, Alberta, Canada

Introduction

Acute severe ulcerative colitis is a medical emergency. Recognition of severe ulcerative colitis is based on a comprehensive clinical assessment. The Truelove and Witts criteria [1] still remain useful in characterizing the severity of this condition (Table 34.1). These patients require hospitalization and urgent management. Acute severe ulcerative colitis may be further sub-classified into severe colitis and fulminant colitis. Clinical disease activity scores such as the Mayo score categorizes severe ulcerative colitis as a score of 9–12 and Mayo endoscopic sub score of 3 characterizes endoscopically severe changes. These scores need to be associated with the systemic symptoms noted in table 34.1 In order to be diagnosed as acute severe ulcerative colitis. Fulminant colitis is associated with abdominal distension, tenderness on palpation and colonic dilatation on plain abdominal radiograph. Most patients will give a history of the gradual onset of diarrhea with the passage of blood and mucus. There may be severe abdominal cramps and tenesmus. Constitutional symptoms may include severe malaise, fever, joint and muscle pain and marked weight loss. Colonic dilatation >6.0 cm in association with constitutional symptoms of toxicity constitutes toxic megacolon. In some cases the onset may be abrupt over 24–48 hours. There is often a history of ulcerative colitis.

Clinical examination should include rectal examination, abdominal radiography and flexible sigmoidoscopy which can usually be carried out on the unprepared colon. This must be followed by stool culture, *Clostridium*

difficile toxin assay and real time PCR If available. Blood tests should include hemoglobin, white cell count, platelet count, C-reactive protein, erythrocyte sedimentation rate, and albumin concentration. A number of intestinal diseases that mimic acute severe ulcerative colitis should be excluded by initial history and investigations (Table 34.2).

Acute severe crohn's colitis

This condition is less common than ulcerative colitis, but may present as severe or fulminant colitis which is difficult to distinguish clinically and is an important differential diagnosis. Approximately 65% of Crohn's disease patients have either colonic involvement alone or ileocecal disease. There may be a previous clinical history of Crohn's disease with small bowel involvement and previous surgical procedures. Perianal disease will point to a diagnosis of Crohn's disease. Initial clinical assessment is identical for these patients, with the exception that there may be concomitant small bowel disease which has to be considered as a potential cause of internal fistulization or abdominal sepsis with abscess formation. If Crohn's colitis is suspected and accompanied by fever, abdominal tenderness or the presence of a mass on palpation, an abdominal computerized tompgraphy (CT) or magnetic resonance imaging (MRI) may be indicated to assist the surgeon in planning management. Active sepsis should also induce caution in commencing immunosuppression or steroids before it is controlled with antibiotic therapy (see later sections).

Gastrointestinal Emergencies, Third Edition. Edited by Tony C. K. Tham, John S. A. Collins, and Roy Soetikno.
© 2016 John Wiley & Sons, Ltd. Published 2016 by John Wiley & Sons, Ltd.

Table 34.1 Truelove and Witts classification of ulcerative colitis.

Mild	Moderate	Severe
<5 bowel motions/ day	Intermediate	>6 bowel motions/ day between mild and severe
Blood in stool (Small amount)		Blood in stool (Visible amounts)
No fever		Temperature >37.5°C
No tachycardia		Pulse >90 beats/min
Hemoglobin $10 g/dL		Hemoglobin 10 g/dL
ESR <30 mm/ 1st hour		ESR >30 mm/1st hour

Table 34.2 Diseases mimicking severe ulcerative colitis.

Acute infectious gastroenteritis	Outbreak related to contaminated food or drinks, recent travel
Radiation proctopathy	History of pelvic radiotherapy
Pseudomembranous colitis (*C. difficile*)	History of antibiotic exposure
Sexually transmitted infections	History of anal sex
Amoebiasis	Recent travel to endemic areas

Table 34.3 Monitoring regimen in acute severe ulcerative colitis.

Detecting impending complications
Daily abdominal radiographs till the patient improves
Watch for colonic dilatation
Watch for colonic perforation (often silent)
Watch for small intestinal dilatation
Assessing course of disease
Stool frequency
Blood in stool
Pulse rate
Temperature
C-reactive protein (CRP)
Albumin
Hemoglobin
Flexible sigmoidoscopy to look for deep ulcerations

Principles of management

Acute severe ulcerative colitis patients require hospitalization and close monitoring. Some patients at presentation may appear to be less ill than the Truelove and Witts criteria suggest. Therefore it is important to monitor the patient in a gastroenterology (not a general) ward with an accurate record of stool frequency, blood in stool, temperature, pulse rate, and abdominal tenderness. Infection must be eliminated by stool culture, but commencement of treatment should not wait until the stool culture reports become available. The management of severe ulcerative colitis patients is a team effort between gastroenterologists, surgeons, inflammatory bowel disease nurses, dieticians, and clinical psychologists. In a patient admitted with acute severe ulcerative colitis and dilatation of the colon, joint assessment by a gastroenterologist and a colorectal surgeon is required urgently. In all other patients admitted with acute severe colitis, a colorectal surgical assessment will be required within 24 hours.

Initial therapy

The standard initial therapy of acute severe ulcerative colitis consists of intravenous corticosteroids [2], fluid and electrolyte replacement with special attention to potassium. Blood transfusion may be required to maintain a hemoglobin concentration above 10 g/L and subcutaneous heparin should be started to prevent thromboembolic complications. Intravenous corticosteroids generally chosen include hydrocortisone 100 mg four times a day or methylprednisolone 60 mg/daily by continuous infusion. Addition of rectal therapy has no clear advantages and is generally poorly tolerated by patients in the acute severe phase. Antibiotics are not necessary unless infection is considered a strong differential diagnosis from history (Table 34.2). However, rapid exclusion of infection, including *Clostridium difficile* is necessary.

Monitoring of such patients needs to be intensive and should be directed at detecting impending complications which may necessitate urgent colectomy (Table 34.3). Plain CT scan or abdominal radiography accurately denotes extent of disease, but colonoscopy to assess extent is unnecessary. The majority of patients with acute severe ulcerative colitis suffer from extensive colitis. Nutritional support is important and most patients can be encouraged to have an adequate oral intake. Rarely, patients may require supportive parenteral nutrition. Codeine and loperamide should not be used and non-steroidal anti-inflammatory drugs avoided.

Overall, patients hospitalized for acute severe colitis and treated with intravenous steroids may have a colectomy rate between 29% and 46% over the next 90 days. The colectomy rates vary between countries, indicating different thresholds for offering surgery.

Managing intravenous steroid refractory acute severe colitis

Close monitoring should lead to early recognition of those patients who fail to respond to intravenous steroids. Such recognition may be aided by formal rules, but clinical judgment is paramount based on the monitoring parameters noted in Table 34.3. The two commonly used rules, which are very similar to each other, are:

1 *Fulminant colitis (Sweden) index*: **This is calculated as:** Number of daily bowel movements × 0.14 × C-reactive protein level (mg/L). A value >8 predicts colectomy with 75% sensitivity and specificity. This index was recently used in a salvage therapy trial discussed below (4).

2 *Travis index*: At day 3 after commencement of intravenous steroids, a stool frequency of more than 8 per day or C-reactive protein concentration of >45 mg/L is 85% predictive of colectomy and therefore may be used to seek surgical team involvement and consider start of salvage therapy with infliximab or ciclosporin (5).

Some patients respond initially to intravenous steroids but continue to have symptoms. These patients should be offered salvage therapy 5–7 days after initiation of intravenous corticosteroids as the colectomy rate is high in this group. This latter group may also benefit from a careful flexible sigmoidoscopy, as demonstration of deep ulceration indicates a poor prognosis and consideration of salvage therapy or surgery (see Fig. 34.4). Overall, a high proportion of patients failing intravenous steroids will undergo colectomy – 67% underwent colectomy within 90 days without salvage therapy in a study reported recently.

It is important in acute severe colitis refractory to intravenous steroids to exclude coinfections with cytomegalovirus (CMV) and *Clostridium difficile* as treatment of these infections with ganciclovir or vancomycin may rescue the patient from possible colectomy (Table 34.4). Such infections are uncommon but important to detect. However, *Clostridium difficile* is increasingly associated with acute severe ulcerative colitis and it is now mandatory to exclude it all patients.

Two principal medical salvage therapies are currently available: ciclosporin and infliximab.

Table 34.4 Principles of salvage therapy in intravenous steroid-refractory patients.

Monitor very carefully
Pulse rate
Temperature
Hemoglobin and albumin
CRP
AXR
In case of non-response
Repeat stool cultures, *C. difficile*
Cytomegalovirus (in tissue and blood)
Colonoscopy
If a patient deteriorates on salvage therapy, move to immediate colectomy

AXR, abdominal X-ray; CRP, C-reactive protein.

Ciclosporin

Ciclosporin, a cyclic peptide of 11 amino acids, acts by binding to cyclophilin and thereby inhibiting calcineurin. Inhibition of calcineurin prevents transcription of interleukin-2 (IL-2) and activation of T-lymphocytes. With the demonstration that treatment with 2 mg/kg of ciclosporin is as effective as the conventional 4 mg/kg with fewer occurrence of some side effects such as hypertension [6], the lower dose is now accepted as standard therapy in most hospitals. The dose is not generally adjusted according to serum ciclosporin levels, unless serum levels are in toxic range. Once the patient has responded and is feeling better, the intravenous preparation may be replaced by oral micro-emulsion ciclosporin 5 mg/kg. It is no longer necessary to exclude patients with low plasma cholesterol due to risk of seizures, as the intravenous preparation does not contain the incriminating chromophore. Ciclosporin may also be used as monotherapy in place of intravenous steroids [7], but this is hardly ever considered in practice, unless steroid therapy is contraindicated. In a patient who responds to ciclosporin, the drug is continued as oral therapy for 3–4 months, while corticosteroids are tapered and discontinued and azathioprine 2.5 mg/kg or 6-mercaptopurine 1.5 mg/kg is introduced at the time of discharge as long-term maintenance therapy. Such patients are quite severely immunosuppressed and therefore a high vigilance for opportunistic infections and prophylaxis for *Pneumocystis carinii* with co-trimoxazole is necessary. Ciclosporin is associated with a number of serious adverse events, including an appreciable mortality (Table 34.5), and therefore the use of ciclosporin as rescue therapy is limited in acute severe colitis – both surgery and infliximab are considered as potentially more attractive options by both physicians and patients. In patients rescued by ciclosporin, 58% eventually have a colectomy over the next 7 years, not surprising as ciclosporin is not considered a long-term therapy due to its adverse effect profile on long-term use. A number of predictive factors for response to ciclosporin have been proposed based on simple clinical criteria such as fever, tachycardia, C-reactive protein >45 mg/l and the presence of severe endoscopic lesions [8]. In patients with acute severe Crohn's colitis there is no evidence that ciclosporin is effective and treatment failure after commencing ciclosporin may be an indication that this condition is in fact causing the patient's illness. In these cases infliximab or other biological agents are indicated (see below as for ulcerative colitis).

Table 34.5 Incidence of adverse events associated with ciclosporin

Tremor/paresthesia	9%
Hypertrichosis	6%
Gingival hyperplasia	6%
Renal insufficiency	6%
Seizures	1%
Anaphylaxis	0.3%
Hypertension	7%
Opportunistic infections	3%

Infliximab

The chimeric anti-tumor necrosis factor (TNF) antibody infliximab was used in intravenous steroid refractory ulcerative colitis in a pivotal Scandinavian study in which a single 5 mg/kg infusion of infliximab was used [4]. The trial design is shown in Fig. 34.1. Patients unresponsive to IV corticosteroids at day 3 were randomized to additional single dose of 5 mg/kg of infliximab or placebo. Patients who were not considered unresponsive at day 3 but remained symptomatic at day 5–7 were also randomized to a single 5 mg/kg dose of infliximab or placebo. Overall, 29% of patients underwent colectomy in the infliximab arm compared with 67% in the placebo arm (Fig. 34.2). In a recent Italian study, patients who had received multiple doses of infliximab had better outcome than those receiving a single dose of infliximab in a group of intravenous steroid resistant acute severe colitis patients [9]. Keeping this in mind, it may be wise to administer infliximab at 0, 2, and 6 weeks and thereafter every 8 weeks till the patient is in remission. Subsequently, in those patients who are azathioprine/6-mercaptopurine naïve, this drug may be used as long-term therapy and infliximab discontinued. In patients who developed acute severe intravenous steroid-resistant colitis while on azathioprine or 6-mercaptopurine, infliximab should preferably be continued long term. The use of infliximab may be associated with opportunistic infections but, in the Swedish randomized controlled trial, adverse effects were similar in those receiving infliximab or placebo. Dose optimization of infliximab at early stages of induction therapy may give better results as therapeutic

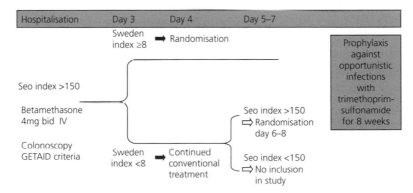

Fig. 34.1 Scandinavian randomized controlled trial of infliximab in acute severe ulcerative colitis. Source: Jarnerot et al. 2005 (4). Reproduced with permission of Elsevier.

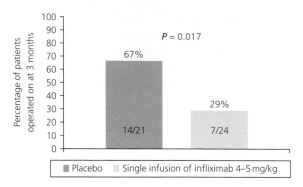

Fig. 34.2 90 day colectomy rate in infliximab arm compared to placebo arm in IV steroid refractory ulcerative colitis. Source: Jarnerot et al. 2005 (4). Reproduced with permission of Elsevier.

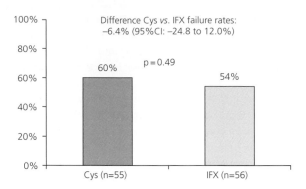

Fig. 34.3 Ciclosporin versus infliximab study (CYSIF) – primary efficacy endpoint of treatment failure at day 98.

drug levels are often low due to increased clearance, colonic drug loss and increased TNF burden due to severe extensive colitis.

Though patients failing ciclosporin may respond to infliximab, repeated salvage therapy generally results in unacceptable delay to surgery and profound immunosuppression. Therefore only one form of salvage therapy should be decided upon after discussion with the patient, and failure of such therapy should lead to surgery. A patient developing acute severe colitis while on therapy with oral corticosteroids should be admitted but may proceed straight to second-line salvage therapy.

Infliximab or ciclosporin?

The question of whether to choose ciclosporin or infliximab as salvage medical therapy in toxic megacolon is important. In a parallel open labelled randomized controlled trial, ciclosporin was not more effective than infliximab over a 14 weeks follow-up period in hospitalized acute severe ulcerative colitis patients refractory to intravenous corticosteroids [10]. Treatment failure defined by pre-determined criteria occurred in 60% of patients who received ciclosporin and in 54% of patients who received infliximab over the 14-week period (Fig. 34.3). The dosing regimen for ciclosporin was 2 mg/kg adjusted subsequently by drug trough levels – patients who responded at 7 days were switched to oral ciclosporin 4 mg/kg. The dosing regimen for infliximab was 5 mg/kg and patients who responded received further doses at week 2 and 6. Both groups received azathioprine started in responders at day 7. The initial clinical response at day 7 was 86% in the

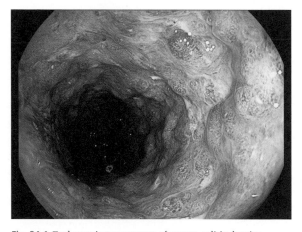

Fig. 34.4 Endoscopic appearance of severe colitis despite treatment with infliximab for 7 days. The patient underwent colectomy. (*see insert for color representation of the figure.*)

ciclosporin group and 84% in the infliximab group. The incidence of serious adverse events was 16% in the ciclosporin group and 25% in the infliximab group. Physician and inflammatory bowel disease center experience should guide the treatment choice but most centers are now more familiar with the use of anti-TNF therapy. In addition, ciclosporin therapy is associated with a 1–2% mortality rate. In a cohort study in Australia, infliximab salvage therapy in acute severe steroid refractory colitis was associated with lower rates of severe adverse events and colectomy compared with ciclosporin salvage therapy [11]. It is important that failure of treatment with infliximab or ciclosporin is rapidly recognized and this may be helped by careful flexible sigmoidoscopy without insufflation (Fig. 34.4).

Experience with other therapies in acute severe colitis

Vedolizumab

The $\alpha_4\beta_7$ monoclonal antibody vedolizumab has recently approved for moderate to severe ulcerative but there is currently no experience in using it in hospitalized acute severe ulcerative colitis.[12]. Future experience of this drug in acute severe ulcerative colitis is awaited though the slow onset of action will require co-treatment with intravenous steroids.

Visilizumab

Humanized IgG2 antibody against CD3 lymphocytes has undergone preliminary trials in intravenous steroid refractory ulcerative colitis [13]. Though initially promising, subsequent phase II studies were prematurely terminated due to lack of efficacy. Anti-CD3 antibodies also have a propensity to cause an acute cytokine release syndrome, which may be minimized by hydration and premedication with acetaminophen (paracetamol) and antihistamines.

Daclizumab

Monoclonal humanized antibody to interleukin-2 receptor (CD25, IL-2R) was considered an attractive potential therapy for ulcerative colitis as the mechanism of action is similar to ciclosporin. However, a randomized controlled trial in 159 patients with moderate active ulcerative colitis showed no evidence of efficacy [14] and therefore it is unlikely that this antibody will have any place in the treatment of severe steroid-refractory ulcerative colitis.

Basiliximab

Monoclonal chimeric antibody to interleukin-2 receptor (CD25, IL-2R) has been shown to act as a steroid sensitizing agent but an uncontrolled trial failed to demonstrate promising efficacy in steroid-refractory severe ulcerative colitis – 4 out of 7 treated patients underwent colectomy [15]. Therefore anti-CD25 monoclonal antibodies cannot be considered effective salvage therapy in severe steroid-refractory ulcerative colitis.

Tacrolimus

A randomized controlled trial of oral tacrolimus in acute moderate-severe steroid-refractory ulcerative colitis has been reported [16]. Encouraging results were obtained in patients treated with a high trough level of tacrolimus (10–15 ng/mL), but the necessity of frequent measurements of trough levels, toxicities and lack of clear evidence of efficacy in hospitalized acute severe colitis make tacrolimus a generally unattractive choice for the majority of such patients.

Leukocyte apheresis

Commercial columns to remove different white cell populations from circulation via an extracorporeal circuit have been used extensively in Japan and some Scandinavian countries, but randomized controlled trials in true acute severe hospitalized patients are lacking. Randomized controlled trials in ambulatory ulcerative colitis in the West have, however, been negative [17]. Only scant anecdotal data exists in the context of response in steroid-refractory acute severe colitis [18] and this intervention is generally not used in most centers.

General management

Prophylaxis of thromboembolic complications

Patients with acute severe colitis are very ill, often confined to bed, dehydrated and have a hypercoagulable state. Active inflammation may play a direct role in producing a thrombophilic state [19] and all patients should receive prophylactic heparin. Administration of heparin is safe and does not increase the incidence of colonic bleeding [20]. Either unfractionated and low molecular weight heparin may be used for prevention of venous thrombosis at least as long as the patient is on intravenous steroids or is confined to bed.

Antibiotics

In the absence of infections, there is no evidence for empiric use of antibiotics. In hospitalized patients with developing toxic megacolon, oral vancomycin may be considered until the stools are negative for *C. difficile*. Real-time PCR on feces might permit a rapid diagnosis of *C. difficile* and early treatment with vancomycin. Broad-spectrum antibiotics are occasionally used in patients with significant abdominal tenderness, however there is no definite evidence for efficacy and there is the risk of *C. difficile* infection. There is scant evidence for fecal microbial transplant in toxic megacolon associated with *C. difficile* in the setting of severe ulcerative colitis.

Management of nutritional status

Bowel rest via total parenteral nutrition has no therapeutic benefit in reducing the inflammation in acute severe ulcerative colitis. However, a number of patients are admitted with very poor nutritional status and are too ill to have adequate oral nutritional intake. A dietician should always be involved in managing such patients, and parenteral nutrition (along with oral nutrition) should be considered on nutritional grounds if oral intake is persistently inadequate, so that emergency surgery in a nutritionally debilitated patient can be avoided. Patients should be nil by mouth in toxic megacolon.

Management of fluid and electrolyte disturbances

Many of these patients are dehydrated and hypokalemic, especially after high doses of steroids, and careful monitoring and replacement are necessary. If the patient is unable to drink adequately, intravenous fluids will be required.

Blood transfusion

Blood transfusion and iron replacement should be considered in patients in order to maintain a hemoglobin concentration above 10 g/dL. This is important in terms of keeping a patient in a fit state for surgery if medical management fails.

Management of abdominal pain

Narcotic analgesics should be avoided as it may worsen colonic dilatation. Severe pain in the setting of toxic megacolon generally represents transmural Inflammation and impending perforation and hence surgical review and emergency colectomy may be required rather than pain management. It is important that adequate vigilance is maintained to trigger surgical intervention as a matter of urgency in the event of severe abdominal pain.

Surgery

A well-timed operation is an invaluable part of appropriate management of acute severe ulcerative colitis and can be life-saving. With the availability of more salvage therapy choices, it is important that these are offered early to patients failing steroid therapy; therefore, in most instances, surgery will be offered after failure of second-line salvage therapy with infliximab or ciclosporin. An exception may be patients presenting with fulminant colitis who may be ill enough to undergo surgery if they do not rapidly improve after intravenous

corticosteroids. Severe hemorrhage, perforation, or toxic megacolon developing on treatment are indications for emergency surgery.

Surgery should be discussed with all patients admitted with acute severe ulcerative colitis as one of the possible options. Colorectal surgeon, gastroenterologist, stoma therapist and inflammatory bowel disease specialist nurse will all play a role in discussing surgery as one of the therapeutic options if intravenous steroid therapy fails. The opportunity to discuss the implications of surgery with a patient who has undergone colectomy in the past is often considered useful by the patient. Some of the potential complications and drawbacks of surgery also require balanced discussion and deliberation:

- sepsis
- small intestinal obstruction
- urinary retention
- pouchitis
- fecundity and impotence
- other forms of pouch dysfunction
- incontinence
- pouch failure.

It is therefore inappropriate to present colectomy as a cure of ulcerative colitis to the patient.

In patients with acute severe colitis, surgery has to be a staged process. Subtotal colectomy with ileostomy is performed initially, increasingly laparoscopy-assisted in specialized centers. After 3–6 months with the patient in much better health, completion proctectomy with ileal pouch anal anastomosis (IPAA) is performed. Use of salvage therapy such as infliximab [4] or ciclosporin [6] in the setting of acute severe colitis does not appear to increase the risks of complications after colectomy. In a minority of patients with poor anal sphincter function, a permanent ileostomy may be preferable to avoid disabling incontinence. Careful psychological support and counselling throughout the process are invaluable, especially in patients who lose their colon after only a short spell of illness.

Conclusion

Acute severe ulcerative colitis is a medical emergency. All patients require hospitalization and precise management, otherwise mortality rates will increase. With optimum medical and surgical management, however, the

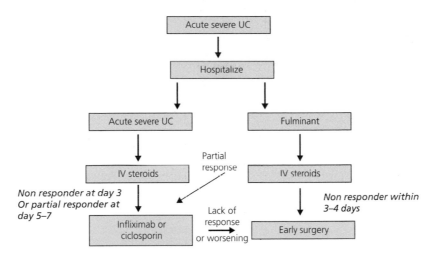

Fig. 34.5 A management algorithm for short-term management of acute severe colitis.

mortality rate should approximate zero. Two golden rules are important in management:

Rule 1

In hospitalized patients with acute severe ulcerative colitis on intravenous corticosteroids, worsening of disease on *any day*, or lack of response by day 3, should result in consideration of salvage therapy or surgery.

Rule 2

In intravenous steroid-refractory acute severe ulcerative colitis on second-line therapy (infliximab or ciclosporin) significant worsening of clinical status on any day compared with previous day should lead to consideration of surgery.

A management algorithm to summarize the approach discussed in this chapter is illustrated in Fig. 34.5. Intravenous steroids remain first-line therapy, but infliximab appears a more acceptable salvage therapy than ciclosporin, though results of randomized trials are awaited.

All patients require assessment by a senior gastroenterologist twice daily to analyze potentially confusing features such as a decrease in stool frequency heralding worsening colonic status. In addition, patients require surgical assessment on a daily basis until the patient is considered to be no longer at a risk for colectomy. With precise medical and surgical management, caring for acute severe ulcerative colitis

patients can be extremely gratifying. Decisions have to be taken quickly and correctly, so that a patient is never put in a life-threatening situation after admission.

References

1. Truelove SC, Witts LJ. Cortisone in ulcerative colitis: final report on a therapeutic trial. *Br. Med. J.* 1955;**ii**:1041–8.
2. Truelove SC, Jewell DP. Intensive intravenous regimen for severe attacks of ulcerative colitis. *Lancet* 1974; **i**:1067–70.
3. Gustavsson A, Halfvarson J, Magnuson A, Sandberg-Gertzen H, Tysk C, Jarnerot G. Long-term colectomy rate after intensive intravenous corticosteroid therapy for ulcerative colitis prior to the immunosuppressive treatment era. *Am. J. Gastroenterol.* 2007;**102**:2513–19.
4. Jarnerot G, Hertervig E, Friis-Liby I, et al. Infliximab as rescue therapy in severe to moderately severe ulcerative colitis: a randomized, placebo-controlled study. *Gastroenterology* 2005; **128**:1805–11.
5. Travis SPL, Farrant JM, Ricketts C. Predicting outcome in severe ulcerative colitis. *Gut* 1996;**38**:905–10.
6. Van Assche G, D'Haens G, Noman M. Randomised, double blind comparison of 4 mg/kg vs 2 mg/kg intravenous cyclosporine in severe ulcerative colitis. *Gastroenterology* 2003; **125**:1025–31.
7. D'Haens G, Lemmens L, Geboes K. Intravenous cyclosporine versus intravenous corticosteroids as a single therapy for severe attacks of ulcerative colitis. *Gastroenterology* 2001; **120**:1323–9.

8. Cacheux W, Seksik P, Lemann M, et al. Predictive factors of response to cyclosporine in steroid-refractory ulcerative colitis. *Am. J. Gastroenterol.* 2008;**103**(3):637–42.

9. Kohn A, Daperno M, Armuzzi A, Capello M, Biancone L, Orlando A. Infliximab in severe ulcerative colitis: short-term results of different infusion regimens and long-term follow-up. *Aliment. Pharmacol. Ther.* 2007;**26**: 747–56.

10. Laharie D, Bourreille B, Branche J, et. al. Ciclosporin versus infliximab in patients with severe ulcerative colitis refractory to intravenous steroids: a parallel, open label randomised controlled trial. *Lancet.* 2012;**380**:1909–15.

11. Croft A, Walsh A, Doecke J, et. al. Outcomes of salvage therapy for steroid- refractory acute severe ulcerative colitis: ciclosporin versus infliximab. *Aliment. Pharmacol. Ther.* 2013; **38**:294–302.

12. Feagan BG, Rutgeerts P, Sands BE, et al.; GEMINI 1 Study Group. Vedolizumab as induction and maintenance therapy for ulcerative colitis. *N. Engl. J. Med.* 2013;**369**(8):699–710.

13. Plevy S, Salzberg B, Van Assche G, Regueiro M, Hommes D, Sandborn W. A phase I study of visilizumab, a humanized anti-CD3 monoclonal antibody, in severe steroid-refractory ulcerative colitis. *Gastroenterology* 2007;**133**:1414–22.

14. Van Assche G, Sandborn WJ, Feagan BG, Salzberg BA, Silvers D, Monroe PS. Daclizumab, a humanised monoclonal antibody to the interleukin 2 receptor (CD25), for the treatment of moderately to severely active ulcerative colitis: a randomised, double blind, placebo controlled, dose ranging trial. *Gut* 2006;**55**:1568–74.

15. Creed TJ, Probert CS, Norman MN, Moorghen M, Shepherd NA, Hearing SD. Basiliximab for the treatment of steroid-resistant ulcerative colitis: further experience in moderate and severe disease. *Aliment. Pharmacol. Ther.* 2006; **23**: 1435–42.

16. Ogata H, Matsui T, Nakamura M, Ida M, Takazoe M, Suzuki Y, Hibi T. A randomised dose finding study of oral tacrolimus (FK506) therapy in refractory ulcerative colitis. *Gut* 2006;**56**:1255–62.

17. Sands BE, Sandborn WJ, Feagan B, et al.; Adacolumn Study Group. A randomized, double-blind, sham-controlled study of granulocyte/monocyte apheresis for active ulcerative colitis. *Gastroenterology* 2008;**135**(2): 400–9.

18. Hanai H, Watanabe F, Saniabadi AR, Matsushitai I, Takeuchi K, Ida T. Therapeutic efficacy of granulocyte and monocyte adsorption apheresis in severe active ulcerative colitis. *Dig. Dis. Sci.* 2002;**47**:2349–53.

19. Danese S, Papa A, Saibeni S, Repici A, Malesci A, Vecchi M. Inflammation and coagulation in inflammatory bowel disease: the clot thickens. *Am. J. Gastroenterol.* 2007; **102**:174–86.

20. Shen J, Ran ZH, Tong JL, Xiao SD. Meta-analysis: the utility and safety of heparin in the treatment of active ulcerative colitis. *Aliment. Pharmacol. Ther.* 2007;**26**:653–63.

CHAPTER 35

Gastrointestinal infections

Graham Morrison[1] and John S. A. Collins[2]

[1] Altnagelvin Hospital, Londonderry, UK

[2] Northern Ireland Medical and Dental Training Agency, Royal Victoria Hospital, Belfast, UK

Introduction

Gastrointestinal infections are a major cause of mortality and morbidity worldwide [1]. The vast majority of these are due to gastroenteritis/infectious diarrhoea which will be the focus of this chapter. The approach to diarrhoea and its definition is discussed elsewhere.

While the mortality rate in developed countries has improved infectious diarrhea continues to affect 1 in 5 people per year [2]. There are an estimated 1.8 billion episodes of childhood diarrhea per year in the developing world, where diarrheal disease is responsible for approximately 3 million deaths each year among children under 5 years of age [1,3]. In both the developed and developing world the young, elderly and immunocompromised are at particular risk.

Gastroenteritis

This is by far the commonest manifestation of gastrointestinal infection. It presents with diarrhea which may be accompanied by nausea, vomiting and abdominal pain. Onset is often abrupt and can range from mild illness to life-threatening sepsis. It is most problematic in high-risk groups (Table 35.1). Most cases do not need hospital admission and can be managed in the community. The pathogen involved is often not isolated but this rarely has an impact upon treatment as most episodes are self-limiting.

Causes

A variety of viral, bacterial and parasitic pathogens can be implicated. Viral infections cause the majority of gastroenteritis in developed countries, especially among children [4]. Pathogens are rarely isolated [5]. Of those identified the most common are: viral, particularly rotavirus and norovirus; *Campylobacter* and *Salmonella* (*see later sections*).

History and examination

The history of infectious diarrhea can provide important clues to the infecting organism and etiology of infection. Relevant history includes foreign travel, contact with carriers (human and animal), contaminated food (unpasteurized dairy produce, uncooked food, seafood, and unwashed or unpeeled fruit), antibiotics, comorbidities, and relevant immune status.

Clinically three syndromes are seen:
- acute watery diarrhea, usually resolving within 5–10 days
- bloody diarrhea
- persistent diarrhea (>14 days) with or without malabsorption.

Although useful, there is considerable overlap between the above making prediction of the pathogen involved unreliable. Crampy abdominal pain, diarrhea, mucus, and pyrexia are common presenting symptoms. Nausea, vomiting, arthralgia, fatigue, and headache may also occur and may precede diarrhoea. Most bacterial and viral illnesses resolve within 5–10 days.

Gastrointestinal Emergencies, Third Edition. Edited by Tony C. K. Tham, John S. A. Collins, and Roy Soetikno.
© 2016 John Wiley & Sons, Ltd. Published 2016 by John Wiley & Sons, Ltd.

Table 35.1 High-risk groups for infectious diarrhea.

Factor	Patients at risk
Age	Infants/children
	Elderly
Immunodeficiency	HIV/AIDS
	Malignancy
	Chemotherapy/drugs
	Genetic disease
	Malnutrition
Low gastric acidity	Elderly
	Achlorhydria
	Medications
	Total gastrectomy
Altered gut flora	Antibiotics
Increased exposure	Hospital or Institutional patients
	Travellers
	Contaminated food or water

Parasitic infections tend to be more insidious, as do those in immunocompromised patients.

Examination findings tend to be nonspecific. Abdominal tenderness and fever are common. Tachycardia and hypotension may occur in severe cases. Peritonism may occur and suggests perforation. Examination findings are rarely useful in distinguishing infectious diarrhea from inflammatory bowel disease. The presence of a self-limiting illness without relapse or identification of the organism are the only reliable indicators of an infectious cause.

Investigations

Mild, self-limiting illness requires no formal investigation unless a more serious condition is suspected. Supportive measures will usually suffice in these cases. Further investigations are needed in the following cases:
• prolonged symptoms
• severe disease
• atypical features
• multiple (more than 1) people affected
• bloody diarrhea
• elderly
• residential or institutional outbreak
• public health reasons.

Generally it is best to start with the simplest, least invasive test and work upwards as required to more invasive testing. General examination and routine blood tests should be done first before proceeding onto looking for a specific pathogen.

Stool microscopy and culture

This is the first-line investigation. It is simple, relatively cheap and can provide an early diagnosis [6]. Three samples are usually examined under the light microscope for parasites by an experienced observer. Samples are then cultured for bacterial pathogens. Microscopy is used for diagnosis of *Giardia lamblia*, *Entamoeba histolytica*, *Cryptosporidium*, and *Cyclospora* species. Rapid enzyme immunoassays are used for detection of *Clostridium difficile* toxins, *Campylobacter*, enterohemorrhagic *Escherichia coli*, and *Shigella*.

Electron microscopy

Useful in diagnosis of viral infection but rarely required. Large outbreaks in institutions or culture negative outbreaks are the main use.

Serological diagnosis

Antibody testing is useful in a limited number of infections. It is particularly useful in amebiasis where antibodies are present in 80–90% of patients. Others include *Yersinia*, *Strongyloides*, and schistosomiasis.

Abdominal imaging

A plain radiograph is useful in severely unwell patients to exclude colonic dilatation and perforation. It can be used to assess the severity and extent of infectious colitis.

Endoscopy

Lower gastrointestinal endoscopy is useful when symptoms persist despite negative cultures. The main indication is to distinguish between infectious colitis and inflammatory bowel disease. Biopsies can be unreliable but may show features in keeping with inflammatory bowel disease and can identify cytomegalovirus, *E. histolytica* and the ova of *Schistosoma* spp. [3]. Pseudomembranes are typical of *C. difficile*. Upper gastrointestinal endoscopy can be useful in patients with persistent diarrhoea. Duodenal biopsies may show villous atrophy in keeping with intestinal protozoa and may even reveal the presence of cysts or trophozoites. Giardiasis and *Strongyloides* can be diagnosed on aspiration of duodenal fluid.

General management

Supportive care is the mainstay of treatment. Mild self-limiting cases can be managed by encouraging oral intake of fluids and electrolytes. In most cases this will be sufficient unless the patient is vomiting or very unwell. Contact precautions should be strictly adhered to and oral intake of both fluids and food should be encouraged.

Maintenance of hydration is critical in management. This is preferably achieved via the oral route with solutions containing water, salt and sugar [7,8]. Oral rehydration solutions are designed to meet this need and have revolutionized the treatment of infectious diarrhea. They are underused in treatment, especially in the developed world [9,10]. Several preparations are available and are shown in Table 35.2.

Most patients can be managed with oral rehydration solutions that can be given via nasogastric tube if required. Patients who are vomiting, unable to tolerate oral fluids or have severe dehydration should receive intravenous fluids until the diarrhea has settled.

Antibiotics are usually reserved for patients who are severely unwell with evidence of systemic upset. They may also be considered for prolonged disease or certain virulent pathogens (see specific conditions below). Antibiotics for specific infections are discussed later and outlined in Table 35.3. If empirical antibiotics are required ciprofloxacin 500 mg twice daily for 5–7 days is a reasonable choice.

Table 35.2 Oral rehydration solutions.

	mmol/L (unless stated)			
	Na1	K1	CL2	CHO
Dioralyte (powder) (Aventis Pharma)	60	20	60	90 (Glucose)
Dioralyte Relief (Aventis Pharma)	60	20	50	30 g (Rice Starch)
Rehydralyte (Abbott)	75	20	65	139 (Glucose)
Electrolade (Baxter)	50	20	40	111 (Glucose)
Rapolyte (Provalis)	60	20	50	110 (Glucose)
Ceralyte (Cera)	70	20	60	30 g (Rice Starch)
WHO Formulation Oral Rehydration Salts	75	20	65	75 (Glucose)

Note: WHO solution is the revised 2002 solution containing less Na.

Antimotility drugs are best avoided but may be used for symptomatic relief in those without fever or bloody stools. Loperamide is most frequently used, 4 mg initially followed by 2 mg after each unformed stool to a maximum of 16 mg/24 hours. Antimotility drugs are best avoided in children.

New antisecretory drugs, such as racecadotril, an enkephalinase inhibitor that potentiates enkephalins in the intestine and increases absorptive activity [11,12] are available for use in some countries.

Specific infections

Viral

Viral pathogens cause the majority of childhood gastroenteritis and a significant proportion of adult cases. They are a significant cause of morbidity in the developing world and although a less common cause of death in the developed world are still responsible for significant morbidity [13,14]. The commonest agents are rotavirus, norovirus, enteric adenovirus, and astrovirus. Rotavirus and norovirus are the commonest and most medically important and will be discussed here.

In recent times norovirus has presented significant problems in the hospital and institutional setting leading to large-scale outbreaks and public health initiatives to reduce infection.

The management of viral cases is supportive with the general measures described above. Other measures will depend on the setting in which the infection occurs, for example institutional outbreaks will require appropriate infection control measures. Enteric precautions should be taken and include hand washing, barrier use and the wearing of gloves. These simple measures can lead to a significant reduction in diarrheal risk [15]. If an outbreak is suspected the relevant public health authority should be involved to identify a source and take appropriate measures.

Rotavirus

This is primarily an infection of children and most will have been infected by age 5 [16]. It is a significant health burden causing over 100 million diarrhea episodes each year and 600 000 deaths in children younger than 5 years worldwide [17], almost all of which are in the developing world. It is uncommon in adults and usually

Table 35.3 Antibiotic treatments for infectious diarrhea.

Organism	1st Line	Alternative	Efficacious
Campylobacter/ Salmonella	Ciprofloxacin 750mg bd 5–7 days Ciprofloxacin 750 mg bd 7 days	Azithromycin 500 mg od 3–5 days 3rd generation cephalosporin	Severe disease Severe disease
E. coli	Ciprofloxacin 500 mg bd	Ciprofloxacin as single dose	Yes
ETEC	3–5 Days		
EIES	As for Shigella		
EHEC	Controversial given risk of HUS		
Shigella	Ciprofloxacin 500 mg bd 3 days	Azithromycin 500 mg od 3–5 days Cotrimoxazole	Yes for dysenteric shigellosis
Yersinia	Ciprofloxacin 500 mg bd 5–7 days	Tetracycline 250 mg qds 7–10 days	Doubtful unless septic
Clostridium difficile	Metronidazole 400 g tds 10–14 days	Vancomycin 125–250 mg qds 10–14 days	Yes
Vibrio cholerae	Ciprofloxacin 1 g single dose or 500 mg bd 3 days	Tetracycline 500 mg tds 3 days Doxycycline Co-trimoxazole	Yes
Gardia	Tinidazole 2 g single dose or metronidazole 750 mg tds 3 days	Mepacrine 100 mg tds 5–7 days	Yes
Entamoeba histolytica	Metronidazole 750 mg tds 5 days	Diloxanide furoate 500 mg tds 10 days	Yes

presents with fever, watery diarrhea, and vomiting. The virus is highly infectious and can occur as and endemic disease or in outbreaks.

Diagnosis can usually be made on clinical grounds but stool analysis for viral antigens is possible. Treatment is supportive and the infection usually resolves within 5 days. A vaccine against rotavirus has been developed and is available in some countries.

Norovirus

Norovirus is the commonest cause of non-bacterial gastroenteritis in adults and is a major cause of epidemic outbreaks throughout a variety of settings [18]. Large-scale outbreaks in hospitals and institutions have increased public awareness of these infections. The virus is readily transmitted via food with uncooked food and shellfish being a particular risk. The illness normally lasts around 24–48 hours and usually presents with acute onset diarrhea and vomiting. Elderly patients are most prone to severe disease.

Diagnosis is usually on clinical grounds but specific viral diagnosis can be achieved by reverse transcriptase polymerase chain reaction (PCR) on stool samples which has superseded electron microscopy [19].

Again, the virus is highly infectious and strict contact precautions should be followed as well as general supportive care and adequate hydration.

The other viral pathogens are managed as outlined above. Of special note are cytomegalovirus and herpes simplex virus. These are discussed later in the chapter.

Bacterial

Bacterial infection can cause severe and even life-threatening gastroenteritis.

Campylobacter

Campylobacter (C. jejuni and C. coli) is an important cause of diarrhea worldwide and one of the commonest causes of bacterial gastroenteritis [20,21]. It is a zoonosis and transmitted via poultry, pigs, cattle, water, unpasteurized milk, and pets. The organism is very sensitive to cooling and drying and large food-borne outbreaks do not usually occur (compare with Salmonella).

The incubation period ranges from 3 to 5 days with a prodrome of fever and malaise that is commonly followed by mild diarrhea. Vomiting is unusual, but enterocolitis with abdominal pain and severe bloody diarrhea with an acute abdomen can occur.

Arthritis (2%), pancreatitis, and septicemia can rarely occur. The diagnosis is usually made on stool culture and most cases will settle on supportive therapy. Ciprofloxacin (750 mg twice daily for 5 days) or azithromycin (500 mg daily for 3–5 days) can be used for severe cases.

Of note the organism can be excreted for up to 5 weeks after infection but no treatment is required unless severe signs are present.

Salmonella

Salmonella can cause a variety of infections in humans that are commonly described as typhoidal and non-typhoidal. These include classical typhoid fever, gastroenteritis, bacteremia, and metastatic infection such as osteomyelitis and abscesses. Non-typhoidal disease tends to be a domestic illness while typhoidal tends to be acquired abroad.

Non-typhoidal salmonella (*S. enteritidis* and *S. typhimurium*) is the commonest cause of food poisoning in the UK and the commonest isolated pathogen in acute foodborne illness [22,23]. It is a zoonosis with a large reservoir in the animal population with poultry, raw eggs, meat, and unpasteurized milk often being implicated [24]. Gastroenteritis is the commonest presentation. The incubation period is 12–36 hours after which diarrhea, vomiting, abdominal pain, and fever occur. Severe infection can cause enterocolitis, which may mimic ulcerative colitis, and can lead to septicemia and death.

Diagnosis is made on stool culture and most cases will settle on supportive therapy. Severe cases and high-risk patients should be treated with ciprofloxacin (750 mg twice daily for 7 days), although multiresistant organisms are now emerging. Feces may be positive for weeks after infection and rarely a chronic carrier state may occur. Treatment for this is not usually required unless a specific indication is present, for example, immunocompromised individuals. Chronic carriers can be treated with 4–6 weeks of antibiotics. Food handlers should be advised to remain at home during the illness and public health advice should be sought.

Typhoidal salmonella (*S. typhi* and *S. paratyphi*) cause a systemic febrile illness, in which diarrhea is less prevalent [25]. In contrast to above *S. typhi* has no animal host and causes disease in humans only. Spread is via contact with those infected or indirectly via contaminated water and food. Infection usually follows an insidious onset with headache, dry cough, malaise and anorexia. This is followed by a bacteremic phase in the first 7–10 days with abdominal pain and fever during which time blood cultures are usually positive. Rose spots, a relative bradycardia and hepatosplenomegaly may occur by the second week. Without treatment this may progress to meningitis, pneumonia, osteomyelitis, and intestinal hemorrhage. Recovery starts in the fourth week but mortality remains high without treatment and up to 10% of patients will relapse and around 2–4% of affected individuals will become chronic carriers (commoner in those with cholelithiasis or biliary tract disease).

Diagnosis may be made on cultures from blood, stool, urine and bone marrow as well as the clinical picture. Supportive treatment and hydration is essential and antibiotic therapy should be instigated. Ciprofloxacin, chloramphenicol or co-trimoxazole (usually for 2 weeks) are suitable choices. Chronic carriage may be treated with longer courses of antibiotics with consideration to cholecystectomy. Of note a vaccine for typhoid is available and should be recommended to those travelling to high-risk areas [26].

Shigella

Shigella (*S. sonnei*, *S. flexneri* and others) is the classic cause of colonic or dysenteric diarrhea and transmission is by person-to-person spread and contaminated food and water. It remains a major problem in institutions and the developing world [27,28]. The infecting dose is low, making transmission easy. Incubation is 2–3 days followed by small bowel invasion and watery diarrhea that progresses to the colonic phase with bloody diarrhea. Most cases tend to be mild and self-limiting. However, severe disease with fever, malaise, and abdominal pain may occur [29]. Toxic megacolon is a rare complication and a reactive arthritis may also occur.

Diagnosis is by stool culture. The majority of cases settle with supportive measures but severe cases may be treated with ciprofloxacin (500 mg twice daily for 3 days) or co-trimoxazole (3-day course).

Escherichia coli

Escherichia coli are common organisms and occur naturally in the human gastrointestinal tract. They can, however, become pathogenic and are a frequent cause of diarrhea [30]. The type of clinical syndrome produced generally classifies them. The three main types to consider are enterotoxigenic *E. coli* (ETEC), enteroinvasive (EIEC), and enterohemorrhagic *E. coli* (EHEC). Two other varieties, enteropathogenic (EPEC) and enteroaggregative (EAEC), also occur less commonly in children and the immunocompromised.

ETEC

Common in the developing world, this organism causes watery diarrhea in children and travellers and is a major cause of traveller's diarrhea [31]. The organism is acquired via contaminated food and water with rapid onset of watery diarrhea, nausea, and crampy abdominal pain. Vomiting may also occur. The classical case is the traveler moving from an area of good to poor hygiene, with subsequent gastroenteritis. Diagnosis can be made on stool culture. Supportive therapy is usually sufficient as the disease is self-limiting in the majority of cases. Severe cases can be treated with ciprofloxacin and advice regarding meticulous attention to food and water consumption should be given to travellers.

EIEC

Enteroinvasive *E. coli* are similar and closely related to *Shigella* spp. and cause a disease similar to bacillary dysentery. Diagnosis is by stool culture and management is as above.

EHEC

EHEC was first described in 1982 after an outbreak in the US [32]. They are responsible for large outbreaks of hemorrhagic colitis around the world and act via production of shiga toxins that play a major role in pathogenesis and development of complications. The main serotype, O157:H7 is responsible for the majority of outbreaks [33]. More recently a new strain, O104:H4 has been identified as a cause of outbreaks in Europe [34].

EHEC is acquired via undercooked beef, meat, milk, and contaminated water. After a short incubation (12–24 hours) it causes diarrhea that is frequently bloody, with associated abdominal pain and nausea. This may progress to septicemia and multiorgan failure. Thrombotic thrombocytopenic purpura (TTP) and hemolytic uremic syndrome (HUS) are recognized complications and are more common in children [35,36].

Treatment is mainly supportive but hospital admission is frequently required. Antibiotics have not been shown to be of benefit and have been suggested as a trigger for release of shiga toxin and possible precipitant of hemolytic uremic syndrome, and for this reason are best avoided [37,38].

Yersinia

Yersinia (*Y. enterocolitica* and *Y. pseudotuberculosis*) infection is common in developed countries with *Y. enterocolitica* being common in the US and *Y. pseudotuberculosis* in Europe [39]. Infection is associated with waterborne or foodborne outbreaks. Presentation ranges from mild watery diarrhea to prolonged diarrhoea, dysentery, and terminal ileitis that may be indistinguishable from Crohn's disease.

Diagnosis is usually on stool culture or serology in delayed presentation. The illness is often self-limiting but ciprofloxacin (500 mg twice daily for 5 days) may be used for severe cases.

Bacillus cereus

Bacillus is usually contracted via infected food; boiled and fried rice are commonly implicated [40]. The incubation period is a matter of hours before abrupt onset of diarrhea and vomiting. The organism can be cultured from stool but recovery is usually rapid and anything more than supportive care is rarely required.

Vibrios (*V. cholerae*)

Cholera is a disease of the tropics, particularly Africa and Asia. It is an important cause of diarrhea in travellers returning from endemic areas. It is a disease of poverty and poor sanitation and remains a significant cause of morbidity and mortality worldwide [41]. It is a waterborne disease and transmission is via the fecal–oral route. Contaminated water is the major carrier of the disease and once ingested the organisms grow on the epithelia of the small bowel, where they produce enterotoxin that leads to a massive secretory diarrhoea.

Incubation is 1–5 days and clinical infection is heralded by the abrupt onset of painless diarrhea sometimes referred to as "rice-water stools".

Fluid and electrolyte losses may be massive and can lead rapidly to death from dehydration [42].

Diagnosis is made by direct stool microscopy for organisms but can often be made on clinical grounds. The cornerstone of treatment is aimed at replacing fluid and electrolytes. Oral rehydration solutions have revolutionized this. Tetracycline (500 mg three times daily for 3 days) or ciprofloxacin (500 mg twice daily for

3 days) can be used to shorten the period of diarrhea and excretion as well as to aid recovery.

Oral cholera vaccination is available and recommended by the World Health Organization in cholera control programs in endemic areas [43].

Clostridium difficile

This is one of the most common nosocomial infections and has become a major problem in hospital practice. *Clostridium difficile*-associated disease (CDAD) is a common cause of morbidity and mortality among hospitalized patients [44,45], and is on the increase in both the inpatient and outpatient setting. More recently specific strains (e.g. ribotypes 027 or 078) have been associated with more severe and refractory Infection.

The organism exerts its effect via toxin production (A and B) that leads to secretory diarrhoea and colonic inflammation. Different strains have varying toxigenicity and some patients will be colonized and become asymptomatic carriers of the organism (approx. 3% of the healthy population but much higher in hospitalized adults). Those who are colonized or infected shed the organism and transmission is most often by contaminated hands and equipment. Colonized individuals are at particular risk of CDAD after treatment with antibiotics but in the absence of symptoms treatment is not usually recommended.

Risk factors for infection include: old age; debilitation; concomitant illness; gastrointestinal surgery; antibiotic use (all but especially penicillins, clindamycin, and cephalosporins); gastric acid suppression; enteral feeding; and non-steroidal anti-inflammatory drug (NSAID) use.

Clinical infection ranges from an asymptomatic carrier state to acute, persistent or recurrent diarrhoea. Pseudomembranous colitis and death may occur. In those who develop diarrhea, symptoms usually begin soon after colonization, with the incubation period normally less than 1 week. Diarrhea is typically loose or watery and while mucus may be present overt blood is rare. Diarrhea may be minimal in severe disease and ileus, toxic dilatation, and pseudomembranous colitis may develop. Protein-losing enteropathy and ascites may occur. *C. difficile* is a common cause of relapse In Inflammatory bowel disease and should be excluded in these patients.

Diagnosis should be directed towards those where clinical suspicion of *C. difficile* exists and is made by demonstration of toxins in stool samples and occasionally endoscopy. Toxin degrades quickly at room temperature and samples should be cooled or sent to the laboratory as soon as possible. Stool toxin may be positive for up to 6 weeks after treatment. Several methods are available for laboratory diagnosis including PCR, enzyme immunoassay (EIA) and culture. PCR detects toxin A & B and is quick, sensitive and specific. Because of the potential for false positive results some institutions will combine PCR with EIA (for glutamate dehydrogenase (GDH) or toxin A & B). GDH is produced by toxigenic and non-toxigenic *C. difficile* and testing is therefore only useful in combination with another method. If initial testing for *C. difficile* is negative repeat testing is usually not of benefit.

General management involves introduction of infection control policies and correction of any of the above risk factors if possible. Supportive treatment is coupled with specific antibiotic therapy. First-line therapy is with oral metronidazole (400–500 mg three times daily for 10–14 days) or vancomycin (125–250 mg four times daily for 14 days). Vancomycin is recommended first line in severe disease.

Relapse may occur in up to one third of patients [46–49] and should be managed as above with Metronidazole or vancomycin (or both in severe disease), while other causes of diarrhea should also be considered. Fidaxomicin, if available, is an alternative choice. Other antibiotics and non-antibiotic therapy (such as fecal transplant, immunoglobulins, and probiotics) should be instigated in conjunction with microbiology advice. An approach to recurrent infection is shown in Table 35.4.

Table 35.4 Approach to recurrent *Clostridium difficile* infection.

First relapse	Second relapse	Further relapse
Confirm diagnosis and exclude other causes	Confirm diagnosis and exclude other causes	Confirm diagnosis and exclude other causes
14 days antibiotics as outlined above	Discuss with local microbiologist and consider	Discuss with local microbiologist and consider
Fidaxomicin alternative drug	Vancomycin taper: 125 mg qds for 7 days 125 mg tds for 7 days 125 mg bd for 7 days 125 mg od for 7 days (Other regimes available)	Vancomycin and rifaximin
	Probiotics	Probiotics
	Fidaxomicin	Fidaxomicin
	Rifaximin	Intravenous Immunoglobulin
		Fecal transplant

Severe disease can be difficult to manage and toxic dilatation may rarely require surgical intervention and resection. Other measures may also be required such as intravenous metronidazole, vancomycin enemas, and those mentioned previously for relapsers. These patients should be discussed with microbiology and a gastroenterologist or infectious disease physician with experience in managing severe *C. difficile* infection.

Parasites/protozoa
Giardiasis
Giardia lamblia is a protozoan parasite and is the most common protozoal infection of the gastrointestinal tract [50]. It causes sporadic, epidemic and endemic diarrheal illness throughout the world and is most common in areas of poor sanitation. It is particularly common in travellers. Cysts (the infectious form) are passed into water supplies by the human host and are then ingested via contaminated food or water. Trophozoites then multiply in the small bowel, causing clinical disease and release of further cysts and so on [51]. Most cases are either asymptomatic or have self-limiting diarrhea and gastrointestinal disturbance. Infection can lead to chronic diarrhea, malabsorption, and growth retardation in children.

Diagnosis is by the identification of trophozoites or cysts on stool examination and three samples may be required. Rarely duodenal fluid aspiration may be required, and giardiasis is a cause of villous atrophy.

Tindazole 2 g in a single dose or metronidazole 750 mg three times daily for 3 days are the treatments of choice. Patients with symptoms, children and those at risk of spreading infection should be treated. Relapse can be treated with a longer course of antibiotics or a second-line agent such mepacrine (alone or in combination with above).

Amebiasis
E. histolytica is another protozoan parasite also occurring worldwide but is more common in developing countries with poor sanitation and lower socioeconomic conditions. Infection is usually seen in migrants from endemic areas as well as travellers to these areas. It is a significant health problem with an estimated 40 000 deaths per year [52–54] and significant complications [55]. As with *Giardia* it is the cysts that are infectious and the trophozoites that cause clinical disease. Cysts are ingested via contaminated food or water.

Most infections are asymptomatic. Of those that develop clinical amebiasis two forms are recognized:
- Amebic dysentery, which occurs over several weeks and can range from diarrhea through to bloody stools, weight loss, and fever. Uncommonly a fulminant colitis with toxic megacolon (mimicking ulcerative colitis) can occur with a high mortality.
- Non-dysenteric, which is less common, and consists of diarrhea, abdominal pain, and weight loss. This form may persist for years and can be confused with Crohn's disease. Localized colonic infection leading to an ameboma can occur, as can strictures, abscesses, and fistulae.

Amebic liver abscesses may also occur and are heralded by right upper quadrant pain and fever. Metastatic spread can develop and rupture can lead to peritonitis.

Diagnosis is made by antigen testing of stool and serum. Serology can also be used but remains positive for years after infection. Stool microscopy is often used but is less sensitive and unable to exclude non-pathogenic strains.

Treatment should be given to all patients to avoid risk of invasive disease. Metronidazole (750 mg three times daily for 5 days) will eliminate trophozoites and should be followed by either paromycin (25 mg/kg/day in three divided doses for 7 days) or diloxanide (500 mg three times daily for 10 days) to eradicate luminal parasites. Follow-up stool examination is required to ensure eradication.

Cryptosporidiosis
Cryptosporidium species are intracellular protozoa, which are associated with gastrointestinal and biliary tract disease [56]. It is a common pathogen in humans and an important cause of persistent diarrhoea in the developing world. Children, the immunocompromised, and those from areas of poor sanitation and lower socioeconomic standing are at particular risk. Clinical disease can range from asymptomatic infection to mild diarrhoea (including water-related outbreaks) or a severe enteric illness with biliary involvement. Transmission is by person-to-person spread and via infected food and water.

Immunocompetent patients typically develop diarrhea, malaise, and occasionally, abdominal pain that usually resolve in 10–14 days without treatment. Oocyst (infectious) excretion can continue for prolonged periods after clinical infection has resolved.

Immunocompromised patients tend to have more prolonged and severe illness. Aquired immune deficiency syndrome (AIDS) patients are particularly at risk and can develop prolonged, large volume diarrhea, and wasting. Cholecysytitis, cholangitis, hepatitis, and pancreatitis may occur.

Diagnosis is based on identification of oocysts in stool, tissue, or aspirates from the gastrointestinal or biliary tract. Treatment depends upon the immune status of the infected patient. Healthy individuals will usually recover spontaneously. For human immunodeficiency virus (HIV)-infected patients the initiation of highly active antiretroviral therapy (HAART) is the crucial step in therapy. This may lead to resolution of infection, but often antibiotics are required. Nitazoxanide (500 mg twice daily for 3 days) is the drug of choice but specialist advice should be sought.

Cyclospora

This parasite is an increasingly recognized cause of diarrhea. It occurs most often in foreign travellers and in patients with AIDS. Large outbreaks can occur and transmission is via contaminated food and water. Diarrhea and malaise are the most frequent symptoms and, while disease may be short and self-limiting, prolonged illness commonly occurs.

Diagnosis is made on stool microscopy and treatment is with double strength co-trimoxazole (800 mg/160 mg twice daily) for 1 week.

Other important gastrointestinal conditions

Tuberculosis (TB)

Intestinal tuberculosis is relatively uncommon in the developed world but increasing as the incidence of TB rises throughout the world [57,58]. This is due, in part, to immigration from high-risk areas and the problems posed by increasing HIV infection rates. The commonest site affected is the ileocecal region but the peritoneum and perianal area may also be involved. Clinical presentation is often vague and nonspecific and can lead to delay in diagnosis. Abdominal pain, anorexia, fever, sweats, weight loss, and altered bowel habit are the commonest symptoms. A right lower quadrant mass may be present. Ascites, obstruction, and perforation may occur.

Diagnosis is usually made in the clinical setting of known TB or in high-risk individuals, such as the immunocompromised, immigrants, intravenous drug abusers, or immunosuppressive therapy. CT scanning and small bowel radiology are useful but colonoscopy and biopsy for histology, culture, and PCR will usually provide a definitive diagnosis. Fine needle biopsy or guided biopsy may occasionally be required. Differential diagnoses include Crohn's, cancer, lymphoma, *Yersinia*, and actinomycosis.

Treatment is as for pulmonary TB. Surgery is occasionally required in the acutely presenting patient.

Schistosomiasis

This is a waterborne fluke infection found in the tropics and subtropics where it is endemic. Of the three species that cause disease *Schistosoma mansoni* affects the large bowel. Infection is acquired via skin penetration by the organism following fresh water exposure in an endemic area. Chronic disease is rare in travellers as time is required for the worm burden to develop. Travellers may develop dermatitis or an acute illness (Katayama fever) with fever, rigors, bloody diarrhea, and hepatosplenomegaly. If not treated eggs may migrate to the liver causing hepatitis followed by periportal fibrosis that can lead to portal hypertension and its complications.

The diagnosis is made by identifying the schistosome ova in feces and this may require repeat samples. Serology can be useful in the symptomatic traveller but indicates previous exposure only.

Treatment is with praziquantel (40 mg/kg as a single dose) but is best managed by infectious diseases or those with experience of the condition.

Infection in the immunocompromised

Opportunistic gastrointestinal infections may occur in the immunocompromised. HIV infection is the commonest cause worldwide, with chemotherapy and the use of other immune-suppressing drugs being common in the developed world. Several infections that are more common in the immunocompromised have already been discussed. Some other important pathogens are outlined below.

Candida

Oral and esophageal candidiasis are common illnesses. They present with a painful mouth, odynophagia, and occasionally dysphagia. Diagnosis is clinically on sight of characteristic white oral plaques and may be confirmed by culture of a swab or biopsy.

Treatment is with nystatin (1 mg four times daily) or fluconazole (50 mg o.d. for 2 weeks). Prophylactic treatment should be given in the setting of AIDS after the first infection.

Cytomegalovirus

Cytomegalovirus (CMV) rarely causes significant disease in the immunocompetent. Most of those infected have no symptoms or a mild mononucleosis syndrome that settles spontaneously. CMV colitis may occur but is rare in healthy subjects.

Immunocompromised patients are at risk of significant CMV gastrointestinal infection. Before the introduction of HAART for HIV it was commonly seen among AIDS sufferers, where it carried a poor prognosis [59,60]. Other patients on immunosuppressive treatment (Including those with inflammatory bowel disease) can also be affected [61].

CMV can affect any part of the gastrointestinal tract, but is seen most often in the esophagus and colon. CMV esophagitis causes nausea and odynophagia. Multiple discrete ulcers are usually seen at endoscopy. CMV colitis is the commonest gastrointestinal manifestation and mimics the presentation of ulcerative colitis. Fever, abdominal pain, anorexia, weight loss, and watery diarrhea are common. Widespread inflammation, ulceration, and even perforation can occur and can be life-threatening.

Diagnosis is usually suspected in those known to be at risk and in whom other causes of symptoms have been excluded. Detection of virus via PCR In blood and tissue with endoscopic biopsy to look for Inclusion bodies can provide a definitive answer.

Treatment involves anti-CMV treatment such as ganciclovir or foscarnet, as well as initiation of HAART if appropriate.

In general these patients should have input from specialists in gastroenterology, infectious diseases and genitourinary medicine.

Herpes simplex virus

Herpes simplex (HSV 1) is rarely a clinical problem in the healthy patient. In the setting of immunosuppression, however, the virus can cause considerable illness and patients infected with HIV who have low CD4 counts are at particular risk. Gastrointestinal infection in these patients can produce esophagitis, hepatitis and colitis. Esophagitis may be severe and should be suspected in susceptible patients with odynophagia or dysphagia.

Diagnosis may be made by viral culture, serology, or identification on histology. Treatment is with acyclovir (400 mg three times daily for 7 days).

References

1. Bern C, Martinez J, de Zoysa I, et al. The magnitude of the global problem of diarrhoeal disease: a ten-year update. *Bull. World Health Organ.* 1992;**70**:705.
2. Wheeler JG, Sethi D, Cowden JM, et al. Study of infectious intestinal disease in England: rates in the community, presenting to general practice, and reported to national surveillance. *BMJ* 1999;**318**:1046–305.
3. Casburn-Jones AC, Farthing MJG. Management of infectious diarrhoea. *Gut* 2004; **53**:296–305.
4. Tam CC, Rodrigues LC, Vivani L, et al. Longitudinal study of infectious intestinal disease in the UK (IID2 study): incidence in the community and presenting to general practice. *Gut* 2012;**61**:69–77.
5. Feldman RA, Banatvala N. The frequency of culturing stools from adults with diarrhoea In Great Britain. *Epidemiol Infect* 1994; **113**:41.
6. Public Health England (2013). Gastroenteritis and Diarrhoea. UK standards for Microbiology Investigations. S7 Issue 1. [Online] https://www.gov.uk/government/uploads/system/uploads/attachment_data/file/344110/S_7i1.pdf (accessed 13 July 2015).
7. Avery ME, Snyder JD. Oral therapy for acute diarrhoea. *N. Engl. J. Med.* 1990;**323**:891–4.
8. World Health Organization. Reduced osmolarity oral rehydration salts (ORS) formulation. [Online] http://apps.who.int/medicinedocs/en/d/Js4950e/2.4.html (accessed 13 July 2015).
9. Santosham K, Keenan EM, Tulloch J, et al. Oral rehydration therapy for diarrhoea: an example of reverse transfer in technology. *Paediatrics* 1997;**100**:E10.
10. Victora CG, Bryce J, Fontaine O, et al. Reducing deaths from diarrhoea through oral rehydration therapy. *Bull. World Health Organ.* 2000;**78**:1246.
11. Turvill JL, Farthing MJG. Enkephalins and enkephalinase inhibitors in intestinal fluid and electrolyte transport. *Eur. J. Gastroenterol. Hepatol.* 1997;**9**:877–80.
12. *Drug Ther. Bull.* 2013; **51**(5):54–7.
13. Parashar UD, Burton A, Lanata, C, et al. Global mortality associated with rotavirus disease among children in 2004. *J. Infect. Dis.* 2009;**200** Suppl 1:S9.
14. Patel MM, Widdowson MA, Glass RI, et al. Systematic literature review of role of noroviruses in sporadic gastroenteritis. *Emerg. Infect. Dis.* 2008;**14**:1224.

15. Curtis V, Cairncross S. Effect of washing hands with soap on diarrhoea risk in the community: a systematic review. *Lancet Infect Dis* 2003; **3**:275–81.

16. Soriano-Gabarro M, Mrukowicz J, et al. Burden of rotavirus disease in European Union countries. *Paediatr. Infect. Dis.* 2006;**25**:S7–S11.

17. Grimwood K, Buttery JP. Clinical update: rotavirus gastroenteritis and its prevention. *Lancet* 2007;**370**:302–4.

18. Lopman B, Vennema H, Kohli E, et al. Increase in viral gastroenteritis outbreaks in Europe and epidemic spread of new Norovirus variant. *Lancet* 2004;**363**:682–8.

19. Marshall JA, Bruggink LD. Laboratory diagnosis of Norovirus. *Clin. Lab.* 2006;**52**:571–81.

20. Peterson MC. Clinical aspects of *Campylobacter jejuni* infection in adults. *West. J. Med.* 1994;**161**:148–52.

21. Kirkpatrick BD, Tribble DR. Update on human *Campylobacter jejuni* infections. *Curr. Opin. Gastroenterol.* 2011; **27**:1–7.

22. Adak GK, Long SM, O'Brien SJ. Trends in indigenous foodborne disease and deaths, England and Wales: 1992 to 2000. *Gut* 2002;**51**(6):832–41.

23. Centers for Disease Control and Prevention (CDC). Preliminary FoodNet data on the incidence of Infection with pathogens transmitted commonly through food-10 states, United States, 2005. *MMWR Morb. Mortal. Wkly Rep.* 2006;**55**:392

24. Hohmann EL. Nontyphoidal salmonellosis. *Clin. Infect. Dis.* 2001;**32**:263–9

25. Bhan MK, Bhatnagar S. Typhoid and paratyphoid fever. *Lancet* 2005;**366**:749–62.

26. Steinberg EB, Bishop R, Haber P, et al. Typhoid fever in travellers: who should be targeted for prevention? *Clin. Infect. Dis.* 2004;**39**:186–91.

27. Niyogi SK. Shigellosis. *J. Microbiol.* 2005;**43**:133–43.

28. Kotloff KL, Winickoff JP, Ivanoff B, et al. Global burden of Shigella Infections: implications for vaccine development and implementation of control strategies. *Bull. World Health Organ.* 1999;**77**:651–66

29. Morduchowicz G, Huminer D, Siegman-Igra Y, Drucker M, Block CS, Pitlik SD. Shigella bacteraemia in adults: a report of five cases and review of the literature. *Arch. Intern. Med.* 1987;**147**(11):2034–7.

30. Nataro JP, Kaper JB. Diarrheagenic *Escherichia coli*. *Clin. Microbiol. Rev.* 1998;**11**:142–201.

31. Von Sonnenberg F, Tornieporth N, Waiyaki P, et al. Risk and aetiology of diarrhoea at various tourist destinations. *Lancet* 2000;**356**:133–4.

32. Riley LW, Remis RS, Helgerson SD, et al. Haemorrhagic colitis associated with a rare *Escherichia coli* serotype. *N. Engl. J. Med.* 1983;**308**:681–5.

33. Slutsker L, Ries AA, Greene KD, et al. *Escherichia coli* O157:H7 diarrhoea in the United States: clinical and epidemiologic features. *Ann. Intern. Med.* 1997;**126**(7): 505–13.

34. Frank C, Werber D, Cramer JP, et al. Epidemic profile of Shiga-toxin-producing *Escherichia coli* O104:H4 outbreak in Germany. *N. Engl. J. Med.* 2011; **365**:1711.

35. Boyce TG, Swerdlow DL, Griffin PM. *Escherichia coli* 0157:H7 and the haemolytic-uraemic syndrome. *N. Engl. J. Med.* 1995;**333**:364–8.

36. Razzaq S. Haemolytic uraemic syndrome: an emerging health risk. *Am. Fam. Physician* 2006;**74**(6):991–6.

37. Safdar N, Said A, Gangon RE, Maki DG. Risk of haemolytic uraemic syndrome after antibiotic treatment of *Escherichia coli* 0157:H7 enteritis: a meta-analysis. *JAMA* 2002;**288**(6): 996–1001.

38. Wong CS, Mooney JC, Brandt JR, et al. Risk factors for the haemolytic uraemic syndrome in children Infected with Escherichia coli O157:H7: a multivariate analysis. *Clin. Infect. Dis.* 2012;**55**:33.

39. Naktin J, Beavis KG. *Yersinia enterocolitica* and *Yersinia pseudotuberculosis*. *Clin. Lab. Med.* 1999;**19**:523–36.

40. Kotiranta A, Lounatmaa K, Haapasalo M. Epidemiology and pathogenesis of *Bacillus cereus* infections. *Microbes Infect.* 2000;**2**:189–98.

41. Griffith DC, Kelly-Hope LA, Miller MA. Review of reported cholera outbreaks worldwide, 1995–2005. *Am. J. Trop. Med. Hyg.* 2006;**75**(5):973–7.

42. Sack DA, Sack RB, Nair GB, Siddique AK. Cholera. *Lancet* 2004;**363**:223–33.

43. Cholera vaccine: WHO position paper. *Wkly Epidemiol. Rec. 2010*; **85**:117–28.

44. Kyne L, Hamel MB, Polavaram R, Kelly CP. Health care costs and mortality associated with nosocomial diarrhoea due to *Clostridium difficile*. *Clin. Infect. Dis.* 2002;**34**:346–53.

45. Bartlett JG. Narrative review: the new epidemic of *Clostridium difficile*-associated enteric disease. *Ann. Intern. Med.* 2006;**145**:758.

46. Fekety R, Mcfarland LV, Surawicz CM, et al. Recurrent *Clostridium difficile* diarrhoea: characteristics of and risk factors for patient enrolled in a prospective, randomized, double-blinded trial. *Clin. Infect. Dis.* 1997;**24**:324.

47. Fekety R. Guidelines for the diagnosis and management of *Clostridium difficile* associated diarrhoea and colitis. American College of Gastroenterology, Practice Parameters Committee. *Am. J. Gastroenterol.* 1997;**92**:739–50.

48. Pepin J, Alary ME, Valiquette L, et al. Increasing risk of relapse after treatment of *Clostridium difficile* colitis in Quebec, Canada. *Clin. Infect. Dis.* 2005;**40**:1591–7.

49. Debast SB, Bauer MP, Kuijper EJ, Committee. European Society of Clinical Microbiology and Infectious Diseases: update of the treatment guidance document for *Clostridium difficile* infection. *Clin. Microbiol. Infect.* 2014;**20** Suppl 2:1.

50. Musher DM, Musher BL. Contagious acute gastrointestinal infections. *N. Engl. J. Med.* 2004;**351**:2417–27.

51. Strickland GT: Giardiasis. In Hunter's Tropical Medicine, Hunter GE, Strickland GT (eds). Saunders, Philadelphia, 1991.

52. Li E, Stanley SL. Amoebiasis. *Gastroenterol Clin North Am* 1996; **25**:471–2.

53. Wright SG. Protozoan infections of the gastrointestinal tract. *Infect. Dis. Clin. N. Am.* 2012;**26**:323–39.

54. Slack A. Parasitic causes of prolonged diarrhoea in travellers - diagnosis and management. *Aust. Fam. Physician.* 2012;**41**:782–6.

55. Haque R, Huston CD, Hughes M, et al. Amoebiasis. *N. Engl. J. Med.* 2003;**348**:1565–73.

56. Chen XM, Keithly JS, Paya CV, LaRusso NF. Cryptosporidiosis. *N. Engl. J. Med.* 2002;**346**:1723–31.

57. Gioulene O, Paschos P, Katsaros M, et al. Intestinal tuberculosis: a diagnostic challenge - case repost and review of the literature. *Eur. J. Gastroenterol. Hepatol.* 2011;**23**:1074–7.

58. Donoghue HD, Holton J. Intestinal tuberculosis. *Curr. Opin. Infect. Dis.* 2009;**22**:490.

59. Dieterich DT, Rahmin M. Cytomegalovirus colitis in AIDS: presentation in 44 patients and a review of the literature. *J. Acquir. Immune Defic. Syndr.* 1991;**4**(suppl 1): S29–35.

60. Feasey NA, Healey P, Gordon MA. Review article: the aetiology, Investigation and management of diarrhoea in the HIV-positive patient. *Aliment. Pharmacol. Ther.* 2011;**34**: 587–603.

61. Lawlor G, Moss AC. Cytomegalovirus in inflammatory bowel disease: pathogen or innocent bystander. *Inflamm. Bowel Dis.* 2010;**16**:1620–7.

Useful links

Centers for Disease Control www.cdc.gov
World Health Organization www.who.int.en/

CHAPTER 36

Diverticular disease

Jennifer M. Kolb[1] and Tonya Kaltenbach[2]

[1] Icahn School of Medicine at Mount Sinai, Internal Medicine, New York, NY, USA
[2] Stanford University, Palo Alto, CA, USA

Introduction

Diverticular disease is common. Diverticula are caused by alterations in colonic wall structure, colonic dysmotility and dietary fiber deficiencies. Diverticula typically occur between the taenia coli due to weaknesses of the circular muscle layer at sites of penetration of the vasa recta (Fig. 36.1), and are most commonly distributed in the left colon in Western and right colon in Asian populations. Most patients with diverticulosis are asymptomatic throughout their lifetime. About 20% of patients, however, may develop complications of diverticulosis such as diverticulitis with infection, abscess, fistula, obstruction, and perforation, or diverticular bleeding.

The definitions of diverticular disease are given in Table 36.1.

The prevalence of diverticular disease increases with age, from less than 20% in persons younger than 40 years of age, to up to 66% in patients over the age of 60 years. In the United States, it is responsible for 312 000 admissions and 1.5 million days of inpatient care per year with increased hospitalizations for acute diverticulitis in younger populations. It has an estimated mortality rate of 2.5 per 100 000 per year. Mortality in acute diverticulitis is about 1% with surgical mortality up to 5%.

Acute diverticulitis

Natural history

Acute diverticulitis is the most common clinical complication of diverticular disease. Hospitalization is required in less than 10% of diverticulitis attacks. With conservative non-operative management, up to 90% of acute diverticulitis will improve and most patients have no future problems. However, about one third of patients are at risk for recurrence.

Elective resection after two attacks of acute diverticulitis was previously recommended, but new guidelines suggest that surgery should be considered on a case-by-case basis. Recent data suggests that recurrent attacks are not more severe than the initial, do not have increased morbidity and mortality, and can be medically managed the same way as the initial attack. Particular groups, such as younger and immunosuppressed patients, should be considered more closely as surgical candidates.

Presentation

- Visceral abdominal pain with tenderness localized to area of maximal inflammation
- Nausea, vomiting, and altered bowel habits
- Rectal tenderness
- Fever
- Leukocytosis.

Evaluation

- Complete blood count – leukocytosis.
- Radiographs
  - Upright chest – assess for pneumoperitoneum
  - Supine abdomen – assess for bowel dilation, ileus, obstruction or soft tissue densities to suggest an abscess
- Urinalysis – assess for colovesicular fistula
- Computerized tomography (CT) abdomen and pelvis with intravenous and oral contrast (94% sensitivity, 99% specificity)

Gastrointestinal Emergencies, Third Edition. Edited by Tony C. K. Tham, John S. A. Collins, and Roy Soetikno.
© 2016 John Wiley & Sons, Ltd. Published 2016 by John Wiley & Sons, Ltd.

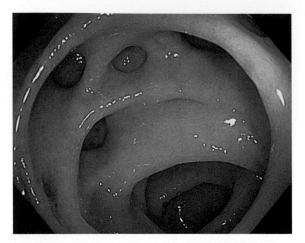

Fig. 36.1 Diverticulosis of the colon. (*see insert for color representation of the figure.*)

Table 36.1 Definitions of diverticular disease.

Diverticulosis	The presence of diverticula in the bowel. 70% asymptomatic 5–15% develop diverticular bleed 15–25% develop diverticulitis
Acute diverticulitis	Inflammation or infection of diverticula
Complicated diverticular disease	Acute diverticulitis with abscess, fistula, obstruction, or perforation
Diverticular bleeding	Painless, arterial bleeding from diverticula Most common cause of lower gastrointestinal hemorrhage

   ○ Pericolic fat infiltration
   ○ Thickened fascia
   ○ Muscular hypertrophy
 • Barium enema and endoscopy are generally avoided due to potential to exacerbate a perforation.

Management
Outpatient
Patients with mild presentation, ability to tolerate oral intake, low severity of illness, and adequate support can be treated as an outpatient with:
 • Clear liquid diet
 • Broad-spectrum oral antibiotics for 10–14 days
   ○ Amoxicillin-clavulanate or
   ○ Fluoroquinolone + metronidazole or
   ○ Trimethoprim-sulfamethoxazole + metronidazole

   ○ Can substitute clindamycin if intolerant to metronidazole.
Symptomatic improvement should be appreciated within several days.

Recent data suggest that antibiotic therapy may not accelerate recovery or prevent complications and recurrence in uncomplicated diverticulitis, but may be helpful for pain control. However, antibiotic therapy is still widely used and further studies are necessary.

Hospitalized
Patients with a more severe attack of diverticulitis may require hospitalization with:
 • Analgesia
 • Bowel rest
 • Intravenous fluid
 • Broad-spectrum antibiotics for 10–14 days, begin with intravenous and transition to oral pending clinical improvement
   ○ Metronidazole or clindamycin + 3rd generation cephalosporin or Fluoroquinolone or
   ○ Monotherapy with a β-lactam/β-lactamase inhibitor (piperacillin/tazobactam or ticarcillin-clavulanate) or
   ○ Monotherapy with carbapenem.

Follow-up
Routine colonoscopy is recommended 2–6 weeks after resolution of presumed diverticulitis in patients who have not had recent evaluation to determine extent of disease and exclude underlying malignancy.

Complicated diverticular disease

Over half of patients who present with complicated diverticulitis do so at their first attack, which include abscess, fistula, obstruction and perforation. The mortality rate of complicated diverticulitis is approximately 10–12%, the highest being with perforation. There is an overall trend toward a more conservative approach to acute complicated diverticulitis utilizing medical management and endoscopic therapy, with surgery as a last resort for patients who are not improving, septic, or with significant stenosis or fistula. Overall mortality for emergency surgery is about 15%. There has been a shift in management away from the traditional two-stage open procedure to a single laparoscopic operation with resection and primary anastomosis.

Abscess
Natural history
Pericolonic or intramesenteric abscesses complicate approximately 15% of acute diverticulitis episodes.

Presentation
- Episodic fevers
- Weight loss
- Leukocytosis
- Pain localized to visceral and parietal innervation of the abscess wall
- Dysuria, urinary frequency, tenesmus, dyspareunia in pelvic collections.

Evaluation
- CT

Management
Small pericolonic
- Conservative:
  - Bowel rest
  - Intravenous fluids
  - Broad-spectrum antibiotics
  - Abscesses <2 cm may resolve without further intervention
- Interventional – if not responsive to conservative
  - CT or ultrasound (US)-guided percutaneous drainage
  - Surgery for failed percutaneous drainage- primary resection and anastomosis (eliminates the need for two stage surgical procedure with interval colostomy).

Distant or un-resolving abscesses
- Interventional
  - CT or US-guided percutaneous palliative drainage
  - Surgery, single-stage.

Fistula
Natural history
A fistula may form when a diverticular abscess extends into an adjacent organ. The most common diverticular fistula involves the bladder. Only about one-half of patients diagnosed with a diverticular fistula have a history of diverticulitis.

Presentation
- Symptoms preceding abscess
  - Abdominal pain
  - Fever
  - Weight loss
- Symptoms by location of fistula
  - Colovesicular present with pneumaturia, fecaluria, dysuria, urosepsis
  - Colovaginal present with perineal irritation, infections or feculent discharge
  - Coloenteric present with malabsorption and diarrhea from bacterial overgrowth
  - Colocutaneous present with abdominal wall irritation.

Evaluation
The diagnostic yield of each modality varies widely:
- Colonoscopy
- Barium enema
- Fistulography
- Cystoscopy
- CT: accurately predicts the presence of a fistula
  - Local colonic thickening adjacent to an area of thickened organ
  - Associated diverticula
  - Oral contrast material or air in the organ.

Management
- Surgical single stage fistula closure with resection of diseased colon and anastomosis and repair of contiguous organ.

Obstruction
Natural history
Intestinal obstruction is uncommon in diverticulitis, occurring in approximately 2% of patients. It may present during an episode of acute diverticulitis due to luminal narrowing caused by inflammation, compression by an abscess, or localized inflammation causing ileus. Recurrent episodes of subclinical diverticulitis can result in progressive fibrosis and stricturing of the colonic wall without associated inflammation.

Presentation
- Nausea
- Vomiting
- Weight loss
- Distention.

Evaluation
- Fluid status
- Electrolytes

- Radiograph
- Endoscopy to assess stricture and exclude malignancy.

Management
- Conservative
  - Bowel rest
  - Intravenous fluids
  - Broad-spectrum antibiotics
- Intervention
  - Endoscopic dilation
  - Endoscopic stenting
    - Palliative
    - Decompression prior to elective surgery
  - Surgical resection.

Perforation
Natural history
Over 20% of patients hospitalized with diverticular disease have peritonitis due to a perforation. It is associated with a mortality rate as high as 35% and requires urgent surgical evaluation. Risk factors include immunosuppression and steroid use.

Presentation
- Severe acute abdominal pain
- Dehydration
- Fever
- Tachycardia
- Generalized tenderness with guarding
- Absent bowel sounds.

Evaluation
- Complete blood count
- Serum electrolytes
- Arterial blood gas
- Radiograph
- Close surgical monitoring.

Management
- Bowel rest
- Aggressive intravenous fluids
- Broad-spectrum antibiotics
- Surgery
  - Preliminary evidence shows that laparoscopic peritoneal lavage with drain placement for perforated diverticulitis with peritonitis is a safe and effective alternative to laparotomy with resection.

Diverticular hemorrhage

Natural history
Diverticulosis remains the most frequent cause of lower gastrointestinal hemorrhage (LGIB; about 30–40%), and presents as acute, painless hematochezia, often in elderly patients with comorbid conditions including hypertension, ischemic heart disease, diabetes, obesity, and who use oral anticoagulation or antiplatelet medication. Diverticulae are located in the colonic wall at the sites of penetrating nutrient vessels. Bleeding is arterial and can occur either at the dome or the neck of the diverticulum. It is important to recognize the various stigmata of diverticular bleeding including large and small vessel, adherent clot, flat pigmented spot and erosion (Fig. 36.2). About 35% of patients will have recurrent hemorrhage with particular risk factors including age >70, hypertension, arteriosclerotic disease, and chronic renal failure.

Presentation
- Abrupt, voluminous, painless hematochezia.

Evaluation
Stratification
Most acute diverticular bleeding is self-limiting. In general, patients with stable vital signs, no recent bloody effluent and no syncope, have a low risk of continued bleeding and elective colonoscopy is appropriate. Urgent interventions should be targeted for patients with

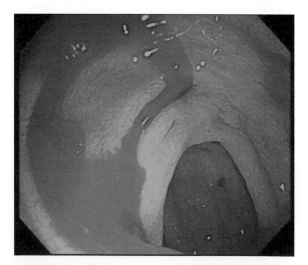

Fig. 36.2 Active diverticular bleed. (*see insert for color representation of the figure.*)

severe bleeding. (See Chapter 6: Acute Severe Lower Gastrointestinal Hemorrhage).

Independent correlates of severe bleeding:

- Bleeding per rectum during the first 4 hours of evaluation
- Vital sign instability
  - Tachycardia (HR >100)
  - Hypotension (SBP <115 mmHg)
- Syncope
- Non-tender abdominal exam
- Aspirin use
- >2 comorbid conditions
  Check complete blood count
  Assess volume status
  Exclude an upper gastrointestinal source
- Upper endoscopy
  - Patients with a positive nasogastric aspirate.

Management

Once the patient has been resuscitated, the severity and acuity of bleeding assessed, and an upper gastrointestinal source of bleeding excluded, urgent colonoscopy should be performed. In cases of continued bleeding not amenable to endoscopic therapy angiography or surgery should be considered.

Colonoscopy

Available data suggest that endoscopic intervention for diverticular hemorrhage is safe and beneficial.

- Rapid purge preparation with polyethylene glycol based solutions
  - Administer by a nasogastric tube or by drinking 1 L every 30–45 min
  - Median dose of 6 L (range 4–14 L) over 3–4 hours
  - Metoclopramide, 10 mg IV, before starting the purge to control nausea and promote gastric emptying.
  - Nasogastric suction immediate prior to colonoscopy
  - Contraindications: bowel obstruction, gastroparesis
- Techniques
  - Mechanical methods are preferred
    - Clip: Marking for future localization, direct application to neck or dome, use of a cap may facilitate therapy
    - Band ligation
  - Coagulation- generally avoided at the dome due to perforation concern
  - Injection – reported with limited success.

Technetium scan

Literature dating since 1990 suggest that technetium scans are not particularly useful to confirm and localize the bleeding site in order to direct further angiographic or surgical intervention.

Angiography

Angiography techniques have been modified over time to use smaller catheters for coiling or gel foam embolization. Using this optimal embolization technique, twelve published small studies, have shown high rates of successful primary hemostasis in patients with active bleeding. Short-term, less than 1 week, rebleeding rates were, however, high, found to be about 25% with a mean of 10–53%; and data on long term rebleeding rates is lacking. Ischemia was notably reported in close to 20% of patients despite using smaller catheter and more directed therapy.

Surgery

Whenever possible, it is preferable to perform surgery on an elective basis rather than emergently. Operative mortality for complicated diverticulitis is approximately 10%, with significantly increased morbidity and mortality for perforation.

Further reading

Chapman J, Davies M, Wolff B, et al. Complicated diverticulitis: is it time to rethink the rules? *Ann. Surg.* 2005;**242**: 576–581.

Chapman J, Dozois E; Wolff B Gullerud R, Larson, DRM. Diverticulitis: a progressive disease?: Do multiple recurrences predict less favorable outcomes? *Ann. Surg.* 2006;**243**:876–83.

Elta GH. Urgent colonoscopy for acute lower-GI bleeding. *Gastrointest. Endosc.* 2004;**59**:402–8.

Etzioni DA, Mack TM, Beart RW Jr, Kaiser AM. Diverticulitis in the United States: 1998–2005: changing patterns of disease and treatment. *Ann. Surg.* 2009;**249**(2):210.

Farrell JJ, Graeme-Cook F, Kelsey PB. Treatment of bleeding colonic diverticula by endoscopic band ligation: an in-vivo and ex-vivo pilot study. *Endoscopy.* 2003;**35**:823–9.

Foutch PG, Zimmerman K. Diverticular bleeding and the pigmented protuberance (sentinel clot): clinical implications, histopathological correlation, and results of endoscopic intervention. *Am. J. Gastroenterol.* 1996;**91**:2589–93.

Hall JF, Roberts PL, Ricciardi R, et al. Long-term follow-up after an initial episode of diverticulitis: what are the predictors of recurrence? *Dis. Colon Rectum* 2011;**54**:283.

Janes SE, Meagher A, Frizelle FA. Management of diverticulitis. *BMJ*. 2006;**332**:271–5.

Jensen DM, Machicado GA, Jutabha R, Kovacs TO. Urgent colonoscopy for the diagnosis and treatment of severe diverticular hemorrhage. *N. Engl. J. Med*. 2000;**342**:78–82.

Khanna A, Ognibene SJ, Koniaris LG. Embolization as first-line therapy for diverticulosis-related massive lower gastrointestinal bleeding: evidence from a meta-analysis. *J. Gastrointest. Surg*. 2005;**9**:343–52.

Klarenbeek BR, Samuels M, van der Wal MA, van der Peet DL, Meijerink WJ, Cuesta MA. Indications for elective sigmoid resection in diverticular disease. *Ann Surg*. 2010;**251**(4):670–4.

Laméris W, van Randen A, Bipat S, et al. Graded compression ultrasonography and computed tomography in acute colonic diverticulitis: meta-analysis of test accuracy. *Eur. Radiol*. 2008;**18**:2498.

Petruzziello L, Iacopini F, Bulajic M, Shah S, Costamagna G. Review article: uncomplicated diverticular disease of the colon. *Aliment. Pharmacol. Ther*. 2006;**23**:1379–91.

Rafferty J, Shellito P, Hyman NH, et al. Practice parameters for sigmoid diverticulitis. *Dis Colon Rectum* 2006;**49**:939–44.

Salzman H, Lillie D. Diverticular disease: diagnosis and treatment. *Am. Fam. Physician* 2005;**72**:1229–34.

Simpson PW, Nguyen MH, Lim JK, Soetikno RM. Use of endoclips in the treatment of massive colonic diverticular bleeding. *Gastrointest. Endosc*. 2004;**59**:433–7.

Stollman N, Raskin JB. Diverticular disease of the colon. *Lancet* 2004;**363**:631–9.

Strate LL, Syngal S. Predictors of utilization of early colonoscopy vs. radiography for severe lower intestinal bleeding. *Gastrointest. Endosc*. 2005;**61**:46–52.

CHAPTER 37

Gastrointestinal complications of HIV disease

Emma McCarty and Wallace Dinsmore

Royal Victoria Hospital, Belfast, UK

Overview of HIV/AIDS

Human immunodeficiency virus (HIV) is a retrovirus that affects T-lymphocyte or CD4 cells. It transmitted through unprotected sexual intercourse, contact with infected blood products (e.g. blood transfusions prior to 1985, drug users sharing needles or "works") or vertically from mother to baby. Approximately 60% of individuals will experience symptoms of primary HIV infection, or "seroconversion", usually within several weeks of acquisition. The severity of symptoms may range from a mild flu-like illness to viral meningitis, but generally resolves within a few weeks. It is during this stage that individuals will be highly infectious and there is increased risk of onward transmission.

Following seroconversion there is an asymptomatic phase which may last several years. In the absence of any signs and symptoms, the infection is likely to remain undiagnosed during this period unless an individual attends for sexually transmitted infection (STI) testing or is screened in circumstances such as blood donation or antenatal booking. Immune function will initially be normal with a CD4 count usually greater than 500 cells/mm³.

As HIV infection progresses, the CD4 count will decline over time at a rate, which varies significantly between individual patients. Patients may begin to experience HIV-related symptoms such as weight loss, malaise, diarrhea, and night sweats. Other conditions such as multi-dermatomal shingles, seborrhoeic dermatitis, or bacterial pneumonia may occur. If HIV remains undiagnosed or untreated, the CD4 count will continue to decline leaving individuals susceptible to opportunistic infections (OI) or an acquired immune deficiency syndrome (AIDS)-defining illness. AIDS defining illnesses such as *Pneumocystis carinii* pneumonia, Kaposi's sarcoma, and esophageal candidiasis generally occur when the CD4 count is below 200 cells/mm³.

The current UK recommendation for starting antiretroviral therapy is at a CD4 count of 350 cells/mm³ [2]. Indications for earlier initiation include coinfection with hepatitis B or C, AIDS-defining illness or non-AIDS related malignancy requiring chemo- or radiotherapy. The aim of treatment is to suppress viral replication and improve CD4 cell count and function. Once antiretroviral therapy is initiated, treatment is life-long and adherence is imperative to prevent viral rebound and subsequent drug resistance. Antiretroviral drugs may have significant interaction with many commonly used medications including proton pump inhibitors, with concomitant use leading to toxicity or treatment failure. Easily accessible information regarding interactions may be found online through the University of Liverpool HIV Interactions Database [3].

HIV testing in the gastrointestinal setting

Diagnosing HIV infection relies on maintaining a high index of clinical suspicion amongst those individuals who may not appear to fall within traditional risk groups. HIV testing is inexpensive and straightforward, with no longer a requirement for specific pre-test

---

Gastrointestinal Emergencies, Third Edition. Edited by Tony C. K. Tham, John S. A. Collins, and Roy Soetikno.

counseling. It should be offered to all patients in whom an HIV-related illness falls within the differential diagnosis. In 2008, UK National Guidelines for HIV testing were developed with the aim of increasing HIV testing and reducing the frequency of late diagnosis. Key clinical indicator diseases for recommending an HIV test are listed by specialty and include: cryptosporidiosis, oral candidiasis, oral hairy leukoplakia, chronic diarrhea of unknown cause, weight loss of unknown cause, hepatitis B & C, and confirmed cases of shigella, campylobacter or salmonella [4].

Upper gastrointestinal diseases associated with HIV

The common gastrointestinal diseases associated with GI infection are summarized in Table 37.1. Dysphagia and/or odynaphagia are symptoms frequently reported by individuals with HIV and may indicate significant underlying eosophageal pathology. The most common cause of dysphagia is esophageal candidiasis, particularly if the CD4 count is <200 cells/mm³. The incidence of candida infection has fallen dramatically since the introduction of highly active antiretroviral therapy (HAART); however, it remains highly prevalent in those with advanced HIV or on failing antiretroviral treatment [5]. Its presence should alert the physician to the likelihood of immunosuppression or (rarely) seroconversion and prompt HIV testing where the status is unknown. Oral thrush is present in up to 80% of patients with esophageal candidiasis but is insufficient to exclude the possibility of another underlying opportunistic infection, especially in patients with moderate-severe symptoms [6]. It is important to note that multiple pathologies often coexist in HIV infection particularly in those with low CD4 counts [7].

Other common causes of esophageal symptoms in HIV patients include cytomegalovirus (CMV), herpes simplex virus (HSV), Epstein–Barr virus (EBV), and idiopathic ulceration. Ulceration may be caused by a number of medications used by HIV-positive patients such as non-steroidal anti-inflammatories, doxycycline and iron supplements [8]. Other conditions that infrequently cause esophageal symptoms include reflux esophagitis, mycobacterial disease, non-Hodgkin's lymphoma, and Kaposi's sarcoma.

Table 37.1 Gastrointestinal manifestations of HIV infection.

GI symptom	Cause	
	Common	**Uncommon**
Esophageal symptoms	Candida	Kaposi's sarcoma
	CMV	Non-Hodgkin's lymphoma
	Idiopathic ulceration	
	HSV	
	GERD	
Diarrhea	Salmonella spp.	Atypical mycobacterium
	Campylobacter spp.	Microsporidia
	Shigella spp.	Isospora
	CMV	Kaposi's sarcoma
	Cryptosporidium spp.	
	Giardia lamblia	
	HIV enteropathy	
Biliary disease	Cholangiopathy	Non-Hodgkin's lymphoma
	(CMV, MAC, cryptosporidia)	Kaposi's sarcoma
	Acalculous cholecystitis	
	Vanishing bile duct syndrome	
Hepatic disease	Viral hepatitis	Atypical mycobacterium
	CMV	Mycobacterium tuberculosis
	Syphilis	Cryptococcus neoformans
	Non-Hodgkin's lymphoma	Castleman's disease

Investigation of upper gastrointestinal symptoms

In those with uncomplicated esophagitis where signs and symptoms are suggestive of candidiasis, empirical treatment with fluconazole 50–100 mg daily for 7–14 days is recommended [9]. If symptoms worsen or fail to respond to treatment within a few days, upper gastrointestinal endoscopy should be conducted. The endoscopic features that are characteristic of opportunistic infection in the upper gastrointestinal tract are

Table 37.2 Upper gastrointestinal endoscopic findings.

Etiology	Endoscopy
Candida	'Cottage cheese', yellow-white plaques, coating the entire esophagus. Pseudomembranous and ulcerative elements
CMV	One or more large well-circumscribed ulcers, biopsy from the base
HSV	Diffuse erosive esophagitis or small discrete, superficial volcano ulcers; biopsy from the margins
IEU	One or more well-circumscribed ulcers of variable depth
Leishmania	Variable from normal mucosa to mucosal edema, nodularity, multiple superficial erosions, and ulcers
Syphilis	Diffuse antral erythema and edema, thickened gastric folds, polypoid lesions, and serpiginous ulcerations
Cryptococcus	Multiple well-circumscribed nodules with central erosions or focal areas of gastritis with central erosions
MAC	Diffuse gastropathy with erythematous and nonulcerated lesions resembling angioectasis, mainly in gastric body
Gastric Karposi's sarcoma	Multiple raised purple-colored sessile polyps anywhere in the stomach
Non-Hodgkin lymphoma	Enlarged gastric folds, the stomach loses its ability to distend (air insufflations) multiple large ulcerated lesions, with a hardened mucosa

CMV cytomegalovirus; HSV herpes simplex virus; IEU idiopathic esophageal ulcers, MAC Mycobacterium avium complex.

presented in Table 37.2. During the procedure, biopsies should be taken for histology, cultures (mycobacterial, fungal) and molecular tests including CMV PCR and HSV PCR. Candida speciation and sensitivities are useful in cases where there has been a failure to respond to empirical fluconazole.

Treatment
Azole-sensitive strains of candida should be treated with oral fluconazole 200 mg initially followed by 50–100 mg daily for 7–14 days; intravenous administration may be necessary if the patient is unable to swallow medication. Maintenance therapy at lower doses can be given until immune recovery occurs with antiretroviral therapy. Alternative agents include caspofungin 70 mg loading dose, followed by 50 mg daily IV or liposomal amphotericin B 3 mg/kg daily IV for 7–14 days.

CMV esophagitis is treated with ganciclovir 5 mg/kg twice daily IV for 2–4 weeks or until symptoms have resolved. Oral valganciclovir 900 mg twice daily can be used if symptoms are not severe enough to impair the swallow. Foscarnet may be used in cases of ganciclovir resistance. All patients with confirmed CMV esophagitis should be referred for ophthalmic assessment to exclude retinitis. Herpes simplex infection should be treated with aciclovir 5–10 mg/kg IV initially followed by oral therapy at a dose of 400 mg 5 times daily for a total of 14 days. The treatment of choice for idiopathic or aphthous ulceration is thalidomide 200mg daily for 4 weeks, which has been shown to induce complete resolution in approximately 70% patients [10]. Prednisolone is an alternative treatment option for aphthous ulcers at an initial dose of 40 mg daily, reducing to 10 mg daily over 4 weeks [11].

The diagnosis of any opportunistic infection warrants prompt initiation of antiretroviral therapy regardless of the CD4 count. There is much data to demonstrate commencing HAART within 2 weeks of OI treatment is associated with reduced morbidity and mortality.

Gastric diseases associated with HIV

Gastroesophageal reflux disease (GERD) is common in HIV positive patients. Infection with *Helicobacter pylori* has been shown to occur in approximately 70% of HIV patients reporting dyspepsia [12]. It is important to note that the use of acid-lowering drugs is contraindicated with antiretroviral regimes containing atazanavir and rilpivirine as absorption of the latter drugs is significantly impaired resulting in potential virological failure and drug resistance.

The gastrointestinal tract is a common site to be affected by Kaposi's sarcoma, particularly the esophagus and stomach. This is often asymptomatic, although lesions may become haemorrhagic and present with hematemesis or melena. OI that may affect the stomach include CMV, *Cryptosporidium, Toxoplasma gondii, Leishmania,* atypical mycobacteria, *Cryptococcus,* and *Treponema pallidum* (syphilis). Isolated involvement of the stomach is however unlikely. Extra-nodal non-Hodgkin's lymphoma can cause upper gastrointestinal symptoms in patients with advanced HIV/AIDS and may be complicated by massive hematemasis, gastric outlet obstruction and perforation [13].

Gastroscopy with biopsies from multiple normal and abnormal sites is the mainstay of diagnosis, as pathologies such as gastric Kaposi sarcoma tend to be submucosal and may be missed in two-third of the cases [13]. Tissue should be sent for histology, viral staining and culture, mycobacterial staining and culture and molecular studies for CMV, EBV, and HSV PCR. A normal endoscopy in a patient with normal CD4 should be followed with empiric proton pump inhibitors (PPI) for non-erosive GERD or a barium swallow to exclude rings or motility disorders.

Hepatobiliary diseases associated with HIV

Viral hepatitis

Coinfection with hepatitis B or C is common in HIV and is often related to the epidemiological risk group of the individual. The prevalence of hepatitis B co-infection within HIV clinics in the UK has been reported as 3–10% [14]. The overall prevalence of hepatitis C co-infection reported in the UK Collaborative HIV Cohort (UK CHIC) is 9%, however this varies between risk groups (83% in IVDU, 7% in men having sex with men) [15]. Sporadic outbreaks of acute hepatitis C have been reported amongst men having sex with men and are associated with particularly high risk sexual behaviors. There is a significant interplay between HIV and viral hepatitis with affected individuals being less likely to clear the infection, having more rapid progression to cirrhosis and liver failure and higher risk of hepatocellular carcinoma. Guidance on best clinical practice in the treatment and management of HIV and viral hepatitis co-infection has been developed by British HIV Association, and include new developments in hepatitis C drugs [16].

Acalculous cholecystitis

Acalculous cholecystitis is a rare complication of advanced HIV disease. It has been associated with various opportunistic organisms including CMV, *Cryptosporidium parvum* and *Campylobacter jejuni*, although no pathogen is

identified in around 15% of individuals [17]. It typically presents with right upper quadrant pain, tenderness and fever. Ultrasound examination may show thickening of the gallbladder wall and pericholecystic fluid. There is little evidence to support the use of antimicrobial agents and cholecystectomy is the mainstay of treatment.

Cholangiopathy

Cholangiopathy is uncommon except in those with profound immunocompromise (CD4 <50 cells/mm³). It occurs as a result of stricture formation following an opportunistic infection, most likely cryptosporidium parvum, CMV or atypical mycobacteria [18]. It has, however, also been reported in association with *Giardia lamblia* and HSV. It presents with right upper quadrant pain, jaundice, fever and obstructive liver function tests. The investigation of choice is endoscopic retrograde cholangiopancreatography (ERCP), which provides an opportunity for spincterotomy in addition to tissue sampling for diagnostics.

Lower gastrointestinal diseases associated with HIV

In the pre-HAART era, diarrhea was experienced by 30–70% of HIV positive individuals and had a significant impact on quality of life [19]. The use of antiretroviral therapy has dramatically reduced the incidence of chronic diarrhea (0.9–14% of patients), with complete resolution of symptoms being reported in 85% patients taking effective therapy [20]. Diarrhea can affect antiretroviral drug absorption, resulting in resistance and treatment failure, therefore it is important to investigate and, where possible, treat the cause.

Acute diarrhea

Acute diarrhea is defined as more than three loose bowel motions in a 24-hour period, with symptoms present for less than 14 days. In those HIV patients with significantly impaired immune function (CD4 <200 cells/mm³), the differential diagnosis is considerable and a detailed history including travel, new sexual contacts and medication should be taken.

Stool samples should be obtained for ova, cysts and parasites to exclude microsporiosis and cryptosporidium. Further samples should be sent for bacterial culture (*Salmonella* spp, *Shigella* spp, *Campylobacter* spp) and *Clostridium difficile* toxin and culture. Blood cultures for atypical mycobacteria (mycobacteria avium intracellulare) should be considered when CD4 count is < 50 cells/mm³.

In individuals with preserved immune function (CD4 >200 cells/mm³) and suspected bacterial diarrhea, specific treatment is not usually required. If, however, the CD4 count is <200 cells/mm³, therapy is indicated and should be guided by stool cultures and antibiotic sensitivities. Empirical treatment is generally avoided due to increasing antibiotic resistance and associations with *C. difficile* and methicillin-resistant *Staphylococcus aureus* (MRSA) colonization. If symptoms are severe or sepsis is present, the majority of pathogens will respond to ciprofloxacin 500 mg twice daily for 5 days. Metronidazole 400 mg three times daily for 10 days or vancomycin 125 mg four times daily for 7–10 days are recommended for *C. difficile* as in the HIV-negative population. There is no specific therapy for cryptosporidium except early initiation of antiretroviral therapy [21]. Nitazoxanide at a dose of 500 mg twice daily for 3 days has been shown to be effective in those without significant immunocompromise. Interestingly, the widespread utilization of trimethoprim sulfamethoxazole for prophylaxis against pneumocystis jirovecii pneumonia has resulted in reduce incidence of pathogens such as *Salmonella*, *Isospora*, and *Cyclosporidium*.

Chronic diarrhea

Chronic diarrhea is defined as symptoms that persist for more than 1 month. The most likely causes include opportunistic infection, fat malabsorption, or side effect of antiretroviral therapy. Alternately HIV infection itself, or HIV enteropathy, may be responsible for refractory diarrhea. There has been much debate regarding the impact which morphological changes in the intestinal mucosa and detection of virus within the lamina propria have on chronic bowel symptoms. Other mechanisms such as altered and dysfunctional mucosal immune function, increased permeability of the mucosa to foreign antigens and subsequent release of detrimental cytokines and abnormal enteric neural and endocrine function have been implicated in the pathogenicity of this condition [22]. HIV enteropathy is a diagnosis of exclusion after extensive investigation for opportunistic infections and malignancy.

The most common opportunistic infection of the lower gastrointestinal tract is CMV colitis. In addition to persistent bloody or mucus diarrhea, patients may also report abdominal pain, anorexia or weight loss. CMV colitis is an AIDS defining condition and usually occurs in HIV patients with CD4 counts <50 cells/mm³. In patients with severe abdominal pain and peritoneal signs, perforated CMV ulcers of the colon or CMV-associated appendicitis should be considered. Some conditions such as Kaposi sarcoma, non-Hodgkin's lymphoma or adenocarcinoma of the colon may present as colon obstruction or perforation [23].

Investigation of lower gastrointestinal symptoms

In large volume watery diarrhea, the initial investigations should include gastroscopy and duodenoscopy to exclude small bowel pathology. If symptoms include crampy pain, blood, or mucus in stools or tenesmus then sigmoidoscopy and/or colonoscopy should be conducted. The advantage of colonoscopy over flexible sigmoidoscopy lies in its ability to diagnose isolated proximal illness with CMV and has been reported to be as high as 46% in various studies [23]. Endoscopy could be normal in up to 25% of the cases and with this in mind biopsies from normal mucosa should be obtained in addition to those from macroscopically abnormal areas. Endoscopic features of various opportunistic infections affecting the lower gastrointestinal tract are outlined in Table 37.3.

Treatment

Treatment of chronic diarrhea should be pathogen specific (see "acute diarrhea"). If it has not been possible to identify a cause, the use of antidiarrheal agents such as loperamide 4–32 mg daily in divided doses, codeine phosphate 30–60 mg four times daily, or diphenoxylate 2.5 mg/atropine 25 µg two tablets four times daily may be useful for symptomatic relief.

Anorectal diseases associated with HIV

Lymphogranuloma venereum

Lymphogranuloma venereum (LGV) has become one of the leading causes of proctitis in HIV-positive patients. It is a systemic disease caused by three invasive and

Table 37.3 Lower gastrointestinal endoscopic findings.

Etiology	Endoscopy
Common bacterial pathogens	Erythema, edema, hemorrhagic and ulcerated mucosal lesions which could mimic ulcerative colitis
(*Salmonella*, *Shigella* and *Campylobacter*)	
C. difficile	Erythema, edema and friability of the mucosa covered by yellow-white pseudomembrane
TB	Nodular mucosa with areas of ulceration, mostly localized in proximal colon
MAC	Granular white nodules 2 to 4 mm in diameter with a surrounding rim of erythema, occasionally completely normal
CMV	Colitis without ulcers, ulcers without colitis, normal looking colon, and occasionally a pseudotumor, typically distal colon
HSV	Erythematous areas with small vesicular lesions, small ulcers coalescing to form larger ulcers
Cryptosporidium, *Isospora*	Colonic cryptitis, colitis
E. histolytica	Non-specific colitis with ulcerations or larger mucosal ulcers associated with yellow-green pseudomembranes
Balantidium	Ulceration with features similar to those of invasive amoebiasis
Histoplasma	Colitis, ulcerations, or most commonly, a mass lesion
Candida albicans	Patchy erythema or discrete ulcers that resemble those caused by CMV
Karposi sarcoma	Violaceous plaque-like macular or nodular lesions, sometimes with central umbilication or ulceration
Lymphoma	Bulky mass lesion, ulcerations, colitis-like picture, and necrotic abscesses

virulent serovars of *Chlamydia trachomatis* (L1–L3). LGV is endemic in tropical areas however cases originating in industrialised settings were rare until a widespread European outbreak in 2003 occurring in men having sex with men (MSM). It has now become one of the most common causes of proctitis in MSM, particularly in those coinfected with HIV or hepatitis C. It presents with severe rectal pain, mucoid or haemorrhagic rectal discharge, tenesmus, and occasionally systemic symptoms. LGV may mimic inflammatory bowel disease both clinically and histologically, therefore it is important to consider this within the differential diagnosis. A rectal swab should be sent for *Chlamydia trachomatis* PCR and, if positive, LGV genotyping should be conducted. LGV is treated effectively with doxycycline 100 mg twice daily for 3 weeks. If left untreated, chronic infection leads to perirectal fistulae, abscesses, and strictures.

Other sexually transmitted causes of proctitis include *Neisseria gonorrhoeae*, *Treponema pallidum* (syphilis), and HSV. Referral should be made to a genitourinary medicine specialist for appropriate testing, treatment and follow-up.

Anal interstitial neoplasia (AIN) and invasive anal carcinoma

The incidence of anal squamous cell carcinoma in HIV-positive individuals is approximately 40–80 times higher than in the general population [24]. Antiretroviral therapy has unfortunately had no impact on the incidence on anal cancer. Factors implicated in anal cancer in HIV positive patients include human papillomavirus (subtype 16) status, smoking and sexual behavior. Over recent years there has been debate regarding the potential to screen HIV-positive men for precursor AIN lesions using anal Pap smears, in a similar manner to cervical screening for CIN in women. In the absence of UK consensus, it is important to maintain a high degree of suspicion regarding anal lesions in HIV-positive patients and have a low threshold for biopsy.

Gastrointestinal complications of antiretroviral therapy

Gastrointestinal symptoms are amongst the most common side effects of antiretroviral drugs. Protease inhibitors in particular are frequently associated with diarrhea, nausea, and bloating. This class of drugs has also been associated with an increased risk of acute pancreatitis.

Isolate hyperbilirubinemia occurs in approximately 10% of patients receiving atazanavir therapy. The increased in unconjugated bilirubin is due to the inhibition of UDP glucuronyl transferase, the enzyme which is deficient in Gilbert's syndrome. The resulting jaundice can be quite marked, although not indicative of hepatic injury.

Lactic acidosis secondary to mitochondrial toxicity is a rare, but serious and occasionally fatal, complication of antiretrovirals, particularly nucleotide reverse transcriptase inhibitors. It may present with malaise, nausea, abdominal discomfort, or weight loss. Early discontinuation of the treatment should be followed by seeking expert advice on reintroduction of the alternative treatments.

Conclusion

Gastrointestinal symptoms are amongst the most common complaints in HIV-positive patients. Although the gastrointestinal manifestations of HIV have changed since the introduction of HAART, opportunistic infections are still frequent amongst individuals who present with advanced HIV or AIDS. It is important to have an awareness of those conditions which may present to gastroenterology physicians indicating undiagnosed underlying HIV infection. The major challenge for today's HIV epidemic is to increase HIV testing in order to reduce late diagnosis and improve clinical outcomes.

References

1. HIV in the United Kingdom: 2013 Report. Public Health England, 2013. [Online] https://www.gov.uk/government/.../HIV_annual_report_2013.pdf (accessed 9 July 2015).
2. British HIV Association Guidelines for the treatment of HIV-1 positive adults with antiretroviral therapy 2012. *HIV Medicine* 2014;**15**(1): 1–85.
3. HIV Drug Interactions Database. University of Liverpool. [Online] Available from www.hiv-druginteractions.org (accessed 2 July 2015).
4. UK National Guidelines for HIV testing 2008. British HIV Association, British Association of Sexual Health and HIV, British Infection Society. [Online] Available from www.bhiva.org (accessed 2 July 2015).
5. Kaplan JE, Hanson D, Dworkin MS, et al. Epidemiology of human immunodeficiency virus-associated opportunistic infections in the United States in the era of highly active antiretroviral therapy. *Clin. Infect. Dis.* 2000;**30**(Suppl.)1:5–14.
6. Laing RBS, Brettle RP, Leen CLS. Clinical predictors of azole resistance, outcome and survival from oesophageal candidiasis in AIDS patients. *Int. J. STD AIDS* 1998;**9**:16–20.
7. Wilcox M. Approach to esophageal disease in AIDS: a primer for the endoscopist. *Techniques Gastrointest. Endosc.* 2002; **4**:59–65.
8. Yap I, Guan R, Kang Jy, Gwee KA, Tan CC. Pill-induced esophageal ulcer. Singapore Med. *J.* 1993;**34**:257–8.
9. Beeching NJ, Jones R, Gazzard B. British HIV Association and British Infection Association Guidelines for the treatment of opportunistic infection in HIV-seropositive individuals 2011. *HIV Medicine* 2011;**12**(Suppl 2):43–54.
10. Jacobson JL, Spritzler J, Fox L, et al. Thalidomide for the treatment of esophageal aphthous ulcers in patients with human immunodeficiency virus infection. National Institute of Allergy and Infectious Disease AIDS Clinical Trials Group. *J. Infect. Dis.* 1999;**180**:61–7.
11. Wilcox CM, Schwarz DA. A pilot of corticosteroid therapy for idiopathic esophageal ulcerations associated with human immunodeficiency virus infection. *Am. J. Med.* 1992;**93**:131–4.
12. Mach T, Skwara P, Biesiada G, Ciesla A, Macura A. Morphological changes of the upper gastrointestinal tract mucosa and Helicobacter pylori infection in HIV-positive patients with severe immunodeficiency and symptoms of dyspepsia. *Med. Sci. Monit.* 2007;**13**(1):14–19.
13. Monkemuller KE, Olmos M. Gastric diseases in AIDS. *Techniques Gastrointest. Endosc.* 2002;**4**:66–9.
14. De Silva S, Brook MG, Curtis H, Johnston M. Survey of HIV and Hepatitis B or C co-infection management in UK. *Int. J. STD AIDS* 2006;**17**:799–801.
15. Turner J, Bansi L, Gilson R, et al. The prevalence of hepatitis C virus infection in HIV positive individuals in the UK – trends in HCV testing and the impact of HCV on HIV treatment outcomes. *J. Virol. Hepat.* 2010;**17**(8):569–77.
16. Wilkins E, Nelson M, Argwal K, et al. BHIVA guidelines for hte management of hepatitis viruses in adults infected with HIV 2013. *HIV Medicine* 2013;**14**(Suppl 4):1–71.
17. French AL, Beaudet LM, Benator DA, Levy CS, Kass M, Orenstein JM. Cholecystectomy in patients with AIDS: clinicopathologic correlations in 107 cases. *Clin. Infect. Dis.* 1995;**21**:852–8.
18. Sharpstone D, Gazzard B. Gastrointestinal manifestations of HIV infection. *Lancet* 1996;**348**:379–81.
19. Call SA, Heudebert G, Saag M, et al. The changing etiology of chronic diarrhea in HIV-infected patients with CD4 counts less than 200 cells/mm³. *Am. J. Gastroenterol.* 2000;**95**:3142–6.
20. Oldfield ED. Evaluation of chronic dirrahea in patients with human immunodeficiency virus infection. *Rev. Gastroenterol. Disord.* 2002;**2**:276–88.
21. Carr A, Marriott D, Field A, Vasak E, Cooper DA. Treatment of HIV-1 associated microsporidiosis and cryptosporidiosis with combination antiretroviral therapy. *Lancet* 1998; **351**:256–9.
22. Sande MA, Volberding PA. The Medical Management of AIDS, 6th edn. WB Saunders, Philadelphia, 1999: 196–216.
23. Bini EJ, Diehl DL. Colonic disease in patients with AIDS. *Techniques Gastrointest. Endosc.* 2002;**4**:77–85.
24. Melbye M, Rabkin C, Frisch M, Biggar RJ. Changing patterns of anal cancer incidence in the United States, 1940–1989. *Am. J. Epidemiol.* 1994;**139**:772–80.

CHAPTER 38

Gastrointestinal complications in the intensive care unit

James J. McNamee[1] and Daniel F. McAuley[2]

[1] Royal Victoria Hospital, Belfast, UK
[2] Royal Victoria Hospital and Queen's University of Belfast, Belfast, UK

Introduction

Gastrointestinal emergencies can present as *a reason* for admission to a critical care environment or as *a result* of the critical illness itself. Additional physiological monitoring and organ support may be required in management of the former and such conditions are covered in other chapters of this book. The latter are a range of gastrointestinal conditions that can complicate a patient's clinical course in intensive care and it is important to keep these in mind when one observes a critically ill patient for an unrelated problem. There are also various medical conditions that may require intensive care that can mimic an acute abdomen such as lower lobe pneumonia, inferior myocardial infarction, diabetic ketoacidosis, or sickle cell crisis.

Abdominal problems occurring during a critical illness are often more difficult to identify than those causing the admission and require a high index of suspicion to diagnose. Sedation, steroids and other coexisting pathologies can mask symptoms such as pain. Due to endotracheal intubation and the use of sedatives patients are often unable to communicate effectively which can make obtaining an accurate history challenging. In the critically ill patient an abdominal disorder may only be heralded by unexplained and persistent tachycardia, agitation, hypotension, pyrexia, or unexpected progressive renal, hepatic, cardiac, and respiratory failure [1]. The type and amount of nasogastric outputs are significant as are the frequency and quantity of bowel movements where

a patient history is lacking. Gastrointestinal symptoms are common in the intensive care unit and in mechanically ventilated patients it has been found that the number of simultaneously occurring symptoms is higher in non-survivors. Studies have confirmed that up to 62% of intensive care patients have at least one gastrointestinal symptom for at least one day during their Intensive Care Unit (ICU) admission and that critically ill patients with three or more gastrointestinal symptoms have a higher mortality although none of the symptoms were independent predictors of mortality [2,3] (Table 38.1).

Imaging the gastrointestinal tract is made difficult because of the requirements in transporting safely a critically unwell patient on complex organ support to the radiology suite and the risk of worsening renal dysfunction with the use of intravenous contrast agents.

Specific gastrointestinal conditions

Gastrointestinal hemorrhage due to acute stress ulceration

There is a well-established relationship between severe physiological stress and gastrointestinal ulceration, which has resulted in the common use of ulcer prophylaxis in intensive care [4]. Acute stress ulceration is associated with some common critical illness conditions such as sepsis, shock, burns, multiple trauma, head injuries, and respiratory failure. Lesions are most commonly seen in the gastric fundus, and can range from mild erosions to

Gastrointestinal Emergencies, Third Edition. Edited by Tony C. K. Tham, John S. A. Collins, and Roy Soetikno.

Table 38.1 GI symptoms associated with mortality.

Gastrointestinal symptoms for mechanically ventilated patients
Absent bowel sounds
Vomiting/regurgitation
Diarrhoea = loose or liquid stool >3 times/day
Bowel distension = suspected or radiologically confirmed in any bowel segment
GI bleeding = visible appearance of blood in vomit/nasogastric aspirate/stool
High gastric residual volume = >500 mL
High intra-abdominal pressure = >12 mmHg

Source: Blaser et al. 2013 [2]. Reproduced with permission of Springer.

Table 38.2 Risk factors for stress ulcer.

Risk factors for stress ulcer related bleeding
Respiratory failure requiring ventilation > 48H
Coagulopathy
Acute renal failure
Sepsis syndrome
Hypotension
Severe head or spinal cord injury
Anticoagulation
History of gastyrointestinal bleeding
Low intragastric pH
Thermal injury involving >35% body surface area
Major surgery
Steroids
Acute lung injury

Source: Adapted from Bersten & Soni 2009 [6].

acute ulceration [5]. The exact mechanism is multi-factorial and not fully understood but it is postulated that hypoperfusion of the gastric mucosa and hypoxia are contributory. During critical illness both administered and endogenous catecholamines cause vasoconstriction within the splanchnic circulation that can cause the mucosal barrier to become compromised. Bleeding can range from minor blood loss to frank hemorrhage and the incidence of clinically important bleeding is reported to range from 0.6 to 6% of the ICU population. This increases length of ICU stay by up to 8 days and increases mortality by up to four-fold compared to patients that do not develop stress ulceration [5]. It is hypothesized that because our management of respiratory and circulatory conditions have improved over the last number of years along with earlier enteral feeding and less "nil by mouth" the incidence of acute stress ulceration has been declining [6].

Evaluation

Coagulopathy and respiratory failure are the strongest independent risk factors for the development of stress ulceration, although others are reported (Table 38.2).

Management

The management of acute upper gastrointestinal hemorrhage in the critically ill patient is managed effectively with prompt resuscitation, early endoscopy, and hemostasis, combined with continuous intravenous infusion of proton pump inhibitors [6].

There are various agents used for stress ulcer prophylaxis of critically ill patients such as sucralfate, histamine 2 receptor antagonists (H2RA), and proton pump inhibitors. Both sucralfate and histamine 2 receptor antagonists have been found to reduce clinically important bleeding [5]. Sucralfate needs to be delivered into the stomach and the accumulation of aluminum ions can occur in renal failure, so it is less commonly used. H2RAs are the most widely used agent in critical care for stress ulcer related bleeding prophylaxis because they are well tolerated and have low cost. Previously, two meta analysis have shown H2RAs to reduce the risk of clinically important bleeding compared to placebo and also failed to show an increase of noscomial pneumonia, which had been feared due to acid suppression [5,7]. Proton pump inhibitors are the most potent antisecretory agents available and are effective in rendering the stomach pH above 6 to prevent rebleeding. They are also well tolerated with few side effects and recent meta-analysis has shown proton pump inhibitors to be superior to H2RAs in terms of preventing clinically important bleeding [8].

Enteral nutrition is encouraged in critically ill patients, as parenteral nutrition is associated with infectious and central venous line complications. Enteral nutrition optimises splanchnic blood flow distribution, buffers stomach acid and reduces macroscopic ulceration [5]. Since a mortality benefit has not been demonstrated many clinicians discontinue stress ulcer prophylaxis when their patients begin oral/enteral nutrition or when they are discharged from the ICU.

Acalculous cholecystitis

Acalculous cholecystitis (ACC) is an uncommon, but serious, condition found in critically ill patients and requires a high index of suspicion in patients who have developed sepsis of an unknown cause. ACC develops insidiously and can often go unrecognised, as the patient may be critically unwell due to other causes such as trauma, surgery, shock or burns. It is defined as an acute necroinflammatory disease of the gallbladder in the absence of cholelithiasis and is multifactorial in origin. It is clinically indistinguishable from calculous cholecystitis in a sedated, critically unwell patient as the symptoms and signs can be very non-specific. Right upper quadrant pain, fever, leucocytosis, elevated liver enzymes and bilirubin may point towards the diagnosis but often the only sign is a systemic inflammatory response and new or progressive organ dysfunction [9,10]. If left unrecognized ACC may progress to gangrene, perforation or abscess formation, all of which are associated with a high mortality in this group of patients.

ACC is hypothesized to be the result of impaired microcirculation of the gallbladder wall leading to inflammation and ischemia, combined with bile stasis, as a result of fasting and obstruction. Histological examination confirms leukocyte infiltration, wall edema, and increased and deeper bile infiltration of the gallbladder wall. Commonly associated risk factors are trauma, blood transfusions, surgery unrelated to the gallbladder, shock, burns, sepsis, prolonged fasting, and total parenteral nutrition.

Evaluation

Ultimately the diagnosis rests on imaging the gall bladder. Abdominal computerized tomography (CT) scan offers little benefit in the diagnosis over ultrasound, although a CT scan has the advantage that it can be useful in identifying other intra-abdominal pathology. Ultrasound has the advantage in that it does not require the transport of a critically ill patient to a radiology suite. The characteristic features, which can be identified with either imaging modality, include a thickened gallbladder wall, pericholecystic fluid, subserosal edema, intramural gas, and bile sludge.

Management

The two treatment options for ACC are cholecystostomy and/or cholecystectomy. Cholecystectomy is definitive and is the preferred option if the gallbladder wall is ischemic, as

drainage would not be sufficient. This procedure can be performed laparoscopically but will often have to be converted to an open procedure due to the inflamed nature of the gallbladder. Ultrasound or CT guided drainage will often suffice if the gallbladder wall is not ischemic, with the advantages of a safe and rapid procedure.

Abdominal compartment syndrome

The incidence of abdominal compartment syndrome (ACS) varies within the intensive care population studied and ranges from 2–5% in medical and 5–35% in surgical and trauma patients. The presence of ACS is associated with a mortality of 50–75% so it is important to diagnose and treat promptly when identified. ACS can be associated with injury or disease in the abdominopelvic region (primary ACS) or with a condition outside the abdomen that results in a capillary leak that requires significant fluid administration (e.g. sepsis or major burns). A vicious cycle is started whereby there is intestinal edema and visceral swelling, raising the intra-abdominal pressure, which causes mesenteric vein compression and venous hypertension. More fluid is administered to counteract the hemodynamic effects that the splinted abdomen creates, which further compounds the problem. If left unchecked, ACS can result in significant physiological impairment to cardiorespiratory, renal, splanchnic, and neurological organ systems.

Evaluation

Intra-abdominal pressure (IAP) is the steady state pressure concealed within the abdominal cavity. It cannot be reliably estimated with clinical examination. The reference standard for measurement is the instillation of 25 mL of sterile saline into the bladder via the urinary catheter and measurement of bladder pressure via a transducer when the patient is in the supine position. Intra-abdominal hypertension (IAH) is the sustained elevation of intra-abdominal pressure equal to or above 12 mmHg, and should not be based on one single measurement but on a trend of repeated values over time. ACS is defined as a sustained IAP >20 mmHg that is associated with new organ dysfunction/failure [11].

It is recommended that patients should be screened for risk factors for IAH/ACS on admission to the ICU and when new or progressive organ failure develops [3,12]. If a patient has two or more risk factors (Table 38.3), then IAP should be measured for a baseline and a management algorithm followed if it is elevated [11].

Table 38.3 Risk factors for IAH.

Risk factors for IAH/ACS
Acidosis
Hypothermia
Polytransfusion
Coagulopathy
Sepsis
Intra-abdominal infection
Peritonitis
Ascites
Mechanical ventilation
Pneumonia
Abdominal surgery
Massive fluid resuscitation
Gastric distension
Volvulus
Major trauma
Major burns
High body mass index
Prone positioning
Peritoneal dialysis
Laparoscopy

Source: Malbrain 2006 [11]. Reproduced with permission of Springer.

Management

The management of intra-abdominal hypertension and abdominal compartment syndrome can be medical and surgical. Less-invasive medical management should be attempted first. The abdominal wall compliance can be increased with the use of sedatives and neuromuscular blocking agents. Simple methods to evacuate abdominal contents can be attempted, such as nasogastric suction and decompression, rectal tube insertion and enemas, prokinetics, and endoscopic colonic decompression. Paracentesis can be carried out on tense ascites and abdominal hematomas and abscesses can be percutaneously drained [12].

If IAH continues to increase or organ failures result despite medical therapies then surgical decompression should be considered. Decompressive laparotomy is the definitive procedure for lowering intra-abdominal pressure but does have its side effects, which have to be balanced against prolonging organ failures. The procedure results in an open abdomen which, until definitively closed requires a temporary abdominal closure. A device such as a vacuum-assisted closure device may be required for this but can cause trauma itself due to the negative pressure it can create within the abdomen.

Gastrointestinal hypomotility

It is standard practice to provide nutritional support to critically ill patients in order to treat existing malnutrition and minimize wasting of lean body mass. Early enteral nutrition, at least 20 kcal/kg/day, started within 24–48 hours after critical illness is recommended [13]. Acute gastrointestinal injury and feeding intolerance syndrome are impediments to attaining daily nutritional goals in the ICU and should be screened for and monitored routinely before and after feeding has commenced [3]. Increased gastric residual volume, which is the volume of fluid aspirated intermittently from the nasogastric tube, is a cardinal sign.

Evaluation

Paralysis of the lower gastrointestinal tract is the inability of the bowel to pass stool due to impaired peristalsis. Clinical signs include the absence of stool for three or more consecutive days without mechanical obstruction [3]. Bowel sounds may or may not be present.

Management

Laxative drugs can be used, but may take a number of days to have an effect. Neostigmine, a cholinesterase inhibitor, acts by increasing the concentration of acetylcholine at the neuromuscular junction thereby increasing contractions of the normal gut. This has been used in the past with some success but caution is advised as it may cause severe bradycardia so is therefore not advised to be used routinely [14].

When the gastrointestinal tract is not able to perform the digestion and absorption adequately to provide the fluid and nutrient requirements for the body, specific interventions may have to be performed to prevent gastrointestinal tract failure altogether. The use of drugs that may impair the ability of the gastrointestinal tract such as opiates and catecholamines should be limited if at all possible and any electrolyte abnormalities should be corrected. Prokinetic agents such as metoclopromide or erythromycin may be used for a limited period in an attempt to improve propulsion of feed down the tract. In cases of gastroparesis, post pyloric feeding should be considered if prokinetics do not work, ensuring enteral feeding is continued and regularly attempted in these situations.

Despite this, gastrointestinal tract function may not be restored and parenteral nutrition may have to be considered to ensure some delivery of energy and nutrients.

The use of parenteral nutrition later (after one week) compared to early (within 2 days) in patients who are not meeting their nutritional goals is associated with faster recovery and fewer infectious complications [15]. Intra-abdominal hypertension should be looked for as a contributing factor and other undiagnosed abdominal conditions such as cholecystitis, peritonitis, and bowel ischemia should be excluded [3]. Laparotomy, or other emergency procedures such as colonoscopy for colon decompression, may be required as a life-preserving intervention.

Clostridium difficile **colitis**

Clostridium difficile, a Gram-positive spore forming anaerobe bacillus, is responsible for most health care-associated diarrheal illnesses. Typically when antibiotics are used to treat infections they reduce the normal flora in the gastrointestinal tract creating an environment where the anaerobe *C. difficile* can flourish. Proton pump inhibitors, which are used for stress ulcer prophylaxis, are thought to contribute to this by reducing the amount of gastric acid, which would normally protect against the spores. The exotoxins produced by the organism cause intestinal fluid secretion that can result in a spectrum of enteric complications from diarrhoea to pseudomembraneous colitis to toxic megacolon [16].

There are several patient populations at risk of developing *C. difficile* infection (CDI) within a critical care environment. Therefore implementing infection control measures such as patient isolation and enforcing hand washing is important to prevent cross infection. The spores are not affected by alcohol-based hand cleansers and require physical removal with soap and scrubbing. Risk factors in the ICU, similar to those in all patients throughout the hospital, include advanced age, residence in long-term care facilities, prolonged antibiotic exposure, immunosuppression, and post surgery [17]. Nearly all antibiotics have been implicated but clindamycin, cephalosporins and the broad-spectrum penicillins pose a greater risk when used. Hospital incidence has increased since the turn of the millennium, as has its severity, particularly in the elderly population. *C. difficile* colitis causes additional morbidity that result in a significant economic burden because of medical and surgical complications, infection control, and prolonged length of stay. The hypervirulent strain emerging in the last 10 years is responsible for the increasing numbers of surgical complications and deaths [18].

Evaluation

A high index of suspicion is required in the diagnosis of CDI, as the onset of symptoms is variable. Non-infectious diarrhea is common in intensive care patients for a number of reasons, such as enteral feeding, ingestion of sorbitol in medications and laxatives, or comorbid diseases such as carcinoid syndrome. CDI is often associated with a white cell count above 15 000/mL in severe disease, which may help to confirm suspicion of an infectious cause for diarrhea [16]. Diagnosis is confirmed by either tissue culture cytotoxic assay (slow), enzyme immunoassay for the detection of toxins (quicker but less sensitive), or antigen assay (rapid, sensitive but less specific).

Management

When a patient is diagnosed it is advisable to try to discontinue the offending antibiotics if possible or change to those from a different class that are not known to cause CDI. Oral metronidazole is used as first-line therapy although one in four will not respond, in which case oral vancomycin is recommended. Vancomycin enemas may be administered if the oral route is compromised and intravenous immunoglobulin may be considered for recurrent cases [18]. Plain abdominal radiography is crucial for the identification of increasing abdominal dilatation and to aid the decision for surgery. From radiography, toxic megacolon can be diagnosed with colonic dilatation more than 7 cm in combination with systemic toxicity. A CT scan may also help to identify the characteristic findings of thickening of the colonic wall [18]. Surgical management may be required for severe cases for complications such septic shock, ileus, toxic megacolon, and perforation.

References

1. Worthley LIG. Acute abdominal disorders in the paralysed patient. *Anaesth. Intensive Care* 1985;**13**:263–71.
2. Reintam Blaser A, Poeze M, Malbrain M, Bjorck M, Oudemans-van Straaten H, Storkopf J. Gastrointestinal symptoms during the first week of intensive care are associated with poor outcome: as prospective multicentre study. *Intensive Care Med.* 2013;**39**(5):899–909.
3. Blaser A, Malbrain M, Starkopf J, et al. Gastrointestinal function in intensive care patients: terminology, definitions and management. Recommendations of the ESICM working group on abdominal problems. *Intensive Care Med.* 2012;**38**: 384–94.

4. Quenot JP, Thiery N, Barbar S. When should stress ulceration be used in the ICU? *Curr. Opin. Crit. Care* 2009;**15**:139–43.

5. Marik P, Vasu T, Hirani A, Pachinburavan M. Stress ulcer prophylaxis in the new millennium: A systematic review and meta-analysis. *Crit. Care Med.* 2010;**38**:2222–28.

6. Bersten A, Soni N. *Oh's Intensive Care Manual*, 6th Edition, Elsevier, Oxford, 2009.

7. Cook DJ, Reeve BK, Guyatt GH, et al. Stress ulcer prophylaxis in critically ill patients: resolving discordant meta-analysis. *JAMA* 1996;**275**:308–14.

8. Alhazzani W, Alenezi F, Jaeschke R, Moayyedi P Cook D. Proton pump inhibitors versus histamine 2 receptor antagonists for stress ulcer prophylaxix in critically ill patients: s systematic review and meta-analysis. *Crit. Care Med.* 2013;**41**(3):693–705.

9. Huffman J, Schenker S. Acute Acalculous cholecystitis: a review. *Clin. Gastroenterol. Hepatol.* 2010;**8**:15–22.

10. Laurila JJ, Ala-Kokko TI, Laurila PA, et al. Histopathology of acute acalculous cholecystitis in critically ill patients. *Histopathology* 2005;**47**:485–92.

11. Malbrain M, Cheatham M, Kirkpatrick A, et al. Results from the international conference of experts on intra-abdominal hypertension and abdominal compartment syndrome. 1 Definitions. *Intensive Care Med.* 2006;**32**:1722–32.

12. Cheatham M, Malbrain M, Kirkpatrick A, et al. Results from the International Conference of Experts on Intra-abdominal Hypertension and Abdominal Compartment Syndrome. 2. Recommendations. *Intensive Care Med.* 2007;**33**:951–62.

13. Doig G, Heighes P, Simpson F, Sweetman E, Davis A. Early enteral nutrition, provided within 24h of injury or intensive care admission, significantly reduces mortality in critically ill patients: a meta-analysis of randomised controlled trials. *Intensive Care Med.* 2009;**35**:2018–27.

14. Van der Spoel J, Oudermans-van Straaten H, Stoutenbeek C, Bosman R, Zandstra D. Neostigmine resolves critical illness related colonic ileus in intensive care patients with multiple organ failure – a prospective, double-blind, placebo-controlled study. *Intensive Care Med.* 2001;**27**:822–27.

15. Casaer M, Mesotten D, Hermans G, et al. Early versus late parenteral nutrition in critically ill adults. *N. Engl. J. Med.* 2011;**365**(6):506–17.

16. Janka J, O'Grady NP. *Clostridium difficile* infection: current perspectives. *Curr. Opin. Crit Care* 2009;**15**:149–53.

17. Wanahita A. Conditions associated with leuococytosis in a tertiary care hospital, with particular attention to the role of infection caused by clostridium difficile. *Clin. Infect. Dis.* 2002;**34**:1585–92.

18. Gould C, McDonald L. Bench-to-bedside review: *Clostridium difficile* colitis. *Crit. Care* 2008;**12**:203.

Index

Gastrointestinal Emergencies, Third Edition. Edited by Tony C. K. Tham, John S. A. Collins, and Roy Soetikno.
© 2016 John Wiley & Sons, Ltd. Published 2016 by John Wiley & Sons, Ltd.